Digestive System 2023

Symptoms, Causes, Diagnostic Procedures and Treatment
Options for most common digestive conditions

CONTENTS

CHAPTER 4
Gut feelings

CHAPTER 5

Diagnostic tests

PART 2
Digestive diseases

CHAPTER 6
Obesity

CHAPTER 7
Constipation and fecal incontinence

CHAPTER 8
Irritable bowel syndrome and food intolerances

CHAPTER 11
Ulcers and stomach pain

CHAPTER 15
Pancreatic disease

CHAPTER 16
Liver disease

CHAPTER 17

Colorectal cancer

APPENDIX

FODMAP eating plan

The elimination phase

The reintroduction phase

The maintenance phase

Preface

Your digestive system may seem easy to understand: You put food in your mouth. Your digestive organs break down the food. Nutrients in the food are absorbed in your intestines, and the rest is eliminated as waste. Sounds pretty simple, doesn't it?

In fact, the human digestive system is incredibly complex. It acts both as food transporter and food processor, requiring the efficient function of many different organs to transform what you eat and drink into a mixture that fuels good health. Sometimes, things can go wrong, or the process doesn't work as well as it should.

This Book covers signs and symptoms, causes, diagnostic procedures, and treatment options for the most common digestive conditions, as well as preventive actions to consider. Perhaps you've experienced temporary discomfort from heartburn, diarrhea, constipation, nausea or excess gas and are trying to determine what may be triggering your symptoms. Maybe you're dealing with a common condition such as gastroesophageal reflux disease, peptic ulcers or gallstones and you want information on treatment. If you have a long-term condition, such as Crohn's disease or celiac disease, you may be seeking coping skills.

In the last decade, we've seen tremendous advancements in the understanding, early recognition and treatment of many digestive conditions. As an example, today we have a much better understanding of the important role your gut plays — specifically, the bacteria that reside within it — in maintaining your overall health. We're also seeing a connection between the health of your gut and that of other systems within your body. All of this has led to a lot of speculation and misinformation surrounding what to eat — and what not to eat — for good gut health.

This book addresses a wide range of topics, providing a context for what it takes to keep your digestive system healthy and how to respond when disease occurs. Too often, people wait too long before seeking help from their doctors. In general, the earlier you address a problem, the easier it is to prevent it from becoming serious.

Here's hoping that this book can help you enjoy a higher quality of life with fewer digestive concerns. And here's wishing you good digestion!

and made numerous presentations. Dr. Khanna serves on the editorial board of several journals and has won numerous awards including the Miles and Shirley Fiterman Award, the Mayo Brothers Distinguished Fellowship Award, the Donald C. Balfour Mayo Clinic Alumni Association Research Award, the Hartz Foundation Young Investigators' Scholarship, and the Most Distinguished Resident Physician Award from the American Association of Physicians of Indian Origin.

PART 1
Digestive health basics

CHAPTER 1
Why your gut matters

Good health and a healthy gut go hand in hand. Digestion is one of the critical functions your body must perform in order to survive and thrive. The food you eat provides necessary nutrients that supply your cells with sustenance and energy so your body can develop, repair and maintain itself.

When you take a bite of food, what enters your mouth must be transformed before it can nourish your body. That's the primary function of digestion — to break down food into smaller components and change it chemically so nutrients can be extracted and absorbed into your bloodstream (while the remainder is eliminated as waste). The breakdown of food occurs primarily through the action of digestive juices in your mouth, stomach and intestines, with assistance from the tearing, grinding action of your teeth.

When things go according to plan, the organs of your digestive tract perform a variety of specialized functions in an efficient and timely manner. But like any complex system that contains integrated parts, sometimes the process gets disrupted, and even a slight malfunction can cause problems.

When this happens, you begin to experience signs and symptoms. That's your body's way of letting you know something isn't quite right. Often, the problems are minor and infrequent, but sometimes they can be complex and chronic.

WARNING SIGNS

Heartburn, pain, cramps, bloating, nausea, vomiting, diarrhea, constipation, bleeding — these are some of the ways your digestive system alerts you to a problem. And try as you may to ignore what's happening (or isn't happening) in your stomach or gut, doing so is virtually impossible.

For some people, the pain, bloating or nausea comes and goes. It may come on sporadically, and sometimes suddenly, and then gradually diminish after a few hours. For others, digestive distress persists and becomes a constant, unwanted companion.

Digestive issues have many possible causes, including infection, inflammation, digestive tract blockages, and lifestyle issues including diet and stress. For many individuals, no matter what they may try to relieve their signs and symptoms, it doesn't work and the problem persists.

It's estimated that 60 million to 70 million Americans — perhaps even more — experience some type of digestive issue. Evidence of this is on display in drugstore and grocery store aisles lined with an impressive array of digestive-related medicines and supplements, including antacids, acid blockers, laxatives and fiber supplements.

Over-the-counter medications often help relieve bothersome signs and symptoms, but they aren't always the answer. If you're regularly affected by periods of indigestion, pain, nausea or cramps, it's important that you see your doctor.

Knowing the root cause of what's ailing you can help reduce your anxiety, put you more at ease in social situations and allow you and your doctor to work together on a plan to manage the condition and possibly even cure it.

Early action on your part may also prevent a serious digestive condition from becoming life-threatening.

● ● ● ● ●

PROBLEMS BY THE NUMBERS

Are digestive problems more common today than they were years ago? The answer appears to be yes.

Why are digestive issues on the rise? There could be many reasons, and it's difficult to point to one or two factors. However, there seems to be a legitimate association between digestion and lifestyle. Some of the increase in digestive-related issues could be linked to increasingly fast-paced lifestyles, unhealthy diets and reduced exercise.

The prevalence of digestive problems is reflected in these general statistics:

- More than 60 million Americans experience heartburn at least once a month, and more than 15 million may have heartburn daily.
- About 36 percent of Americans have trouble digesting dairy products, a condition called lactose intolerance.
- An estimated 15 million Americans experience abdominal pain, gas, and diarrhea or constipation associated with irritable bowel syndrome.
- More than 3 million clinic and hospital visits each year are

for constipation.

- Just under 6 percent of U.S. adults have ulcers.
- About 3.5 million Americans are living with hepatitis C, a viral liver infection.
- An estimated 135,000 Americans are diagnosed each year with colorectal cancer.

● ● ● ● ●

DIGESTION AT WORK

Your digestive tract is a series of hollow, connected organs including the esophagus, stomach, small intestine and colon. Together they form a long, convoluted passageway extending from the mouth to the anus, where solid waste exits the body. Organs such as the salivary glands, pancreas, liver and gallbladder also serve essential functions in the digestive process.

Along this tract, muscular contractions move food along through successive stages of the digestive process. Valves at critical junctures control the amount of food that can be moved forward and prevent food from moving backward. A network of nerves and glandular cells regulates much of this activity, including the release of enzymes and digestive juices. When food is broken down, nutrients are absorbed into your blood via tiny pores in the intestinal wall. The nutrients are transported in the bloodstream to nourish your body's cells.

When problems occur, certain signs and symptoms may point to any number of possible causes, making a diagnosis difficult (and your life miserable). The tasks at hand for you and your doctor during a medical visit are to identify all the possibilities and — often through a process of elimination — focus on the most likely cause.

In the sections that follow, we describe the different digestive organs and their relationships to one another. This knowledge may help you better understand the complexities of the digestive process and why problems develop.

Salivary glands

Digestion actually starts even before you take your first bite. The aroma of the food you're about to eat — or are thinking about eating — is enough to get saliva in your mouth flowing. You have three pairs of large salivary glands, in addition to smaller glands in the lining of your mouth.

When you take a bite of food, your glands pump out saliva containing the enzyme amylase that begins to chemically break down the food. Your teeth crunch and grind the food, while your tongue mixes it with the saliva. These actions transform a bite of food into a bolus — a soft, moist, rounded mixture suitable for swallowing.

You control many aspects of the digestive process at the beginning — what you put into your mouth, how long you chew it and when you swallow. But once you swallow, the rest of the digestive process is controlled by your nervous system.

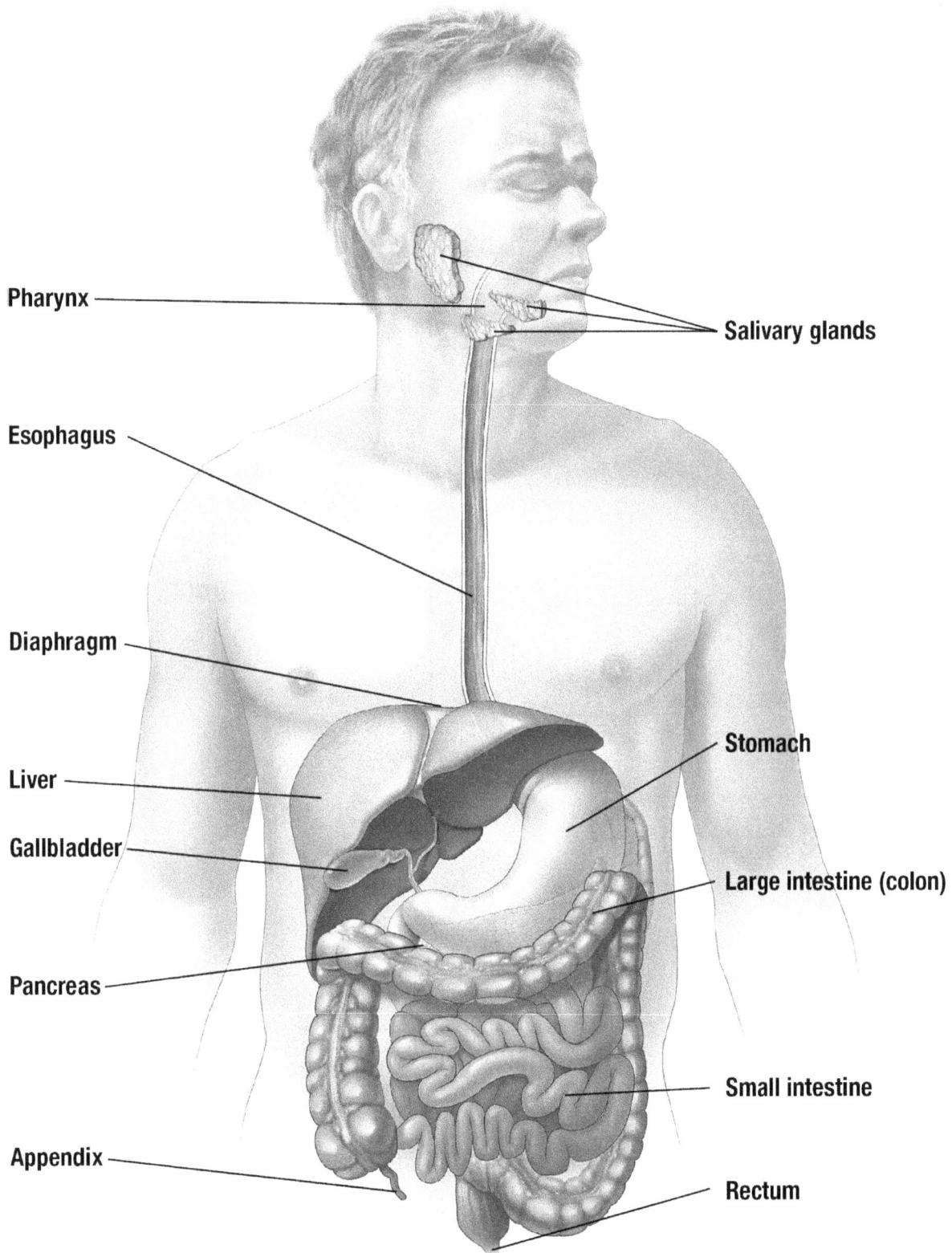

Pharynx

Salivary glands

Esophagus

Diaphragm

Liver

Gallbladder

Pancreas

Stomach

Large intestine (colon)

Small intestine

Appendix

Rectum

The digestive tract begins at the mouth and ends at the rectum and includes several internal organs. Food moves through your body along the digestive tract.

Esophagus

When you swallow, muscles in your mouth and throat propel food through a relaxed ring of muscle (upper esophageal sphincter) that connects the back of your throat (pharynx) to your upper esophagus. The esophagus, commonly referred to as the food pipe, is a tube about 10 inches long that connects your throat and stomach.

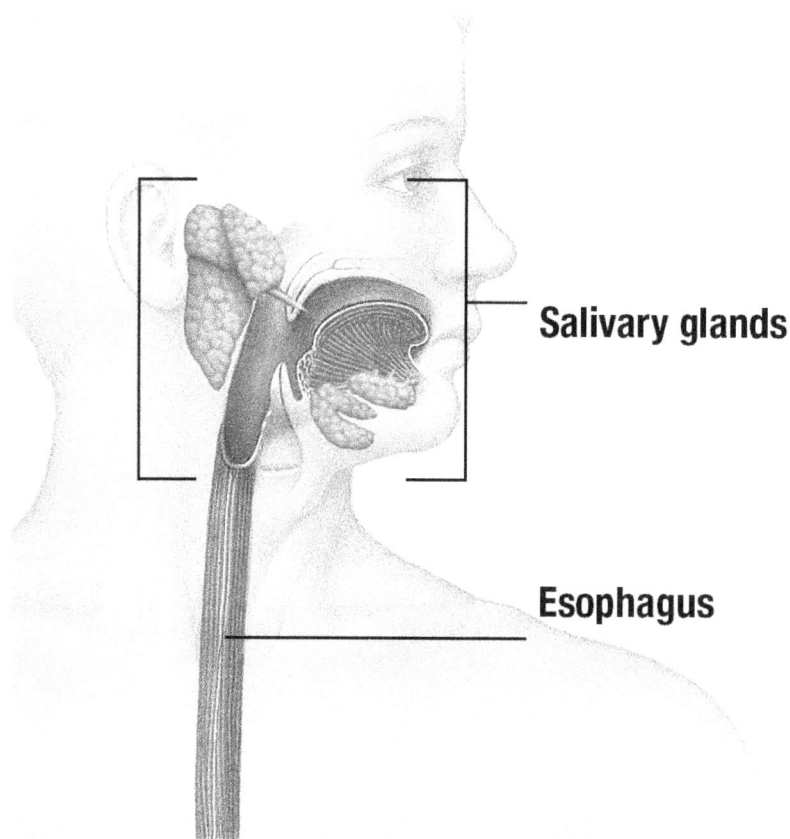

Salivary glands

Esophagus

Gravity alone isn't sufficient to move food through the esophagus. Help comes from muscles in the wall of the esophagus that move in synchronized waves — one after another — propelling the food toward your stomach. Muscles above the swallowed food contract, squeezing it downward, while muscles below the food relax to allow it to advance without resistance. This pattern of progressive contraction and relaxation is called peristalsis.

Peristalsis is a coordinated muscular action that continues through your entire digestive tract.

As food reaches the lower portion of your esophagus, it approaches the lower esophageal sphincter (LES). When you're not eating, this muscle valve remains tightly closed to keep stomach acid from flowing backward (regurgitating) into your esophagus and causing heartburn. The act of swallowing signals the valve to relax and open in order to let food pass through on its way to your stomach.

In some people, food doesn't move down the tract as it should or the LES doesn't relax, resulting in swallowing difficulties (dysphagia). Dysphagia most often occurs because the esophagus has become narrowed, often due to excessive acid exposure. Narrowing of the esophagus is known as a stricture.

Stomach

Your stomach sits in the upper area of your abdomen, just under your rib cage. A hollow, muscular sac, the typical stomach can expand to hold about a gallon of food and liquid. When your stomach is empty, its tissues fold in on themselves, a bit like a closed accordion. As your stomach fills, the folds disappear.

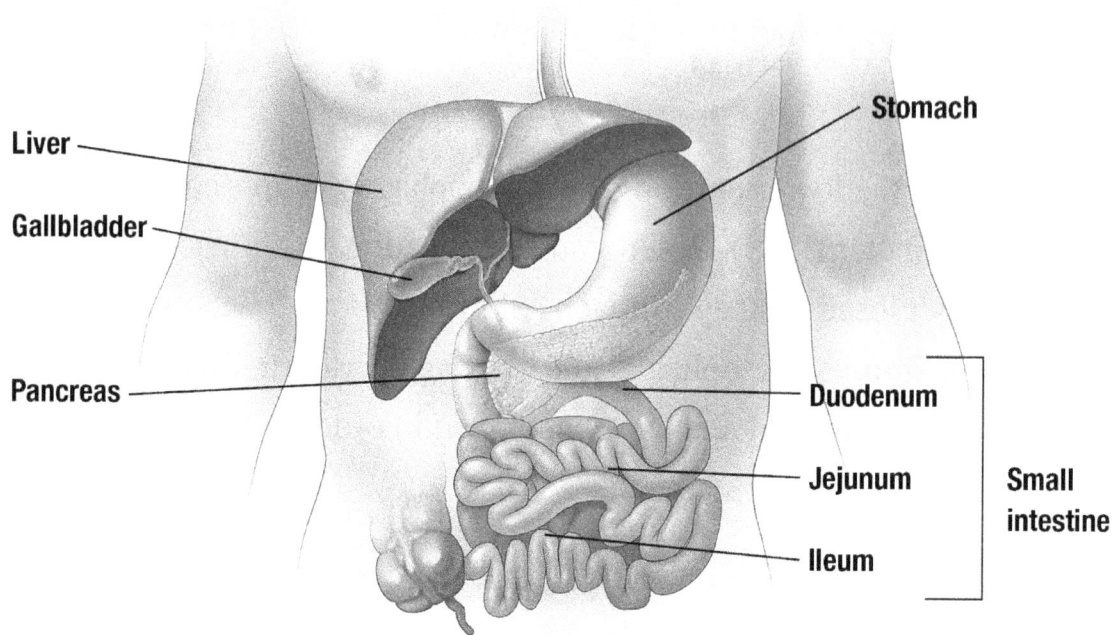

Your stomach performs two functions in the digestive process. It continues to break food down into smaller pieces, and it acts as a storehouse, gradually releasing food into the small intestine — where most chemical digestion and absorption take place.

Generally, it takes your stomach about four hours to empty after a nutritious meal. It may take six hours or more if the meal has a lot of fat.

Even before food arrives, digestive juices in the stomach begin flowing. At the first sight, smell and taste of food, your brain sends messages along the vagus nerve indicating that food will be arriving soon. The messages trigger the release of a chemical called acetylcholine along the nerves and muscles lining the stomach. This chemical sets off a chain reaction that causes your stomach muscles to start contracting and signals your gastric glands to produce digestive juices.

• • • • •

APPETITE, HUNGER AND FEELING FULL

Appetite is that pleasant feeling that lets you know it's time to eat. Hunger comes later, perhaps when you've gone past your normal mealtime and your body tells you so with unpleasant hunger pangs. Appetite and hunger work together to keep you eating regularly.

Your sensations of appetite and hunger are controlled by a part of your brain called the hypothalamus. A portion of the food you eat is converted into blood sugar (glucose). When your blood sugar level drops, the hypothalamus notices and sends nerve impulses along the vagus nerve to your stomach. These impulses trigger the release of gastric juices and set in motion the muscle contractions that produce hunger pangs. You may hear your stomach rumbling as juices and air pass through your intestines. This rumbling sound is normal.

If you aren't able to eat right away, these sensations gradually wear off and you may not feel hungry again for several hours. But later in the day, when it's time for your next meal, you may feel famished.

Once you've eaten, your brain recognizes when you're full. As your stomach fills and stretches to its normal capacity, it signals that your hunger has been satisfied (satiety).

• • • • •

By the time food arrives from your esophagus, conditions are ready for the next stage of digestion. The muscles in your upper stomach relax to allow food and liquid to enter. The stomach walls, which are lined with three layers of powerful muscles, then begin churning the food, mixing it into smaller and smaller pieces. Gastric juices released from glands lining the walls of your stomach help break down food into a thick, creamy fluid called chyme. In a normal day, your stomach produces 2 to 3 quarts of gastric juices.

Hydrochloric acid is one of many kinds of gastric juices. This acid would be very corrosive in your stomach if it weren't for a layer of sticky mucus that acts as a protective force clinging to your stomach walls. Hydrochloric acid kills harmful bacteria and microorganisms swallowed with the food. Gastric juices also contain pepsin, a protein-digesting enzyme. An imbalance in protective forces and damaging forces in the stomach lining can damage the lining, resulting in conditions such as erosion or an ulcer.

Two products that are absorbed directly into your bloodstream from your stomach are aspirin and alcohol, both of which pass quickly through the stomach lining with little trouble.

Once your food is well mixed, rippling waves of muscles in your stomach walls push the stomach contents down toward the pyloric valve, which opens into your small intestine. The pyloric valve, another ringlike sphincter muscle, opens just enough to allow your stomach to release less than an eighth of an ounce of food at a time into the small intestine. The rest of the contents is held back for more mixing.

Small intestine, pancreas, liver and gallbladder

The small intestine is a winding tube about 20 feet long that fills much of your abdomen. It's here that the chemical breakdown of the food you eat is completed, and where most nutrients are absorbed into your bloodstream. The small intestine is divided into three parts: duodenum, jejunum and ileum (<u>see this illustration</u>).

Duodenum Food released from your stomach passes into the duodenum. This is the location where the chemical breakdown of food is the most intensive. Here, digestive juices converge from the pancreas, liver and gallbladder and mix with juices secreted from the walls of the small intestine to carry out the breakdown.

The lining of the duodenum contains enzymes — for example, lactase — that can break down simple sugars, such as lactose, into double sugars, such as glucose and galactose. The duodenum, however, absorbs only small amounts of nutrients through its intestinal walls. Muscular contractions continue moving food waste through the digestive tract.

Pancreas The pancreas is a soft, pink-colored gland that's located behind the stomach. The pancreas is shaped a bit like a fish, with a wide head, a tapering body and a narrow tail.

In addition to other secretions, the pancreas produces two important types of digestive substances. They are:

- Digestive enzymes that are secreted into your upper duodenum and help break down your main energy sources — proteins, carbohydrates and fats
- The hormones insulin and glucagon, which are secreted into your bloodstream and help regulate your metabolism, including levels of

blood sugar (glucose)

Liver The liver is a large organ located just under your rib cage on the right side of your abdomen. It's a virtual chemical factory that performs hundreds of functions. Those functions include storing the nutrients from digested food, as well as filtering and processing potentially toxic substances you consume, such as alcohol, chemicals and most medications.

The liver also produces bile, a yellowish-green solution that helps break down fat so that it can be absorbed into your blood. Bile is what gives your stools their brown, green or yellowish color. This variation in color is normal. Stools that appear red or black, however, may indicate bleeding within the digestive tract.

Gallbladder Your gallbladder is a small, translucent sac that lies adjacent to your liver. The organ is a key part of the biliary tract, a system for transporting bile to the small intestine. The gallbladder functions as a reservoir for bile produced in your liver before the fluid drains into the duodenum.

Bile is produced continuously in your liver, even when your body isn't digesting food. Excess bile is turned into a more concentrated, potent solution in the gallbladder when some of the water that makes up bile is absorbed. When food passes into your duodenum, a hormone signals the gallbladder to release its stored bile.

Jejunum and ileum The middle section of the small intestine is called the jejunum. It is within this middle section where many nutrients are absorbed from food and pass into your bloodstream.

The final section of the small intestine is called the ileum. The primary duty of the ileum is to absorb remaining nutrients from food waste. Absorption of vitamin B-12, an essential vitamin, occurs in the last few feet of the ileum, called the terminal ileum. Bile acids also are absorbed in the terminal ileum. When bile acids aren't removed, they pass into the large intestine and may cause diarrhea.

The jejunum and ileum contain a variety of bacteria that aid in food digestion and nutrient absorption. Researchers are finding that a healthy balance of bacteria is beneficial not only to good digestion but also to your health in general (see Chapter 2).

The journey of food through the small intestine generally takes between 30 minutes and three hours, depending on the composition of your meal.

Colon

The colon is also known as the large intestine. Its job is to store and remove all food waste that your body can't digest.

Transverse

Descending

Ascending

Sigmoid

Colon

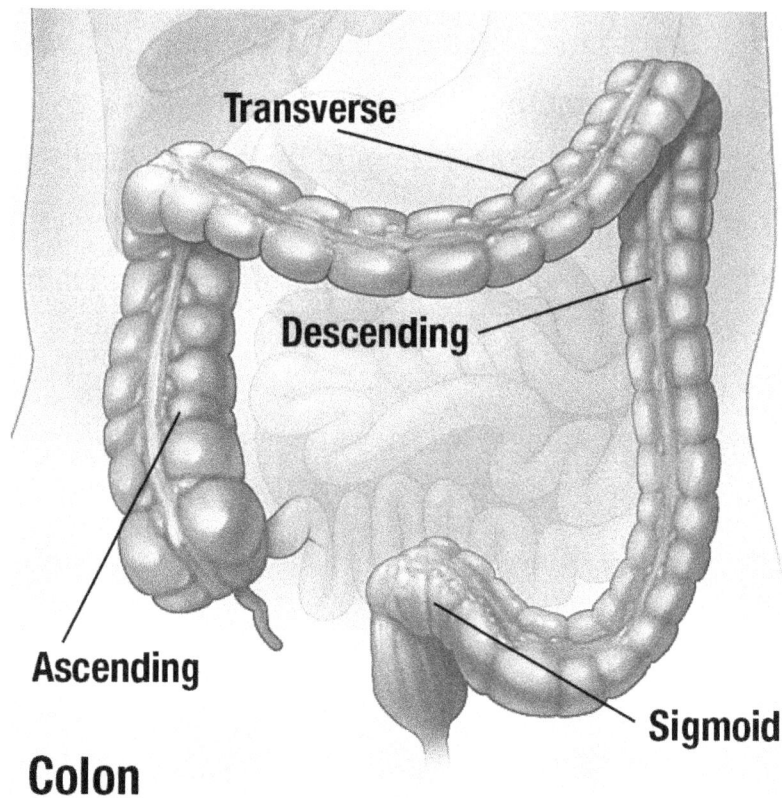

The colon is shorter than the small intestine but its diameter is greater and almost completely frames your small intestine. There are four sections of the colon: ascending, transverse, descending and sigmoid.

Food enters your colon through what's known as the ileocecal valve, located at the end of your small intestine. This muscular valve prevents food waste from returning to the ileum. By the time food waste reaches the colon, your body has absorbed nearly all of the nutrients it can.

What remains are water, electrolytes such as sodium and chloride, and waste products such as plant fiber, bacteria and dead cells shed from the lining of your digestive tract.

During the time that food waste passes through your colon, your body absorbs nearly all of the water from the waste. The remaining residue (stool) is usually soft but formed. It's also loaded with bacteria, which are useful to your body as long as your colon wall remains intact.

These bacteria cause certain food products to ferment, producing gas. This gas (flatus) is mainly an odorless mixture. The odors come from certain foods, especially those rich in sulfur, such as garlic and cabbage, or those with sulfur-based preservatives, such as bread, beer and potato chips.

As the food residue moves through your colon, muscle contractions separate and condense the waste into smaller segments. After each meal, considerable movement takes place in the descending colon, pushing the segments through your lower colon and into the rectum.

As your rectum begins to fill and stretch with waste, it signals your brain that it's time to release stool. Sphincter muscles in your anus, along with the muscles that make up your pelvic floor, serve as a final valve. The sphincter muscles relax as the muscles in your pelvic floor and rectum contract to increase pressure and expel stool from your body.

Sometimes, you need to exert additional pressure on the colon and rectum by using your abdominal muscles. If the muscle groups don't function in synchronization, it can become difficult to expel stool, a condition that leads to constipation.

You can learn more about constipation and how to manage it in Chapter 7.

DIGESTIVE PROBLEMS

As you read earlier in this chapter, digestive problems are among the most common reasons people see their doctors. They're also a leading reason why people take medication. The next time you visit a pharmacy or grocery store, take note of the many medications being sold to treat some type of digestive complaint.

Gastrointestinal woes — whether it's heartburn, diarrhea, constipation or gas — can wreak havoc on your daily routine and keep you from doing the things you enjoy.

In the chapters that follow, you'll learn more about the functions of your stomach, intestines and other digestive organs, including the gallbladder, pancreas and liver. You'll also learn about a variety of factors that can interfere with normal digestion.

With each condition discussed, we list common signs and symptoms associated with the condition and indications as to when you should see a doctor. In addition, we provide helpful information regarding diagnosis and treatment.

The human digestive system is incredibly complex. However, doctors and researchers continue to make new discoveries in regard to common gastrointestinal problems — why they occur, who's most at risk and the best ways to treat them.

Too often, people live with their problems for a long time before seeking medical advice because they believe that what they're experiencing is a normal part of digestion. As an example, if you take antacids regularly, perhaps daily, and have been doing so for several months, or even years, see your doctor. Daily heartburn isn't normal. Plus, the earlier you address a problem, the easier it is to treat and to keep from becoming serious.

In addition to discussing specific diseases and their treatments, this book addresses prevention. You'll learn about steps that you can take to keep your digestive system healthy, reducing your risk of disease. For many individuals, simple lifestyle changes can go a long way toward maintaining healthy digestion.

● ● ● ● ●

UNDERSTANDING THE LANGUAGE

Doctors and other medical professionals use a lot of terms to describe various parts of the digestive tract and conditions that can develop within it. Sometimes a doctor may use terminology that you don't understand. Or you may read an update to your electronic medical record and not really get what it means.

To help you out a bit, here are some terms doctors commonly use and an explanation of what they mean.

abscess. Collection of pus within part of the body

acquired. Developed after birth

acute. Symptoms that occur suddenly and generally last a short time

adjuvant. Additional therapy that follows the main treatment

asymptomatic. No symptoms

atrophy. Organ or tissue shrinks in size

benign. Not cancerous

bowel. Intestines

chronic. Longstanding or comes and goes frequently

contraindication. Situation where a treatment shouldn't be used

diaphragm. Dome-shaped muscular structure that separates the chest and abdominal cavities

distention. Swelling of the abdomen

duodenum. First (upper) part of the small intestine

dyspepsia. Another term for indigestion

dysphagia. Difficulty swallowing

edema. Swelling from excessive fluid buildup

etiology. Cause or origin of an illness or disease

gastric. Related to the stomach

hepatic. Related to the liver

idiopathic. Cause is unknown

ileum. Last part of the small intestine

indolent. Not active or growing slowly

jejunum. Middle part of the small intestine

lesion. Abnormal spot on tissue or skin

malabsorption. Inability to absorb essential nutrients from food

malignant. Cancerous

motility. Movement of food through digestive tract

necrosis. Death of tissue

negative. Means no disease or abnormality is present

noninvasive. Doesn't require entering the body with any instruments

pathogen. Anything that causes disease, normally refers to microorganisms

positive. Means disease or an abnormality is present

prognosis. Likely outcome based on the current situation

satiety. Feeling of fullness

● ● ● ● ●

CHAPTER 2
The gut microbiome

You've probably heard the saying, "You are what you eat." We've known for many years that what we put into our bodies can impact our health. But as science evolves, it's becoming clearer that our health may also be defined by the trillions of microorganisms that live inside of us.

In various parts of our bodies — in the mouth, vagina or respiratory tract, for example — we host a wide variety of micro-organisms. But nowhere are these micro-organisms greater in number and diversity than the gut. Diversity refers to how many different species of microorganisms are living in our gut and how evenly distributed they are in this area. Diversity is crucial, as it's a hallmark of a healthy gut.

Most of the time, the right kind and the right amounts of microorganisms are living in our guts, communicating with almost every area of our body and helping us maintain good overall health. But sometimes the balance of these microorganisms can be disrupted, causing a reduction in good bacteria and an increase in potentially harmful bacteria. Research is continuing to explore how this imbalance may be related to disease, from conditions that probably aren't so surprising, such as digestive disorders, to those you may not expect, such as autism.

Over the last several years, much research has been published looking at all aspects of the subject, thanks to improved testing that can better analyze our microbiome. One of the largest undertakings is the National Institutes of Health's Human Microbiome Project. Launched in 2007, it has helped catalog bacteria present in humans at various sites in the body, with the goal of learning what a healthy human gut is and whether human health could be improved by changing the gut's makeup of these microorganisms.

Despite increased research, many questions still linger. Perhaps the biggest: Are these imbalances actually causing disease, or are they the result of disease? The gut microbiome is complex and difficult to study, so finding an answer isn't easy. As you read through this chapter, keep in mind that for most of the conditions discussed there's only an association between the condition and an unhealthy gut microbiome; gut imbalances have not yet been proved to be the cause.

THE MICROBIOME EXPLAINED

In discussions of how the digestive system impacts our health, you'll see the terms *microbiota* and *microbiome* used a lot. Microbiota refers to all of the different microorganisms that live in a particular environment. For example, your gut houses mainly bacteria, but microorganisms such as viruses and fungi also call it home. These microorganisms provide many benefits, including strengthening the digestive tract, providing nutrients such as vitamins, regulating metabolism and protecting you from invaders that can cause disease. Gut microorganisms also play a role in communication with your immune system and regulating immunity.

The gut microbiome is the total environment of your gut, which includes not only specific microorganisms, but also their genetic components and their surroundings. Think of it as an ecosystem, and much like the ecosystem of Iceland varies from that of Brazil, so, too, does the environment of the gut vary from person to person.

The formation of this microbial ecosystem begins early on. Research suggests that prior to being born, our digestive tracts are almost like a blank slate. With birth, many outside influences begin to help shape the makeup of our guts. For example, an infant born via a vaginal delivery will have gut bacteria that differs from an infant born via a cesarean section. This is because the mother passes along bacteria to her child during a vaginal delivery. Babies who are breast-fed will have a different gut makeup from babies who consume formula. By the time a child is a toddler, he or she will have gut microbiota that resembles and is as diverse as an adult's. All told, our bodies house about 100 trillion gut microorganisms, including several hundred different species of bacteria.

For the most part, gut microbiota remain stable. But certain factors can change this — for example, medications or a change in diet. Aging also can have an impact because the gut's microbiota tend to become less diverse as we get older. This increases the chances of conditions resulting from decreased diversity in the gut, such as *Clostridium difficile* infections. An imbalance may also be linked to other gastrointestinal illnesses, such as irritable bowel syndrome, allergies, obesity and other metabolic problems, and neurological issues, such as autism. These will be discussed later in this chapter.

THE CHANGING GUT

When something changes the balance of your gut bacteria with the potential to cause harm, this is known as dysbiosis. This imbalance can lead to the gut being overpopulated by potentially damaging microbiota, which can interfere with the normal functioning of beneficial gut microbiota in charge of maintaining your health, and lead to the gut being overpopulated by potentially harmful microbiota.

Diet

As you might expect, diet plays a huge part in the makeup of our gut microbiota. Today, it's becoming more common for people around the world to follow a Westernized diet, or a diet that features increased amounts of fast foods and sugar, and decreased amounts of fiber, fruits and vegetables. Researchers have noted that with an increase in people following a Western diet, there's been an uptick in incidence of disease, including cancer, obesity, autoimmune disorders, inflammatory bowel disease and allergies. This may be associated with alterations in the gut bacteria related to diet. Some research has shown that diets high in saturated fats can change the structure and diversity of the gut microbiota, reducing certain bacteria that help prevent obesity. Such diets may also lead to gut inflammation.

Problems can also arise when we restrict our diets. For example, in recent years, people who don't have a gluten intolerance or celiac disease have been avoiding foods containing gluten. One study found that after four weeks of a gluten-free diet, the makeup of participants' gut microbiota had changed, with most having lower numbers of several vital beneficial microbiota species.

Food additives may also play a part in harming gut microbiota. Sweeteners such as sucralose, aspartame and saccharin are much sweeter and have minimal calories compared to sugar. But they may disturb the balance and diversity of your gut. In one study, rats given sucralose had much higher proportions of potentially harmful bacteria in their guts than rats that didn't eat sucralose. Emulsifiers, which are added to processed foods to increase shelf life, have also been shown to decrease gut diversity. Both artificial sweeteners and emulsifiers may increase inflammatory responses in the gut. One cornstarch-based sweetener called trehalose was thought by some researchers to be behind a *Clostridium difficile* epidemic.

On the opposite end of the spectrum, high-fiber, plant-based diets have been shown to be the most gut-friendly. One example is the Mediterranean diet, which focuses on fruits, vegetables, whole grains, legumes, nuts and healthy fats such as olive oil and canola oil. Red meat, if eaten, is limited to just a few times a month with this diet. Fiber, in particular, is important because it can boost diversity in the gut.

Medication

Almost all medications can affect gut microbiota, primarily by altering the gut environment. Some examples include antibiotics and proton pump inhibitors (PPIs) that can produce harmful changes.

Antibiotics, in particular, are known for their ability to affect the gut microbiome, causing a shift that favors the colonization of certain bacteria that can lead to antibiotic- associated diarrhea and the debilitating infection *Clostridium difficile*. There are many different types of antibiotics, dosages and lengths of treatment, and each of these factors will impact the gut in their own way.

Oftentimes, the gut microbiome will return to its original state after taking antibiotics. However, some research has found that exposure to antibiotics, especially in the prenatal or early life stage, can cause a long-term shift in your gut's microbiome and can increase the risk of infection, metabolic conditions, allergies and antibiotic resistance. These effects may last years after medication exposure.

Smoking

Smoking is harmful to many aspects of human health. It can also negatively impact microbiota composition and cause intestinal inflammation. Quitting smoking can reverse this and increase diversity in your gut.

Stress

Your gut and your brain are connected by a shared pathway that allows them to communicate with one another about things such as hormones, inflammation and brain chemicals. Stress can negatively impact this line of communication and increase the risk of a gut imbalance.

Home environment

In particular, having pets or farm animals may influence your gut makeup, though typically in a positive way. Studies have noted a lower incidence in pediatric allergies in homes where there are pets or where children live on farms. The theory is that animals may help to desensitize young, developing immune systems. Microbiota diversity has been shown in some studies to be more diverse and rich in infants whose households contain pets. How animals affect adults isn't known.

WHEN A GOOD GUT GOES BAD

A gut imbalance is thought to play some part in the development of a number of conditions. However, research hasn't been able to prove a definitive link in most cases.

When conducting research on how the state of the gut microbiome affects our health, many studies are conducted in mice, specifically germ-free mice, meaning the mice have no microorganisms living in or on them. More research is needed in humans. Following are some of the conditions that have been linked to gut problems.

Clostridium difficile

Clostridium difficile (*C. diff.*) is an organism that lives in normal gut microbiota. When it grows out of control, it's also the most common cause of hospital-acquired diarrhea, which affects about 450,000 people in the United States every year. In the most severe cases, *C. diff.* infections can cause life-threatening organ dysfunction (sepsis) and death. It is one of the only conditions where a definitive link has been established between an unhealthy gut microbiome and development of infection.

The majority of *C. diff.* infections are caused by taking an antibiotic — particularly a broad-spectrum antibiotic, which disrupts the normal gut microbiota balance and leads to decreased microbiota diversity. This is thought to occur because your digestive system is prevented from producing specific bile acids that keep *C. diff.* growth in check, while at the same time creating nutrients that encourage its proliferation. *C. diff.* growth leads to production of a toxin that damages the intestinal barrier and produces absorption problems, in turn, leading to diarrhea.

Many people who experience a *C. diff.* infection may have repeated infections in spite of being successfully treated. This may be because the gut microbiota haven't completely recovered. For these individuals, traditional treatment with a different antibiotic is often unsuccessful. A procedure called fecal microbiota transplantation (see here) may be used to restore a healthy microbiota. It often produces high cure rates.

Obesity

Obesity is an ever-worsening epidemic worldwide. It's associated with high blood pressure, high cholesterol, fatty liver, diabetes, heart disease and chronic inflammation throughout the body. Considerable research has linked an unhealthy gut microbiome to the development of obesity in humans and animals.

Studies often associate an imbalance of the bacteria *Bacteroidetes* and *Firmicutes* with weight gain, though some recent research doesn't support this link. Mouse studies have shown that transplanting the microbiota of an obese mouse into a germ-free mouse can cause rapid and larger amounts of weight gain not seen when a germ-free mouse receives microbiota from lean a mouse. However, a definitive link hasn't yet been proved. This is an active area of research.

Inflammatory bowel disease

The term *inflammatory bowel disease* includes ulcerative colitis and Crohn's disease, two conditions associated with gastrointestinal inflammation (see Chapter 12). The two conditions can cause frequent diarrhea, fever and abdominal pain. Both ulcerative colitis and Crohn's disease can run in families, but altered microorganisms in the gut are thought to play a role, as well.

A microbial gut imbalance may impair the function of the gut barrier, the lining of the intestine that protects the intestinal tract from harmful invaders and also serves as a filter. The microbiome may also be a critical component in the triggering of inflammatory bowel syndrome. Research suggests an individual's genes and microbiota can interact to promote development of the disease among people who are genetically predisposed.

Irritable bowel syndrome

Though the subject of debate, research suggests irritable bowel syndrome (IBS) may be triggered by a disturbance in the micro-biome because IBS sometimes follows an intestinal infection. In addition, some individuals with IBS respond to treatments that help alter microbiota, such as antibiotics and probiotics, further suggesting potential involvement of the microbiome in development of the disease.

Colorectal cancer

Diet and nutrition are strongly linked to colorectal cancer. While eating fruits, vegetables and whole grains reduces cancer risk, a diet high in saturated fat has been linked to cancer development. In addition, research indicates the diversity of microbiota often is reduced within cancerous tissue, compared to noncancerous tissue, and that cancerous tissue often contains increased amounts of potentially harmful bacteria and less beneficial bacteria. Bacteria may play a role in cancer development in other ways, including the development of inflammation within tissues and the production of toxins that damage DNA.

Autism

Autism spectrum disorders are a collection of complex disorders that negatively impact social interaction and communication. While cases of autism have been increasing, what causes the disorders is poorly understood. Only about 20 percent of autism cases are thought to be related to genetics.

Research suggests a potential link between the gut microbiome and autism spectrum disorders. However, further study is needed and it will likely be several years before researchers know more about a possible relationship.

The gut and the brain share a complex, two-way communication pathway, referred to as the gut-brain axis, which influences each in a number of ways. For example, the gut microbiome can influence the development of chemicals in the brain that are important components of memory, and the brain can impact the gut microbiome with a direct influence on gut functions, such as acid production and movement of food through the digestive tract.

Any disruption in this communication link could trigger problems, particularly if that disruption involves the blood-brain barrier, a system that protects the brain by filtering out harmful substances from the blood.

Many children and adults with autism spectrum disorders experience significant gastrointestinal symptoms, such as constipation and diarrhea. A number of studies have reported altered gut bacteria in children with autism compared to children without autism, although not all research has noted this. Studies have found that children with autism tend to have lower amounts of beneficial bacteria, as well as less diversity of bacteria, in their guts. Some researchers believe this could affect neurological health.

Studies conducted in mice suggest that adding bacteria called *Bacteroides fragilis* may change gut microbiota, helping to correct gut function and possibly improving autism behavior. Another promising area of research is fecal microbiota transplantation (see here). A recent study looking at the effectiveness of the treatment in children found that it was safe, well-tolerated and led to significant improvement in gastrointestinal symptoms and symptoms of autism, such as problems with social skills. However, research is still in its early stages, and fecal microbiota transplantation is considered an experimental treatment.

What role, if any, gut microbiota might play in the development of other neuropsychiatric conditions such as anxiety and depression is also under study. It will likely be several years before results are available.

Allergies

Over the past few decades, food allergies and allergic diseases such as asthma and eczema have become more common. One theory called "hygiene hypothesis" suggests that exposure to microorganisms during childhood are vital to strengthening your immune system. Any change to this process — particularly regular antibiotic use — could lead to changes in the gut microbiota and inappropriate immune responses, resulting in allergies.

● ● ● ● ●

WHAT IS FECAL TRANSPLANTATION?

The concept may seem a bit strange: Treat a condition by transferring gut microbiota from a healthy person to someone who is sick. But fecal microbiota transplantation (FMT) is proving to be highly successful at treating recurrent *Clostridium difficile* (*C. diff.*) infections that aren't responding to standard therapy.

Fecal microbiota transplantation restores healthy intestinal bacteria by placing another person's (donor's) stool in your colon, using a colonoscope or nasogastric tube. Donors are screened for medical conditions, their blood is tested for infections, and stools are carefully screened for parasites, viruses and other infectious bacteria. After being taken from the donor and before being transplanted in your colon, the stool is mixed with a liquid and any solid matter is removed.

Studies of the gut after the procedure show that healthy bacteria quickly take up residence in their new environment and the gut mirrors that of the donor stool. Currently, fecal transplantation is most successful in treating *C. diff.* infections, with success rates reported from 85 percent to more than 90 percent. How exactly it works isn't completely understood, but one hypothesis is that by restoring the normal bacterial populations, there's increased competition for nutrients, which can stop *C. diff.* growth.

Fecal transplantation has also been used in inflammatory bowel disease with mixed success. Researchers are interested in exploring other potential applications of fecal microbiota transplantation, which could possibly include the treatment of obesity, chronic fatigue syndrome and fibromyalgia. One small study found that fecal transplants might reduce autism spectrum disorder symptoms in up to 24 percent of participants, with benefits continuing for at least eight weeks.

As with any procedure, there are risks, including injury, infection and a worsening of existing conditions. Potential long-term risks aren't known at this time. In the treatment of *C. diff.* infection, fecal transplantation is performed after a detailed discussion about the procedure and its risks and benefits. For other diseases, fecal transplantation is only used in research studies.

● ● ● ● ●

NURTURING A HEALTHY GUT

Defining what encompasses a healthy human gut microbiome hasn't been easy. Scientists know that diversity is a good thing. But complicating matters is the variety of microorganisms that live in the gut, even among healthy individuals. So, instead, researchers have tried to identify certain patterns of stable microorganisms in healthy individuals.

In fact, you may see advertisements for microbiome tests that promise insight into the makeup of your gut by analyzing a stool sample. While these tests can tell you the microorganisms that call your gut home, they can't really advise you or your doctor what to do with this information. Gut microbiome research is still in the early stages, and the science isn't at the point where it can definitively determine if an unbalanced gut microbiome causes disease, or if the disease or the medications used to treat it are to blame — bringing us back to the "association doesn't prove causation" problem.

We do know, though, that certain foods and lifestyle habits seem to help promote gut health. For example, moderate to vigorously intense aerobic exercise has been shown to improve the composition of microbiota in your gut.

Research also suggests that eating plant-based foods, such as fruits and vegetables, peas and beans (legumes), and whole grains supply good bacteria to our guts. These foods contain complex carbohydrates. Our bodies can't digest complex carbohydrates, so they become food for gut bacteria, allowing them to thrive. Foods that contain active cultures, such as yogurt, kimchi and kombucha, also may provide helpful bacteria.

In the future, it's possible we may be able to tailor diets to individuals based on their specific gut microbiota. Until that day, the best strategy is to exercise and eat a variety of healthy foods to keep your gut happy. For more information on what foods to eat for good gut health, see the next chapter.

CHAPTER 3
Recipe for healthy digestion

What you put on your plate has a lot to do with good digestion. But it's not only what you eat that's important. How much you eat, and the manner in which you eat — relaxed or hurried, focused or distracted — also play key roles. Your daily food choices and eating habits go a long way toward keeping your digestive system strong and healthy.

Of course, you can't prevent or manage all digestive problems simply by following a healthy lifestyle. Some digestive disorders are hereditary or occur for unknown reasons, and their treatment may require help from a medical professional. Still, there are many digestive signs and symptoms that you can control, and a few changes in your daily habits may help ease your discomfort.

Adopting a healthier diet, eating slowly, managing stress and getting regular physical activity — these are some important lifestyle changes that may have a significant impact on your digestive health.

If you can stick with these changes, gradually they become habits. Those habits, in turn, become a routine, and eventually that routine becomes your new lifestyle. The benefits are many. In addition to improving your digestive health, healthier habits can reduce your risk of disease and help you look and feel better.

WHAT TO EAT

The human body is designed to digest many types of foods, but everyone is different. Certain foods may trigger digestive-related signs and symptoms in some people but not in others. That's why there isn't one recipe for keeping your gut happy. But there are a few basic principles of good digestion — foods to eat and foods to limit — that apply to most people.

For good gut health, you want to eat plenty of foods containing fiber and prebiotics, and fewer processed foods or foods high in sugar or fat. It's also important to get enough fluids.

If you have irritable bowel syndrome or you may be sensitive to certain foods, you may benefit from a special diet called a low-FODMAP diet (see here).

Foods high in fiber

Plant foods — vegetables, fruits and foods made from whole grains — are excellent sources of fiber. Think peas and beans, berries, leafy greens, whole-wheat pasta, and brown rice (see here).

Your digestive tract will accept almost any food you send its way. However, certain foods tend to pass more easily and quickly through your digestive system and help it function properly. These foods are rich in dietary fiber, a nutrient that's an important part of a healthy diet and is especially important to digestion.

Fiber is the part of plant food that's indigestible and your body doesn't absorb. Fiber comes in two forms: soluble and insoluble, and fiber-rich foods usually contain both forms. Soluble fiber absorbs up to 15 times its weight in water as it moves through your digestive tract, producing softer stools. Insoluble fiber gives stool its bulk.

• • • • •

WHAT ABOUT FIBER SUPPLEMENTS?

It's best to get your fiber from food because supplements don't provide the vitamins, minerals and other nutrients that fiber-rich foods do. But if you can't get enough fiber from diet alone, supplements can help you reach the daily recommended amount.

Regular use of fiber supplements — such as psyllium (Metamucil, Konsyl, others) or methylcellulose (Citrucel) — hasn't been found to be harmful. However, fiber supplements may cause abdominal bloating and gas, at least initially. So, if you have intestinal problems, talk to your doctor before adding a fiber supplement to your diet.

It's also a good idea to ask your doctor or pharmacist whether fiber supplements interact with any medications you take. The supplements could possibly decrease the absorption of certain medications. They can also reduce blood sugar levels, which may require an adjustment in your medications or insulin if you have diabetes.

If you plan to take a fiber supplement, start with a small amount to minimize gas and bloating. Also, be sure to drink plenty of fluids.

• • • • •

A healthy amount of fiber in your diet can prevent constipation, lessen signs and symptoms of irritable bowel syndrome, and reduce your risk of hemorrhoids and diverticular disease, a condition in which pouches form in intestinal walls. Fiber also helps encourage the growth of healthy and diverse bacteria in your gut (see Chapter 2).

How much fiber should you get? The National Academies of Sciences, Engineering, and Medicine recommends the following:

- Adult men age 50 and younger should consume 38 grams of fiber daily, and men older than age 50 should get 30 grams each day.
- Adult women age 50 and younger should consume 25 grams of fiber daily, and women older than 50 should get 21 grams each day.

Unfortunately, most of us don't get enough fiber. Over time, westernized diets have evolved to include fewer plant-based foods, such as fruits and vegetables, and more refined grains, such as white bread, white pasta and white rice. And these changes have resulted in decreased consumption of fiber. Typical westernized diets include about 15 grams of fiber daily.

As you add more fiber to your diet, remember to take it slow. Too much fiber all at once can create its own set of bellyaches, including gas and cramps. Drinking plenty of water can help prevent these symptoms. Also keep in mind that some individuals need to limit fiber. If you have a bowel obstruction, it's best to eat a low-fiber diet to prevent a bowel blockage. And if you have celiac disease or gluten sensitivity, you want to eat whole grains that don't contain gluten.

Foods containing probiotics

Probiotics are often called "friendly bacteria" or "good bacteria." They're beneficial microorganisms created through the fermentation process.

It's been suggested that foods containing probiotics may be good for your digestive system because they contain good microbes that help combat and crowd out any bad bacteria that may be lurking in your gut. At this point, the evidence in favor of probiotics is more suggestive than proved.

Probiotics can be found in yogurt that contains "active" or "live" cultures. Yogurt is made by fermenting milk with different bacteria, which are left behind in the final product. Other sources of probiotics include some cheeses, sauerkraut, a fermented milk drink called kefir, Korean fermented vegetables known as kimchi, and kombucha, a tea.

Your intestinal tract, especially your colon, is filled with a complex and diverse array of bacteria. You need bacteria to digest the food you eat. But an unhealthy balance — not enough "good" bacteria or too many "bad" bacteria can create problems (see Chapter 2).

Probiotic foods may help improve diarrhea and constipation and promote overall gut health. Some studies suggest probiotics also may be beneficial in managing other health conditions including irritable bowel syndrome.

● ● ● ● ●

WHAT ABOUT PROBIOTIC SUPPLEMENTS?

A few studies have suggested that probiotic supplements might be good for your health, but other studies haven't found any benefit. Also keep in mind that manufacturers of probiotic supplements aren't held to the same rules and regulations as drug companies are, so you can't always be sure probiotic supplements contain exactly what's on the label.

It's best to get your probiotics from food if you can. If you choose to take a probiotic supplement, a good place to start is with a combination that contains strains from the *Lactobacillus* family and *Bifidobacterium* family, strains normally found in the human gastrointestinal tract.

Not all probiotic supplements are the same. Each type — and each strain of each type — can work in different ways and have different effects, influencing individuals differently.

Probiotic supplements are generally considered safe, but before taking a probiotic supplement, check with your doctor or pharmacist, especially if you're pregnant or you have a health condition. Individuals with a weakened immune system, such as from cancer treatment or an organ transplant, are at higher risk of having an adverse reaction to a probiotic supplement.

● ● ● ● ●

● ● ● ● ●

WHERE TO FIND FIBER

To avoid digestive upset and gas that can come from eating too much fiber too quickly, gradually increase the amount you eat over a period of several weeks. Here's how much fiber is in some common foods.

Grains, cereal and pasta	Serving size	Total fiber* (grams)
Bran flakes	1 cup	7
Barley, pearled, cooked	1 cup	6
Oatmeal, cooked	1 packet or 1 cup	4
Spaghetti, whole-wheat, cooked	1 cup	3.9
Brown rice, cooked	1 cup	3.5
Bread, 100% whole-wheat	1 slice	2

Legumes and nuts	Serving size	Total fiber* (grams)
Split peas, boiled	1 cup	16.3
Lentils, boiled	1 cup	15.6
Black beans, canned	1 cup	12
Baked beans, vegetarian, canned	1 cup	10
Almonds	1 ounce	3.5
Pistachio nuts	1 ounce	3

Fruits	Serving size	Total fiber* (grams)
Raspberries	1 cup	8
Pear, with skin	1 medium	5.5
Apple, with skin	1 medium	4.4
Blueberries	1 cup	3.6
Banana	1 medium	3.1
Orange	1 medium	3.1
Strawberries (halves)	1 cup	3.0

Vegetables	Serving size	Total fiber* (grams)
Green peas, boiled	1 cup	8.8
Squash, winter, baked	1 cup	5.7
Broccoli, cooked	1 cup	5.1
Brussels sprouts, boiled	1 cup	4.1
Potato with skin, baked	1 medium	3.8
Sweet potato with skin, baked	1 medium	3.7
Sweet corn, boiled	1 cup	3.6

Carrot, raw	1 large	2.1

Sources: USDA National Nutrient Database for Standard Reference, Legacy Release, April 2018 and Mayo Clinic Dietetics Department.

* Fiber content can vary among brands.

● ● ● ● ●

Foods rich in prebiotics

Prebiotics are found in a variety of foods such as asparagus, yams, bananas, onions, garlic, artichokes, legumes and whole-wheat products.

Think of prebiotics as food for the good bacteria (probiotics) that reside in your gut. Prebiotics are natural food components that help probiotics flourish. They are in essence the fertilizer that stimulates the growth of healthy bacteria.

Research suggests prebiotics can help prevent and manage infectious and antibiotic-resistant diarrhea and reduce symptoms associated with inflammatory bowel disease. As part of a healthy diet, prebiotics may even play a role in weight loss.

The best way to get enough prebiotics in your diet is to eat plenty of fruits, vegetables, beans and peas (legumes), and whole grains. Similar to probiotic supplements, it's better to get your prebiotics from food rather than supplements because most foods that contain prebiotics are loaded with other healthy nutrients. And as with probiotic supplements, the regulation of prebiotic supplements is limited.

When it comes to vitamins and supplements, food is best. Eating a healthy diet plentiful in vitamins and minerals is the best route for good health. If you feel that your diet might not be as healthy as it could be, you might consider taking a daily multivitamin. When it comes to specific digestive-related products, talk to your doctor. You don't want to take a supplement that may be a waste of your money, or worse, be potentially dangerous to your health.

Fluids

Fluids are important because they help dissolve nutrients in the food you eat, making them easier to absorb. Fluids also soften stool and lubricate food waste so the waste passes more easily through your digestive tract, helping to prevent constipation.

To make sure all your body systems function properly — including your digestive system — it's important to get enough fluids each day. How much fluid you need depends on a variety of factors, including your health, where you live, how active you are and how much you perspire. You may have heard the advice to drink eight 8-ounce glasses of fluid a day — the 8x8 rule.

The 8x8 rule is easy to remember and a close-enough goal for most people. For some people, fewer than eight glasses might be adequate. Others might need more fluid. Also keep in mind that if you have a specific medical condition, you may need to limit your fluid intake or drink more than is recommended for healthy adults.

Most people can get the recommended amount of fluid by letting thirst be their guide. While water is a good choice, you can also get fluid from juice, milk, coffee, tea, and fruits and vegetables. Most vegetables and fruits are at least 80 percent water.

In the past, caffeinated beverages generally weren't counted as fluids because they were thought to have a diuretic effect, increasing urination and fluid loss. More recent evidence indicates this isn't true. Alcohol, however, doesn't count as a fluid because of its diuretic properties. Alcohol and caffeine may also contribute to heartburn and indigestion.

You may find a warm beverage in the morning preferable to a cold one, especially if you're bothered by constipation. About 30 minutes after drinking warm liquid, your body may have a natural urge to pass stool. Drinking a caffeinated beverage also may stimulate a bowel movement. Because it's a stimulant, caffeine can cause diarrhea in some people.

WHAT TO LIMIT

You know what foods are good for your gut, those that you should eat more of. But are there foods that are harmful to digestion, those you should limit or avoid? The answer is yes; but keeping them out of your mouth can be difficult.

Highly processed foods and foods laden with sugar or fat aren't good for your gut. The problem is, they taste good and they're everywhere. While you may not be able to completely stay away from such foods, do your best to limit them.

Processed foods

Processed foods are foods that have been changed by a manufacturing process so that they appear different from their natural state. Compare an ear of sweet corn, an unprocessed food, and a bag of corn chips or a dessert containing high fructose corn syrup, highly processed products. Corn is found in all three, but they aren't at all alike.

The manufacturing process often removes beneficial food components, such as vitamins, minerals and fiber. At the same time, it adds in unhealthy ingredients, such as preservatives and other artificial ingredients intended to enhance the product's taste, texture or shelf life.

Foods high in sugar

A common additive in processed foods is sugar or high fructose corn syrup. In addition to tasting sweet, sugar is often used as a food stabilizer, bulking agent or preservative.

When you consume more sugar than your bloodstream can absorb, the excess sugar passes through your digestive system. Bacteria in your bowels feast on the sugar, producing gas. This can lead to abdominal pain, bloating and flatulence. Too much sugar also may cause an overgrowth of harmful bacteria. And because it's high in calories, excess sugar can lead to obesity, a common cause of type 2 diabetes.

Artificial sweeteners, such as mannitol, sorbitol and xylitol, aren't digestive-friendly either. These sweeteners, known as sugar alcohols, are found primarily in sugar-free gum and candies. In people who consume a lot, the sweeteners can produce abdominal gas, bloating and diarrhea. Some sugar additives, such as the dietary sugar trehalose, have been linked to a bacterial infection of the intestine called *Clostridium difficile* (*C. diff.*) infection.

Foods high in fat

Too much fat isn't good for you because fat can slow the digestive process. Foods high in fat tend to sit in your stomach longer, increasing the production of gastric acids, causing bloating and triggering heartburn.

Some people experience diarrhea after eating high-fat, greasy foods. This may be because their bodies can't adequately digest or absorb the fat, causing the food to move through the digestive tract more quickly than normal.

● ● ● ● ●

THE EFFECTS OF ALCOHOL

Too much alcohol — anything above a moderate amount — can cause digestive problems. Alcohol can inflame your stomach lining. It can also relax the valve (lower esophageal sphincter) that prevents stomach acid from backing up into your esophagus. This can increase your risk of heartburn or esophageal bleeding.

People who drink excessively are more likely to experience inflammation of the digestive tract and internal bleeding. People who consume too much alcohol may also be at increased risk of liver disease and pancreatitis, as well as cancer of the mouth, throat, esophagus, stomach, colon or liver. Individuals who regularly drink alcohol and also use tobacco have an even greater risk of cancers of the mouth, throat and esophagus.

Women may be more susceptible to alcohol-related disorders because their bodies produce fewer enzymes to break down alcohol. In addition, as people age, their tolerance for alcohol often decreases. An older person isn't able to metabolize alcohol as readily, making him or her more vulnerable to alcohol's effects.

Limit alcohol to a moderate amount — up to one drink a day for nonpregnant women and men older than age 65, and up to two drinks a day for men age 65 and younger. A drink is defined as 12 ounces of beer, 8 ounces of malt liquor, 5 ounces of wine or 1.5 ounces of 80-proof distilled spirits.

If you don't drink alcohol during the week, it isn't OK to drink excessive amounts on the weekend, in essence making up for the drinks you missed during the week. This can lead to serious liver damage.

● ● ● ● ●

YOUR EATING HABITS

How you eat can be just as important for good digestion as what you eat. Poor digestion may simply be due to the unhealthy habits you practice during or between meals. To help improve your digestion, follow these tips:

Eat moderate proportions

Large meals put increased demands on your digestive system. Your body is able to produce only a certain amount of digestive juices. If you eat too much, not enough digestive juices may be available to meet the task. Large amounts of food also increase the amount of waste moving through your digestive tract, which may lead to bloating.

Moderate portions, on the other hand, are digested more comfortably. Plus, if you eat smaller portions, you reduce the risk of overeating and may find it easier to control your weight.

Eat in the morning

The morning is one of the best times of day to take advantage of regular muscle contractions taking place in your colon (gastrocolic reflex). This reflex helps move waste from the colon to the rectum, triggering an urge to expel stool. Eating breakfast loads your digestive system with food — and ultimately food waste — helping to promote regular bowel movements.

Eat at regular times

Your digestive organs operate best when you follow a regular schedule — such as eating three meals a day versus eating whenever you feel like it. With a regular schedule, your digestive system also has time to rest between meals. Skipping meals isn't good for you because it can lead to excessive hunger, which often results in overeating.

Relax while you eat

Hectic schedules seem to have more people rushing through their meals or eating on the go. When you eat fast, you often overeat before your stomach can signal that it's full — which often leads to overconsumption and weight gain. In addition, you tend not to chew your food long enough or to grind it into small enough pieces, forcing your digestive system to work harder. When you gulp down food rapidly, you also swallow more air than you would if you were eating slowly. This can lead to belching, bloating and intestinal gas.

Your state of mind while you eat — whether you're hurried, stressed or relaxed — affects your digestion. When you're relaxed, you tend to chew your food more completely, gastric and intestinal juices flow more freely, and digestive muscles contract and relax normally. Eating when you feel stressed interferes with the normal functioning of your intestines, and can result in stomach upset, bloating, heartburn, constipation or diarrhea.

Sit up when you eat

To make sure food digests properly and stomach acid doesn't regurgitate into your esophagus, don't eat while lying down. And don't lie down right after a meal. Wait at least three hours after eating before lying down or going to bed.

PHYSICAL ACTIVITY

You might wonder why we mention physical activity. The fact is, physical activity is very important to digestion. Daily physical activity helps speed the movement of food through your digestive tract in addition to helping you maintain a healthy weight.

Physical activity refers to any movement you do that burns calories, such as gardening, cleaning the house, or taking a stretch break from your office desk. Exercise is a structured, repetitive form of physical activity, such as swimming laps, bicycling, brisk walking and lifting weights.

Aerobic exercise — exercise that increases your breathing and heart rate — is the most beneficial for healthy digestion. Aerobic exercise stimulates the activity of your stomach and intestinal muscles, helping to move food and waste through your digestive tract. Aerobic exercise also promotes weight loss.

Unfortunately, Americans have become increasingly sedentary. We don't participate in recreational sports or exercise regularly. In fact, a recent report by the Centers for Disease Control and Prevention found that only 23 percent of American adults get the recommended amount of physical activity.

If you aren't active, there's no better time to get started. If you have health problems, are significantly overweight or haven't been active for several years, it's important that you talk to your doctor beforehand. He or she can help you choose activities that are safe and appropriate.

Aim for at least 30 minutes of physical activity most, if not all, days of the week. If you're not sure how to start, walking is a good activity to begin with because it's easy, convenient and inexpensive. All you need is a good pair of walking shoes.

Here are some tips as you take steps to become more active.

Walk before you run

Being overly enthused can lead you to the "terrible toos" of physical activity — too much, too hard, too often, too soon. This all-or-nothing approach is a recipe for discouragement, not to mention injury. The best approach is to start slowly and gradually build up.

Look for opportunities

Try to build more activity into your regular schedule. One way to be more active is to place your treadmill or exercise bike in front of the TV and walk or bike while watching your favorite programs. Or you might take the stairs instead of the elevator or park farther from work and walk a few additional blocks. Consider wearing an activity tracker to motivate you to take more steps.

Listen to your body

Activity shouldn't cause discomfort. If you feel pain, shortness of breath, dizziness or nausea, take a break — you may be pushing yourself too hard. If you're not feeling well, take a day or two off and resume the activity as soon as you can. And make sure to warm up before exercise with easy walking and gentle stretching. Also, allow time to cool down after exercise.

Do what you enjoy

If you want to develop a more formal exercise program that you'll stick with, try to include activities that are fun for you. Many different types of activities can increase your fitness level. The trick is choosing ones that also stimulate and entertain you.

Pick a time and stick with it

Schedule a specific time to exercise, whether it's a one-hour workout or short, regular intervals throughout the day. Don't try to exercise in your "spare time." If you don't make it a priority, exercise will be pushed aside for other concerns.

STRESS

Have you ever had a "gut-wrenching" experience or felt the "butterflies" in your stomach? Most people have. That's because the body's brain and gastrointestinal system are intimately connected, and they "talk" to each other a lot. This link between those cells that control your digestive functions and those that regulate your brain's emotional center is called the gut-brain axis.

What this means in regard to digestion is that when you're anxious, worried or feeling stressed you don't digest food well. Not surprisingly, a lot of gastrointestinal disorders are associated with stress and anxiety.

When you're under stress, your body reacts as if you're in danger. It pumps extra blood to your muscles so that you'll have more energy either to fight off an attack or to run away. This leaves less blood volume to support digestion. Your digestive muscles exert less effort, your body secretes fewer enzymes to aid digestion, and the passage of food and waste through your digestive tract shifts into low gear. This produces symptoms such as heartburn, bloating and constipation.

Sometimes stress does the opposite. It speeds passage of food through your intestines, causing abdominal pain and diarrhea. Stress may also worsen symptoms of digestive conditions such as ulcers, irritable bowel syndrome and ulcerative colitis.

Getting help

Everyone experiences stress. What's important is to recognize when you're feeling stressed and take steps to relieve the tension. Left untreated, stress can take a major toll on your health. It can lead to weight loss or weight gain, cause headaches, create sleep troubles, and negatively affect your digestion.

One of the best ways to help reduce and manage the stress is with exercise. Exercise often serves as a sort of timeout from your problems — you tend to focus on the immediate task at hand and not on the tensions of the day. As you exert your body, your mind senses a feeling of calm and control.

Other tools for combating stress include techniques such as relaxed breathing and progressive muscle relaxation, as well as therapies such as meditation and yoga. Medications also can help.

If you're having difficulty controlling the stress in your life, don't be afraid to seek professional help. Your doctor can connect you to appropriate individuals trained in stress management. One method that therapists often use to help manage stress is called cognitive behavioral therapy. It focuses on identifying specific factors that contribute to your distress, learning how to change your thoughts and emotions, and developing strategies to manage stress.

MEDICATIONS

Almost all medications affect digestion in one way or another. Often the effects are mild and go unnoticed, but some medications produce moderate to severe signs and symptoms, especially if you take them regularly.

For example, opioids taken to relieve pain can produce constipation, medications taken for high blood pressure can cause diarrhea or constipation, and antibiotics taken to fight infection can result in nausea or diarrhea. Antibiotic diarrhea can affect the balance of bacteria normally present in the large intestine, causing some forms to overgrow.

Aspirin and nonsteroidal anti-inflammatory drugs (NSAIDs) are some of the most potentially damaging medications. NSAIDs include the over-the-counter drugs ibuprofen (Advil, Motrin IB, others) and naproxen sodium (Aleve). When taken occasionally and as directed, aspirin and NSAIDs are generally safe. But if taken regularly, or if you take more than the recommended amounts, the drugs may cause nausea, stomach pain, stomach bleeding or ulcers. If you take any of these medications regularly, discuss this with your doctor.

Certain medications — including some antidepressants, sedatives and tranquilizers, asthma medications, and specific drugs to treat nausea — can interfere with the action of the sphincter muscle located between the esophagus and stomach that allows food to pass into the stomach after swallowing. If the muscle isn't functioning properly, stomach acid can back up into the esophagus, causing acid reflux.

In addition, some people have difficulty swallowing tablets or capsules, or they take medicines without liquid. Tablets or capsules that stay in the esophagus may release chemicals that can irritate the lining of the esophagus (see here). This may cause ulcers, bleeding and narrowing (stricture) of the esophagus. It's important to swallow medications with plenty of liquids and stay upright after swallowing.

Talk to your doctor

If you think that your digestive issues might be related to the medications you take, make an appointment to see your doctor and bring your medications with you. Your doctor might suggest you take a different drug that's less damaging to your digestive tract, or possibly a smaller dose of your current medication. For some medications, taking them with food also might help reduce their side effects.

But don't stop taking a medication, especially a prescription drug, without first talking to your doctor or a pharmacist. Abruptly stopping certain medications can cause severe side effects.

UNDERSTANDING DIGESTIVE DISEASE

We've touched on a lot of topics in this chapter, and they're all important. The health of your digestive tract has a lot to do with your lifestyle — the type of food you eat, how much food you eat, how physically active you are, the pace of your day, the amount of stress in your life and the medications you take.

Remarkably adaptive, the human digestive system can adjust to a wide variety of situations. It can also tolerate an astonishing amount of stress, as well as abuse from hurried or poorly planned meals.

Over time, though, an unhealthy diet, poor eating habits, stress and inactivity may take their toll. Occasional symptoms, such as heartburn or abdominal pain, may eventually become more frequent and severe.

Not all digestive problems, however, stem from lifestyle. Some conditions are thought to be hereditary or related to inflammation or an infection. And for some digestive issues, there's no known cause.

Information in the chapters that follow can help you understand some of the most common digestive conditions. You'll also learn more about steps you can take to be good to your gut and improve your digestive health.

CHAPTER 4
Gut feelings

You know the feeling. You've had it before, and you'll most likely encounter it again. It may be an uneasy sense of nausea or an attack of diarrhea urging you to the nearest bathroom. Perhaps it's that all-too-familiar sear of heartburn after a heavy meal.

Almost everyone on occasion experiences signs and symptoms that suggest something isn't quite right in his or her gut.

Often, two or more signs and symptoms occur at the same time, making it hard to describe exactly what the feeling is. When you complain of "indigestion," for example, you may actually be referring to a range of signs and symptoms, such as bloating, belching, nausea and mild cramping.

In addition, the cause of many digestive problems often is unclear. There are several complex organs, functions and interconnections in your digestive tract. Certain signs and symptoms, such as difficulty swallowing, almost always signal a digestive disorder, while others, such as nausea, can be more vague and don't always point to a gastrointestinal problem.

Often, digestive problems are temporary. And sometimes, they're caused by things you eat or do — which may give you some control over fixing them.

Behaviors that can trigger digestive problems include:

- Eating spicy foods or fatty foods
- Eating too much at one meal

- Eating too fast
- Drinking too much caffeine or alcohol
- Smoking tobacco
- Experiencing stress or anxiety

The discomfort that can occur from any one of these behaviors varies — some people are affected a lot, while others experience only minor irritations. Often, signs and symptoms start to diminish soon after stopping the behavior that's triggering them and they gradually disappear.

It's when digestive signs and symptoms quickly become severe and debilitating or they persist or worsen over days or weeks that you have more reason to be concerned. Your signs and symptoms could signal a condition that deserves medical attention.

Don't forget that sometimes what you think is a digestive problem could actually be something else, such as a heart or lung condition. For instance, one of the symptoms of a heart attack is indigestion. If you have severe or persistent indigestion, especially if it comes on quickly or is accompanied by other symptoms, don't delay in seeing a doctor.

The purpose of this chapter is to help you better understand the most common digestive signs and symptoms and what may — or may not — be producing them. But it's still important to see your doctor, especially if your problem is severe or persistent. Together, you may be able to identify a cause. A physical examination, along with questions about your signs and symptoms, eating and exercise habits, and daily routine, may be all that's necessary to allay your worries. Further testing (described in Chapter 5) may be necessary to explore more-serious problems.

• • • • •

COMMON DIGESTIVE COMPLAINTS

It's not uncommon for people to see a doctor for digestive concerns. Reasons people seek medical help include:

- Difficulty swallowing
- Chest pain and heartburn
- Indigestion
- Nausea and vomiting
- Abdominal pain
- Belching, bloating and intestinal gas
- Diarrhea or constipation
- Bleeding
- Weight loss

• • • • •

DIFFICULTY SWALLOWING

Most people take swallowing for granted. They take a bite of food, chew, swallow and don't give it a second thought. For others, swallowing can be a daily problem.

If you get the feeling when you swallow that food is sticking in your throat or chest, you may have dysphagia. The term comes from the Greek words *dys* ("difficult") and *phagia* ("to eat"). Dysphagia can occur in two locations in your upper digestive tract — the pharynx and esophagus.

Pharynx

The pharynx is located at the back of the throat and leads into your food pipe (esophagus). If you have pharyngeal dysphagia, you have trouble moving food from your mouth and throat into your upper esophagus. The problem often, but not always, stems from weakened throat muscles because of a stroke or a neuromuscular disorder, such as muscular dystrophy or Parkinson's disease.

Sometimes, swallowing difficulty may stem from what's called Zenker's diverticulum. In this condition, a small pouch forms in the upper part of the esophagus, where food particles collect and can impede swallowing.

Other signs and symptoms may include:

- Choking or coughing while swallowing
- Regurgitating fluid (or sometimes food) through the nose
- Bad breath
- Repeated throat clearing or coughing
- A weak voice
- Weight loss

Esophagus

Esophageal dysphagia refers to the sensation of food sticking or getting hung up in your food pipe (esophagus). This form is more common than pharyngeal dysphagia and is often accompanied by pressure or pain in your chest. Other signs and symptoms may include:

- Painful swallowing

- A sore throat
- A persistent cough
- Gurgling sounds

There are many reasons for esophageal dysphagia. One of the most common is a narrowing of the lower esophagus due to the formation of scar tissue. Scar tissue may develop when stomach acid backs up into the esophagus and inflames esophageal tissues. Other conditions such as a viral or fungal infection also can produce esophageal inflammation.

An allergy-like condition of the esophagus called eosinophilic esophagitis can lead to swallowing difficulty, especially in children and young adults. In this condition, white blood cells called eosinophils build up in the lining of the esophagus. The buildup can inflame esophageal tissue, causing swallowing difficulty.

Additional causes of dysphagia include radiation burns from cancer treatment and a thin area of narrowing in the lower esophagus. With age, esophageal muscles that propel food to your stomach can weaken, making it more difficult to swallow. Diseases such as achalasia or scleroderma can damage esophageal nerves or muscles, causing swallowing difficulties. Rarely, tumors (noncancerous or cancerous) may produce dysphagia.

Swallowing difficulty that occurs only occasionally often isn't a serious problem and may simply stem from not chewing your food well enough or eating too fast. But if the episodes are frequent or your symptoms are severe, see your doctor.

Treating dysphagia

How dysphagia is treated generally depends on its cause.

Physical therapy If your swallowing difficulty is a result of weakened muscles around the pharynx, a physical therapist may assist you with techniques that help you swallow better.

Medication For dysphagia stemming from gastroesophageal reflux disease (GERD), prescription medications are often effective in preventing reflux of stomach acid into the esophagus. Medications may also improve swallowing difficulty associated with an infection or inflammation. For the treatment of eosinophilic esophagitis, a short course of steroids may be prescribed.

Tissue stretching If your esophagus is narrowed by scar tissue interfering with the passage of food, your doctor may use a device to stretch (dilate) the tissue. The device is threaded through a slender, flexible tube (endoscope) that's inserted down your esophagus. Often, the device is a deflated balloon that's placed in the narrowed section and then inflated to widen the passageway.

Surgery In case of a diverticulum, severe narrowing or a tumor, surgery may be necessary to fix the problem or clear the esophageal path.

Change in diet Sometimes it's necessary to modify the consistency of your diet until a diagnosis is made and a treatment plan developed. Depending on the severity of your signs and symptoms, you may need to limit your diet to soft, puréed or liquid foods. Eating smaller meals more frequently also may reduce dysphagia symptoms. In the case of eosinophilic esophagitis, eliminating certain foods my help treat the problem.

To learn more

For additional information on conditions that may lead to swallowing difficulty, see Chapter 10 on gastroesophageal reflux disease (GERD).

CHEST PAIN AND HEARTBURN

Chest pain can occur for any number of reasons: a warning of a heart attack, lack of oxygen to your heart muscle (angina pectoris), a lung condition or inflammation of cartilage in your rib cage.

Many times, though, chest pain isn't heart- or lung-related. Rather, it stems from a digestive problem. For example, pain associated with gallbladder inflammation (a gallbladder attack) can spread to your chest. The most common source of digestive-related chest pain is heartburn.

Heartburn is a commonly used term to describe a burning sensation in your chest that may start in your upper abdomen and radiate all the way up into your neck. Heartburn isn't a disease; rather, it's a symptom. At times, especially when you're lying down, heartburn may be associated with a sour taste in your mouth stemming from stomach acid that backs up into your upper esophagus and mouth.

Normally, stomach acid stays in your stomach, kept there by the lower esophageal sphincter. This ring of muscle functions as a valve, opening only when you swallow, belch or vomit. But sometimes the valve relaxes or weakens, allowing stomach acid to regurgitate into your esophagus, producing a burning sensation.

Among adults, occasional bouts of heartburn can occur for many reasons. Being overweight, overeating or lying down too soon after a meal puts pressure on the sphincter valve, causing it to open slightly and stomach acid to flow into the esophagus. Too much alcohol or caffeine, as well as certain foods, also can relax the sphincter or increase production of stomach acid.

If you have heartburn several times a week or you need to take antacids frequently, see your doctor. Your heartburn may be a symptom of a more serious condition, such as GERD. If your heartburn seems to be getting worse or is different from normal — especially if it's accompanied by radiating pain in an arm — seek medical help immediately. Instead of heartburn, your pain may be the warning of a heart attack.

To learn more

For additional information on conditions that may produce heartburn or chest pain see Chapter 10 on gastroesophageal reflux disease (GERD).

INDIGESTION

A common complaint of people who see a doctor is indigestion. Indigestion is a general term that describes discomfort in the upper abdomen. It's actually a collection of signs and symptoms — uncomfortable fullness, nausea, heartburn and bloating accompanied by belching. Most commonly, though, people associate indigestion with stomach pain (dyspepsia).

While indigestion may be common, how people experience it differs. Some people have occasional signs and symptoms, while others are bothered every day. Common causes of stomach pain include:

- Peptic ulcers
- Stomach inflammation (gastritis) from medications, alcohol or infection
- Nonulcer dyspepsia, a condition whose symptoms resemble those of an ulcer but an ulcer doesn't exist

Less commonly, indigestion can be a symptom of other digestive disorders, such as gallbladder inflammation or pancreatic disease.

An occasional episode of indigestion generally isn't anything to worry about. It may even be related to hunger pangs. But if you're having persistent, recurrent or severe abdominal pain or discomfort, see your doctor.

To learn more

For additional information on conditions that may produce stomach pain or discomfort, see Chapter 11 on ulcers and stomach pain, Chapter 14 on gallbladder disease or Chapter 15 on pancreatic disease.

NAUSEA AND VOMITING

Most everyone has experienced an occasional bout of nausea, a feeling of stomach distress accompanied by the urge to vomit. Vomiting — forcefully expelling stomach contents — is a natural response to invading organisms and irritants that enter the digestive tract.

Common causes of nausea and vomiting are:

- A viral infection
- Bacteria from spoiled food
- High levels of toxins in blood, including alcohol and drugs
- Increased hormone levels during pregnancy or extended periods of intense stress
- An intense headache or inner ear disturbance, including motion sickness
- An obstruction in the intestines

Nausea and vomiting generally aren't signs and symptoms of serious disease unless they persist or are accompanied by pain. If you can see blood in the vomit or it looks like coffee grounds (partially digested blood), you should see your doctor promptly.

Depending on other signs and symptoms you may be experiencing, nausea and vomiting could be related to a digestive condition that requires medical attention, such as an ulcer, gallstones, pancreatitis, liver disease or an intestinal obstruction.

Self-care

For infrequent nausea and vomiting due to a virus or bacterium, the following may help limit your discomfort and prevent dehydration:

- Stop eating and drinking for several hours until your stomach has had a chance to settle.
- Avoid food odors. Eat cold foods or those that don't require cooking.
- When you begin to feel better, suck on ice chips or take small sips of water, weak tea, clear soft drinks, noncaffeinated sports drinks or broth. Sip beverages often to prevent dehydration.
- When you're ready to start eating, begin with foods that are easily digested, such as gelatin, crackers and dry toast. Once you can tolerate these, try mild-flavored, nonfatty foods, such as cereal, rice and fruits.
- For several days, avoid fatty or spicy foods, caffeine, alcohol, and aspirin or other nonsteroidal anti-inflammatory drugs (NSAIDs).

To learn more

For additional information on conditions that may produce nausea and vomiting, see Chapter 11 on ulcers and stomach pain, Chapter 14 on gallbladder disease, Chapter 15 on pancreatic disease and Chapter 16 on liver disease.

BELCHING, BLOATING AND INTESTINAL GAS

Belching, bloating and intestinal gas are common complaints related to the buildup of air or gas in your digestive tract. While these conditions can leave you frustrated, uncomfortable or embarrassed, they generally aren't a cause for concern.

Some people complain of constantly having too much gas in their digestive systems. Their complaints usually involve one of three forms of distress: excessive belching, bloating or frequently needing to pass intestinal gas from the rectum (flatulence).

Belching

Burping (belching) is a way for your body to expel excess air that you swallow while eating or drinking. The buildup can happen from eating too fast, talking while you eat or drinking carbonated beverages.

When you belch, air that has accumulated in your stomach is forced up into your esophagus and out of your mouth. An occasional belch is normal to relieve stomach fullness, but if you belch frequently, it may indicate that you're swallowing too much air. Some people who belch repeatedly — even when they're not eating or drinking — are swallowing air as a nervous habit.

Belching also can result from the reflux of stomach acid into your esophagus. You may swallow frequently to clear the acid, which leads to more air intake and further belching.

● ● ● ● ●

COMMON FOODS THAT MAY CAUSE GAS

Limiting how much you eat of the foods on this list may help you reduce intestinal gas. But remember that different foods affect different people. Don't eliminate these foods from your diet all at once. Many of the items provide many beneficial nutrients. Plus, if you quit eating them all, you won't know which ones are the real offenders.

Instead, try eliminating one food at a time for a period of a couple of weeks. If your symptoms get better, that particular food may be gas forming for you. Experiment with the food to see if you can tolerate just a small amount or if you need to keep it from your diet.

Legumes and certain vegetables

- Baked beans
- Dried beans
- Lima beans
- Broccoli
- Brussels sprouts

- Cabbage
- Cauliflower
- Lentils
- Onions
- Dried peas
- Radishes
- Sauerkraut

Fruits and fruit juices, in excessive amounts

- Apple juice
- Apples
- Bananas
- Prune juice
- Prunes
- Grape juice
- Raisins

Dairy products

- Ice cream
- Milk

Wheat bran

- Bran flakes and other items that contain wheat bran

Others

Additional foods and products that can produce gas in some people include:

- High-fiber foods (see here)
- High-fat foods such as cream sauces, gravies, pastries, fatty meats and fried foods
- Certain sugar substitutes, such as sorbitol, mannitol, xylitol, erythritol and isomalt, used in sugar-free gum, candies, desserts and some liquid medications

• • • • •

The best way to reduce belching is to swallow less air. If you're not sure how to do that, here are some suggestions that may help you.

- ***Eat and drink slowly.*** Typically, the more time you take to chew your food and drink your beverage, the less air you swallow.
- ***Avoid gum and hard candy.*** When you suck on hard candy or chew gum, you swallow more often than normal. Part of what you're swallowing is air.
- ***Don't use a straw.*** You swallow more air when you suck on a straw than you do sipping from a glass.
- ***Quit smoking.*** If you smoke, there are many reasons why you should quit. Another reason to add to the list is less belching. When you inhale smoke from tobacco products, you also inhale and swallow air.
- ***Drink fewer carbonated beverages.*** Soft drinks and beer release carbon dioxide gas, increasing the volume of air in your digestive system.

At times, a deep-breathing exercise known as diaphragmatic breathing may help reduce belching. If breathing exercises or the steps listed above don't help reduce excess air in your stomach, see your doctor to rule out more-serious conditions associated with belching, such as GERD or stomach inflammation (gastritis).

Bloating

Bloating is a common term for the buildup of gas in your stomach and intestines. Many times, bloating is accompanied by abdominal pain that may be mild and dull or sharp and intense. Passing gas or having a bowel movement may help to relieve the bloating.

Most often, bloating results from eating a lot of fatty foods. During the digestive process, fat delays how quickly your stomach empties its contents, which can increase the sensation of being full. Bloating also can result from gulping air while eating too fast.

Occasionally, bloating may be associated with an intestinal abnormality, such as celiac disease or lactose intolerance — conditions in which your intestines aren't able to absorb certain food components. Another cause may be fructose intolerance, in which you're unable to properly absorb simple sugars found in fruit and many processed foods.

Bloating also may accompany conditions such as irritable bowel syndrome or may be related to stress and anxiety. Less commonly, bloating may be associated with delayed stomach emptying (gastroparesis), a problem for some people with diabetes, or result from a gastrointestinal infection or blockage in the intestines. If your bloating is accompanied by pain or vomiting, see a doctor.

Intestinal gas

Sometimes air you swallow makes it all the way to your colon and is expelled through your anus. Most often, though, intestinal gas (flatus) results from the fermentation of undigested food after it reaches your colon. Gas can also form when your intestines have difficulty breaking down certain components in foods, including the sugars in milk products and fruit.

Constipation can produce intestinal gas. The longer food waste remains in your colon, the more time it has to ferment. Intestinal gas is composed primarily of odorless substances. The foul smells that may accompany flatulence come from gases containing sulfur produced by the decomposing food particles in your colon.

To help reduce intestinal gas:

Limit foods that produce gas Try to identify which foods may be gas forming for you. Certain foods that produce gas for one person may not produce gas for another. See this list of foods that commonly produce gas.

In attempting to relieve your problem, don't eliminate all nutritious foods from your diet, such as vegetables and fruits, just because they may cause gas. Generally, you can find ways to reduce gas while eating a healthy diet. For example, eat smaller amounts of a particular food or prepare it in a different way that's less likely to be gas forming.

Discuss your diet and gas-forming foods with your doctor or a registered dietitian. You may try over-the-counter products containing alpha-galactosidase (Beano, Bean- Assist, others), which reduce gas formation, or one of the many products containing simethicone (Gas-X, Mylanta Gas Minis, others), intended to relieve gas.

Add fiber gradually High-fiber foods are good for digestion and health, but eating too much fiber too quickly can cause gas. If you want to increase the fiber in your diet, do it gradually over a period of several weeks. A dietitian can advise you on which high-fiber foods are less likely to produce gas.

Exercise regularly Physical activity reduces intestinal gas by helping to prevent constipation. Aim for 30 to 60 minutes of physical activity each day. Physical activity may also help reduce bloating.

Drink plenty of water Like exercise, water helps to prevent constipation, thereby reducing gas. Drink eight 8-ounce glasses of water a day, unless you have a medical condition in which you need to limit fluid consumption.

To learn more

For additional information on conditions that may produce belching, bloating or gas, see Chapter 8 on irritable bowel syndrome, Chapter 9 on celiac disease and Chapter 10 on gastroesophageal reflux disease (GERD).

ABDOMINAL PAIN

Abdominal pain can occur on its own, or it may accompany other signs and symptoms, such as gas or bloating. Occasional episodes of pain can stem from overeating or eating too much of the wrong foods, such as fatty foods, gas-forming foods or, for people with lactose intolerance, dairy products. Usually the pain goes away within a few hours. In case of a viral or bacterial infection, discomfort may linger for one or two days.

Some people have a lowered threshold for abdominal pain and experience pain associated with pressure, stimulation or bloating at a level that's more intense than normal. This is known as visceral hypersensitivity, and it's associated with irritable bowel syndrome.

Abdominal pain that's recurrent, persistent, severe, or accompanied by other signs and symptoms may signal a potentially serious condition and should be evaluated by a doctor.

Where the pain is located in your abdomen may help your doctor narrow the list of possible causes; however, it's possible the problem may not be digestive related. Other conditions, including vascular or reproductive disorders, also may trigger abdominal pain. And sometimes the location can be misleading (see "Migrating pain" below).

For digestive-related conditions, here's where pain is most likely to occur:

● ● ● ● ●

MIGRATING PAIN

An unusual characteristic of abdominal pain is its ability to travel along deep nerve pathways and emerge at locations that are some distance away from the true source of the problem. For example, pain from gallbladder inflammation may spread to your chest and up to your right shoulder. Pain from a pancreatic disorder may radiate up between your shoulder blades. Your doctor may call this referred pain.

Because of the number of vital organs in your abdomen and the complex signals they send, it's a good idea to consult your doctor if you experience any of the following pain symptoms:

- Severe, recurrent or persistent pain
- Pain that seems to worsen
- Pain accompanied by fever, bleeding or vomiting

● ● ● ● ●

Navel area

Pain near your navel is often associated with a disorder of the small intestine or inflammation of the appendix (appendicitis). The appendix is a worm-shaped pouch that projects out from your colon. It can become clogged with food waste that causes it to inflame, swell and fill with pus.

Above the navel

The epigastric area is located in the center of your abdomen and directly above the navel. This is where you should expect to feel pain associated with stomach disorders. Persistent pain in this area also may signal a problem with your upper small intestine (duodenum), pancreas or gallbladder.

Below the navel

Pain located below the navel and spreading out to either side may signify a disorder of the large intestine (colon). Pain in this area may also stem from an infection or, in women, pelvic inflammatory disease or an ovarian condition.

Upper left abdomen

It's uncommon to experience pain in the upper left area of the abdomen. If you do, it could suggest a problem in the colon, stomach or pancreas.

Upper right abdomen

Intense pain in the upper right abdomen is often related to an inflammation of the gallbladder (gallbladder attack). The pain may spread to the center of your abdomen and penetrate to your back. Occasionally, inflammation in the pancreas or upper small intestine (duodenum) and some liver disorders can produce intense pain in this area.

Lower left abdomen

Pain in the lower left abdomen most often suggests a problem of the descending sigmoid colon, the section just above the rectum. Possible disorders include an infection (diverticulitis), inflammation (Crohn's disease or ulcerative colitis) or, rarely, cancer.

Lower right abdomen

Pain in the lower right abdomen may indicate an inflammation of the colon or lower small intestine (terminal ileum). Or it may be associated with Crohn's disease or, rarely, colon cancer. Sometimes appendicitis can produce pain in this area.

Abdominal wall

Sometimes, abdominal pain may result from a dysfunction in the configuration of muscles in the abdominal wall (musculature). This condition, called abdominal wall pain, may stem from trauma, a muscle sprain or strain, or scarring and the formation of benign nerve tissue (neuroma) after abdominal surgery. Treatment to alleviate abdominal wall pain may include physical therapy, topical anesthetics or ultrasound-guided trigger point injections.

DIARRHEA AND CONSTIPATION

Diarrhea and constipation are common digestive issues that almost everyone experiences at one time or another. Typically, they last for a short period and then disappear. But sometimes these conditions can be persistent. A continued problem generally signals a digestive disorder.

Diarrhea

The term *diarrhea* describes watery, loose and more-frequent bowel movements. It generally results when the lining of your small intestine becomes inflamed, hampering the ability of your intestinal tract to absorb nutrients and fluids.

After a meal, nutrients from the food and liquid you've consumed are processed and absorbed in your small intestine. Your colon absorbs the remaining liquid from digested food, and waste forms into semisolid stools. Diarrhea results when this process is disrupted.

Various agents can interrupt the digestive process, impeding the absorption of nutrients and fluids:

Viral infection This is the most common cause of diarrhea. An invading virus damages the mucous membrane that lines your small intestine, disrupting fluid and nutrient absorption. Typically, after one to three days, symptoms begin to improve and the diarrhea gradually disappears.

Bacterial infection Bacteria in contaminated food or water may form a toxin that causes the intestines to secrete salt and water. This overwhelms the capacity of your small intestine and colon to absorb fluid. Similar to a viral infection, the diarrhea usually disappears within a few days.

Clostridium difficile, often called *C. difficile* or *C. diff.*, is a bacterium that can cause symptoms ranging from prolonged diarrhea to life-threatening inflammation of the colon. *C. diff.* typically happens after taking an antibiotic.

Other infectious agents Though much less common, diarrhea may result from a parasite. Once the parasite is eliminated, the diarrhea usually disappears. A common parasite that can lead to prolonged diarrhea is called giardia. You can get giardia from drinking contaminated water from a well or stream.

Food related Sometimes diarrhea stems from an intolerance or sensitivity to certain foods. For example, some people have an intolerance to milk and are unable to digest the sugar (lactose) in milk and milk products. If they eat or drink products containing lactose, the lactose can cause cramping, gas and diarrhea. Other components of foods, including food additives and artificial sweeteners, can cause similar problems (see Chapter 3).

Excessive caffeine or alcohol Caffeinated and alcoholic beverages can stimulate the passage of stool. If you drink them in excess, they may cause food waste to move through your small intestine and colon too quickly.

Medications Diarrhea may result from medications. Medications that can cause diarrhea include some antibiotics and certain antacids that contain magnesium hydroxide. Once the medication is discontinued, the diarrhea usually goes away.

Intestinal disorders Diarrhea that persists or recurs frequently is usually related to some form of intestinal disorder. Possible causes include irritable bowel syndrome, an inflammatory disease such as ulcerative colitis or Crohn's disease, or a malabsorption condition such as lactose intolerance or celiac disease. Rarely, diarrhea is associated with a tumor.

Self-care

Diarrhea typically clears up on its own, without the need for antibiotics or other medications. There are some over-the-counter products, such as

Imodium, Pepto- Bismol and Kaopectate, that may slow diarrhea, but these products won't always speed your recovery. See your doctor if you experience severe or persistent diarrhea, persistent or recurrent abdominal pain, or bleeding.

Dehydration often is a concern because diarrhea greatly increases the amount of fluid you would typically lose in a day. Take these measures to prevent dehydration and relieve symptoms as you recover.

- ***Drink plenty of fluids.*** Drink at least eight to 10 glasses of clear liquid daily. This includes water, weak tea, diluted juices or beverages containing electrolytes, such as Pedialyte or Gatorade.
- ***Gradually add solid foods.*** Start your recovery with easily digestible food, such as crackers, toast, rice, cereal and chicken.
- ***Avoid certain foods and beverages.*** Wait a few days before consuming dairy products, fatty foods, spicy foods, or beverages containing caffeine or alcohol. They can prolong diarrhea.
- ***Don't take certain antacids.*** Magnesium hydroxide can cause diarrhea, so avoid any products that contain this substance.
- ***Reduce stress.*** For some forms of chronic diarrhea, therapies such as acupuncture, acupressure or massage may reduce symptoms by relieving stress and stimulating your body's natural defense systems. However, none of these therapies has been scientifically proved.

Constipation

One of your colon's main responsibilities is to absorb water from food residue (waste) as it passes through the colon. The longer food residue remains in your colon, the more water it loses. If it stays for a long time, the waste becomes very dry and difficult to pass as stool. Frequently passing small, solidly formed stools also can be an indication of constipation.

Constipation can occur for many reasons, and it tends to be more common with age. As you get older, the muscles in your digestive tract become less active, which means food residue doesn't move through as easily as before. Your lifestyle also may change. Factors that increase your risk of constipation include not drinking enough liquids, eating too little fiber and not getting enough physical activity.

In addition, certain medications can slow digestion, producing constipation. They include narcotics and antacids containing aluminum. Some people with irritable bowel syndrome experience alternating episodes of diarrhea and constipation.

Generally, constipation is a temporary condition that can be easily corrected. However, there are times when constipation may point to a more serious problem.

See your doctor if you experience:

- Recent, unexplained constipation
- Recent, unexplained changes in bowel patterns or habits
- Constipation that lasts longer than seven days, despite changes in diet or exercise
- Blood in stool or intense abdominal pain

To learn more

For more information on constipation and how to manage it, see Chapter 7. For additional information on conditions that may produce diarrhea, see Chapter 8 on irritable bowel syndrome, Chapter 9 on celiac disease, Chapter 12 on Crohn's disease and ulcerative colitis, Chapter 13 on diverticular disease, and Chapter 15 on pancreatic disease.

BLEEDING

You can easily become alarmed if you notice traces of blood coming from either your mouth or your anus — the two endpoints of your digestive tract. Sometimes the bleeding may be a minor problem, such as gum disease or hemorrhoids. At other times, the bleeding is warning of a more serious condition, such as an ulcer or cancer. The safest course of action is to see your doctor as soon as possible.

Blood in saliva or vomit

Blood may come from many sources, including injury to the mouth, gums or nose. If you cough up blood, the source is usually the lungs or windpipe. Digestive conditions that may cause blood to exit from your mouth in saliva or vomit include:

- A peptic ulcer
- A tear in the lining of your esophagus
- Inflamed tissue in your esophagus, stomach or small intestine
- Cancer of the esophagus or stomach

The blood is usually bright red. Occasionally, it may appear black or dark brown and resemble coffee grounds, which means it's been partly digested in your stomach or upper small intestine. This often indicates a serious problem that should be investigated.

Call for emergency assistance if you vomit blood. While waiting for help, lie down with your legs elevated, if possible. Don't eat or drink anything.

Rectal bleeding

Bleeding from the rectum and anus can result for many reasons. The blood may show up mixed in your stool, on toilet paper or in the toilet bowel. See your doctor to determine what's causing your symptoms.

An anal tear (fissure) and hemorrhoids are the most frequent causes of rectal bleeding. Blood associated with an anal tear or hemorrhoids is usually bright red.

Other causes of rectal bleeding include inflammation of the colon caused by ulcerative colitis or Crohn's disease. Rectal bleeding can also be a warning of noncancerous growths (polyps) or cancer in the colon.

Sometimes, the blood is darker in color and mixed in with stool, producing black, maroon or mahogany-colored stools. Black stools may indicate bleeding from the upper intestine.

To learn more

For additional information on conditions that may produce bleeding, see Chapter 11 on ulcers and stomach pain, Chapter 12 on Crohn's disease and ulcerative colitis, or Chapter 17 on colorectal cancer.

UNINTENDED WEIGHT LOSS

For people who spend years struggling to lose weight, unintentional weight loss might seem like a gift. However, losing a significant amount of weight without really trying can indicate a serious medical disorder, and should be discussed with your doctor.

Everyone's weight tends to fluctuate from day to day and week to week. You should expect a little variation whenever you step on a bathroom scale to weigh yourself.

But what if you notice you're losing weight even though your daily routine is unchanged — you're eating and exercising just as you always have and you're not on a diet? Involuntary weight loss is defined as a loss of more than 5 percent of your body weight over a six-month span. If you typically weigh around 160 pounds, a 5 percent loss would be about 8 pounds.

If you're unsure what your original weight was, other clues may indicate that you're losing weight. For example, you may notice that your clothes fit more loosely, or that you're fastening your belt at a tighter notch.

The list of potential causes for involuntary weight loss is extensive. The first thing many people worry about is cancer, but a majority won't have it. Digestive conditions that may lead to involuntary weight loss include:

- Difficulty swallowing
- Malabsorption disorders
- Pancreatic or liver disease
- Cancer

If you have digestive issues, it's a good idea to weigh yourself regularly. If you find that you're losing weight and you're not sure why, see your doctor.

In preparing for the visit, list any other signs and symptoms you may be experiencing. The management of involuntary weight loss involves determining what's producing the loss. Once a cause has been identified, your doctor will be better able to treat the problem. If you and your doctor think that the weight loss is significant, you may need to undergo some diagnostic testing.

To learn more

For additional information on conditions that may produce weight loss, see Chapter 9 on celiac disease, Chapter 12 on Crohn's disease and ulcerative colitis, Chapter 15 on pancreatic disease, Chapter 16 on liver disease and Chapter 17 on colorectal cancer.

CHAPTER 5

Diagnostic tests

Sometimes a doctor can determine the cause of a digestive problem fairly quickly by asking a few questions and performing a physical examination. Many times, though, before your doctor is able to diagnose your condition and begin treatment, you may need to undergo one or more tests. Diagnostic tests are especially helpful when a number of possible causes could be producing your symptoms. The results may point to or eliminate one or more of the possibilities.

When examining the digestive tract, a doctor is generally looking at three main factors:

- ***Is it built correctly?*** Does food residue flow easily through the digestive tract or are there narrowed areas (strictures) or hernias interfering with the normal passage of residue and waste? Also, are there small pouches along the tract where food can collect?
- ***Is it functioning correctly?*** Are digestive juices being produced and released correctly? Are the nerves and muscles that propel food residue through the digestive tract functioning normally? Are the sphincter muscles that keep food residue from flowing backward working properly?
- ***Is it inflamed or infected?*** Does the lining of the digestive tract appear inflamed or infected, preventing adequate absorption of fluid and nutrients? Does the stomach or small intestine harbor an ulcer?

There are many different types of tests for digestive conditions. Which tests you may have depend, in part, on what your signs and symptoms are, as well as their location, severity and frequency. Other factors may include your age, general health and personal and family medical history. Sometimes, a test may need to be repeated.

The diagnostic tests described in this chapter are the most common ones. Some of these tests generate detailed pictures of the inside of your body, allowing the doctor to see the size and structure of your internal organs. Other tests track how different parts of your digestive system are performing.

While they provide valuable information, these tests aren't always able to identify the exact cause of a problem. For example, it may be difficult to pinpoint what's triggering abdominal pain or nausea. Sometimes, a diagnosis is reached through a process of elimination, guided by the results of mul-tiple tests.

BLOOD TESTS

Blood tests often are a first step in the diagnostic process because they're relatively simple to do and they provide a general idea of what's going on inside your body. A blood test requires little preparation, but you may need to fast before the test.

For the test, a sample of blood is taken from one of your veins — usually a vein in your arm — and the sample is sent to a laboratory for analysis. Depending on your signs and symptoms, one or more of following blood tests may be performed.

Complete blood count (CBC)

This test measures several properties of blood, including levels of red cells, white cells and platelets. Fewer red blood cells (anemia), and lower hemoglobin found within the red cells, may be associated with gastrointestinal bleeding. An elevated level of white blood cells may indicate infection or inflammation.

Liver tests

Liver tests measure levels of certain enzymes and proteins in your blood. If your liver isn't functioning properly, these levels often are abnormal. For more on liver disease, see Chapter 16.

Creatinine measurement

Creatinine is a waste product that comes from the normal breakdown of muscle tissue. An increase in the level of creatinine in your blood can be a sign of kidney disease. Creatinine may be measured to check for disease and medication side effects. It may also be measured to help determine medication dosages.

Albumin, vitamins D, A and B-12, and folate measurements

Low levels of these substances in your blood suggest that your intestines may not be absorbing certain nutrients from food properly — typically, a malabsorption problem.

Electrolyte measurements

Severe vomiting or diarrhea can cause abnormal blood levels of the electrolytes sodium, potassium and magnesium. Abnormal electrolyte levels can put you at risk of heart or brain problems.

● ● ● ● ●

Q. WHY DOES MY DOCTOR REQUEST THAT I NOT EAT BEFORE MY APPOINTMENT?

A. If there's a possibility that you may need some tests as part of your initial evaluation or return visit, your health care provider may request that you not eat before the appointment. This is because some tests, such as blood tests, X-rays or ultrasounds, require fasting to be performed safely and in order to get accurate results. If you've eaten before your appointment, you'll have to come back another day just to have the tests performed.

● ● ● ● ●

URINE AND STOOL TESTS

A urine test can help identify abnormal levels of hormones, proteins, minerals or salts in your urine, or the presence of substances not normally found in urine, such as blood. There are different types of urine tests. For some tests, you just need to provide a small sample, which usually involves urinating into a cup. Other tests require that you collect all of your urine for a period of 24 to 48 hours.

Your doctor may request a stool sample to check for infections or malabsorption of bile acids, which can cause diarrhea. Stool tests can also identify increased levels of fat in your stool, suggesting a malabsorption problem.

Another common stool test is the fecal immunochemical test (FIT). It checks for hidden (occult) blood in your stool, which may be linked to cancer or other diseases that can cause intestinal bleeding, such as ulcers or inflammatory bowel disease. For the test, small amounts of stool are collected on cards or in tubes and tested for the presence of blood. An older and less commonly used version of the test is the fecal occult blood test (FOBT).

Not all cancer lesions or precancerous polyps bleed, however. Therefore, it's possible to get a negative test result on an occult blood test even though cancer is present. That's why most doctors recommend other screening methods for colorectal cancer instead of or in addition to FIT.

A newer stool test measures a type of protein (calprotectin) normally found in white blood cells. People with inflammatory bowel disease (IBD) tend to have higher amounts of calprotectin in their stools than do people who don't have IBD.

Depending on what your doctor is looking for, you may need to provide just one stool sample or you may need to collect your stool for up to 48 hours. Collection of stool is most often done when checking for a malabsorption disorder.

* * * * *

STOOL DNA TEST

A stool DNA test is a newer screening approach for the detection of colorectal cancer. You may have seen advertisements for such a test on television or in the newspaper.

The lining of your colon continually sheds cells that leave your body through your stools. In addition to normal cells, precancerous polyps or cancerous tumors slough off cells that collect in stool. These cancerous and precancerous cells display DNA changes (DNA markers) that make them different from normal cells.

A stool DNA test looks for several DNA markers indicating the possibility of colorectal polyps or colon cancer. It also detects hidden blood in stool, which can indicate the presence of cancer. When DNA markers or blood is identified, other tests, such as a colonoscopy, must be performed to verify the presence of polyps or cancer in the colon.

Unlike more commonly used colorectal cancer screening tests, the stool test doesn't require any preparation. You eat and drink normally, collect a stool sample in a specialized container, and then bring the sample to your doctor's office or mail it to a designated laboratory.

Currently, the stool DNA test Cologuard has been approved for colon cancer screening in the United States for individuals who aren't at increased risk of colon cancer — people with no family history of the disease and no personal history of colon polyps. Stool DNA testing has been endorsed by various institutions, including the American Cancer Society.

• • • • •

X-RAYS

X-ray imaging tests involve exposing a part of your body to a small dose of electromagnetic radiation, which passes through organs and soft tissue. Special film positioned on the other side of your body collects the electromagnetic signals, generating a 2D image of your internal structures.

There are different kinds of X-rays. The kind you have will depend on a variety of factors, including the location of your symptoms. At times, you may be asked to drink a liquid, such as barium, before the X-ray to make your digestive tract easier to see.

Upper gastrointestinal X-ray

This test can help identify problems in your esophagus, stomach and upper portion of your small intestine (duodenum). Fasting before the procedure helps clear food and eliminate liquid from your stomach, making it easier to detect abnormalities.

At the beginning of the procedure, you swallow a white liquid called barium. The barium temporarily coats the lining of your digestive tract so that the lining shows up more clearly on X-ray films. You may also be asked to swallow gas-producing liquid or pills, such as sodium bicarbonate. This stretches your stomach, separating its folds and providing a better view of the inner lining.

A radiologist will position an X-ray machine above you if you're lying down, or in front of you if you're standing. He or she will follow the progress of the barium through your upper gastrointestinal tract on a video monitor, looking for abnormalities or problems.

X-ray images can detect a narrowing (stricture) of your esophagus, as well as growths and other abnormalities in your stomach and duodenum.

Small intestine (small bowel) X-ray

If your doctor suspects a problem in your small intestine, such as an obstruction, a barium X-ray may be expanded to include the entire small intestine. Images are generally taken at 15- to 30-minute intervals as the barium moves through each section. It can take up to four hours for the barium to reach the end of the small intestine. Once the barium reaches your colon, the test is finished.

Large intestine (colon) X-ray

A barium enema is a name commonly used for an X-ray of the large intestine (colon). The test allows your doctor to examine part of your colon, looking for ulcers, narrowed areas (strictures), polyps, small pouches in the lining (diverticula), tumors and other abnormalities.

Your colon needs to be empty for this procedure, so for one to two days beforehand you may need to restrict your diet to clear liquids. You may also be given laxatives, and perhaps enemas, before the test to help empty your colon.

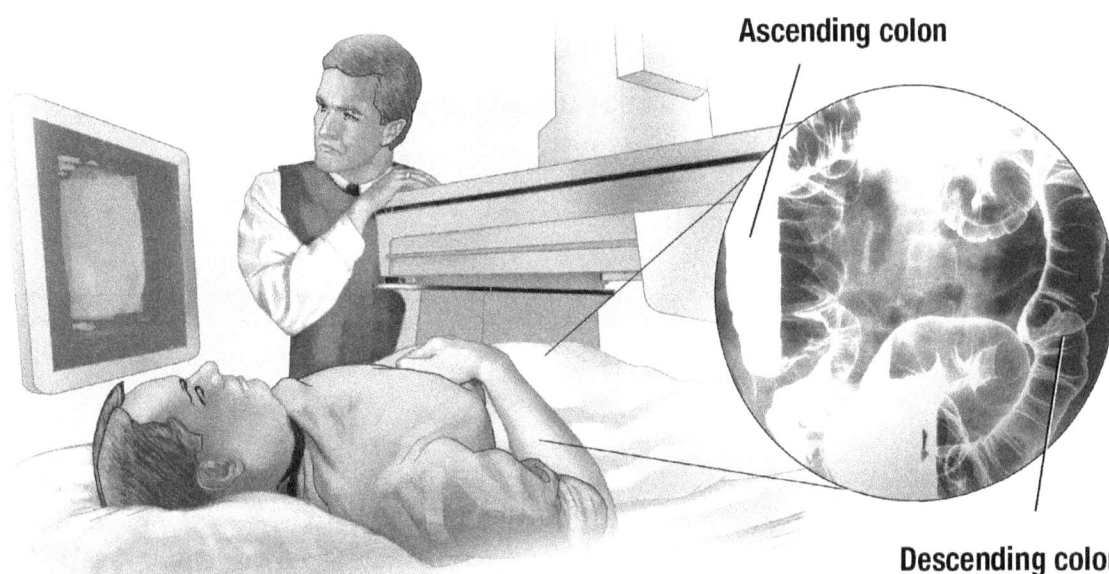

Ascending colon

Descending colon

During a colon X-ray, also known as a barium enema, a small tube containing barium is inserted into your rectum. When the barium is released, it highlights the colon's inner lining, making it more visible on X-ray.

During the procedure you lie on an examination table beneath an X-ray machine. The radiologist places a slender, lubricated tube into your rectum. This tube is connected to a bag of barium that coats the walls of your colon so that its lining will show up more clearly on the X-ray. A small balloon attached to the tube, located in your lower colon, helps keep the barium from leaking back out.

The radiologist will study your colon's shape and condition on a monitor attached to the X-ray machine. As barium fills your colon, you may be asked to turn and hold several positions to provide different views of your colon. At times, the radiologist may press firmly on your abdomen and pelvis to manipulate your colon for better viewing. The radiologist may also inject air through the tubing to expand your colon and improve the image. This is called a double- or air-contrast barium enema.

COMPUTERIZED TOMOGRAPHY

Computerized tomography (CT) combines X-rays with computer technology to produce 3D images of your internal organs and tissues. In contrast to a standard X-ray, a CT scan detects many different levels of tissue density, providing greater detail and clarity.

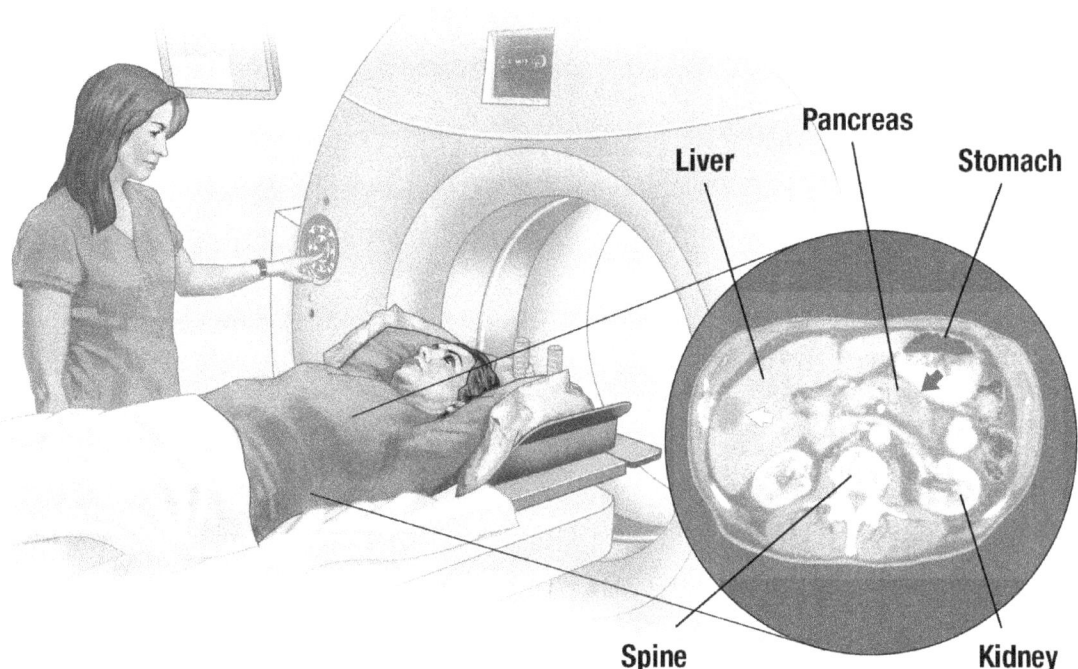

During a computerized tomography (CT) exam, an X-ray scanner rotates around you, taking scans from different angles. At right is a cross-sectional CT image that reveals a tumor in the pancreas (black arrow) that has spread to the liver (white arrow).

CT is an effective imaging procedure for diagnosing narrowed areas (strictures); accumulations of blood or other fluids; infections (abscesses); intestinal hernias, obstructions and perforations; and tumors.

For the procedure, you lie on an examination table that slides into a doughnut-shaped X-ray scanner. The scanner rotates around you, taking a sequence of scans from many different angles. A detector rotates opposite the scanner, on the other side of your body, collecting the X-ray signals. A computer collects and combines the signals into a 3D image of your internal structures that a radiologist can examine from any angle or dissect into cross-sectional layers.

CT scans of your abdomen and pelvis can help identify abnormalities in your pancreas, spleen, liver and kidneys, and sometimes your stomach, intestines, gallbladder, bile ducts and other pelvic organs. You may need to fast before the scan, which helps clear your gastrointestinal tract, making it easier to see the digestive organs and detect any abnormalities.

The most uncomfortable part of the abdominal CT procedure may be drinking (or receiving by injection) a liquid containing io- dine — the taste of which may be unpleasant. The liquid serves as a contrast agent during the procedure, making your organs and tissues show up more clearly on the scan.

Because some people are allergic to iodine, before the test you'll be asked if you've ever had an allergic reaction to iodine or similar agents used in radiologic tests.

ULTRASOUND

Ultrasound (sonography) uses the reflection of high-frequency sound waves to produce pictures of your internal organs — similar in principle to the underwater sonar technology that's used on board ships.

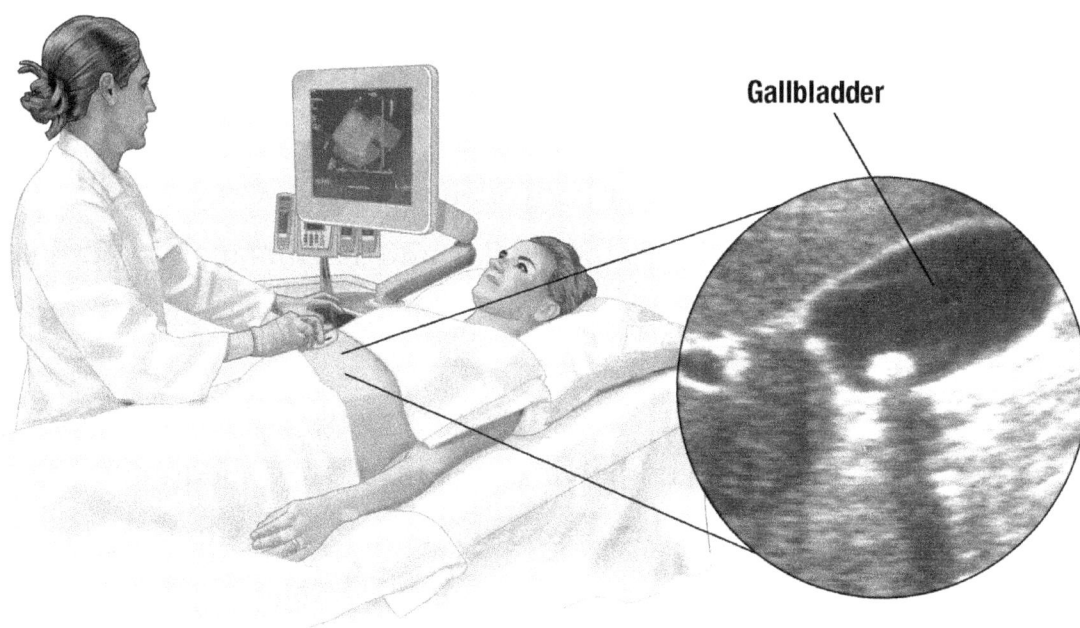

During an ultrasound exam, reflected sound waves emitted from a hand-held transducer are collected and turned into a moving picture displayed on an external monitor. The scan at the right reveals a gallstone (white arrow) in the gallbladder.

While you lie on an examination table, a jelly is rubbed onto your skin and wandlike device (transducer) is pressed against your abdomen. The transducer transmits inaudible sound waves into your body that bounce off internal structures with different tissue densities. The reflected waves are captured by the transducer. A computer translates this data into a moving, 3D image that's displayed on an external monitor.

Ultrasound is especially useful in detecting gallstones and excess fluid (ascites) within the abdominal cavity. Using special techniques, an ultrasound can also help identify a blockage or obstruction.

Another type of ultrasound exam is called endoscopic ultrasound (see here). Endoscopic ultrasound may be used to view organs that are close to the stomach and intestines, such as the liver, pancreas, gallbladder and bile ducts.

ENDOSCOPY

One of the most effective ways for a doctor to diagnose a digestive problem is to look directly inside the digestive tract. To do this, a thin, flexible tube equipped with a fiber-optic light and tiny electronic camera is inserted into your body.

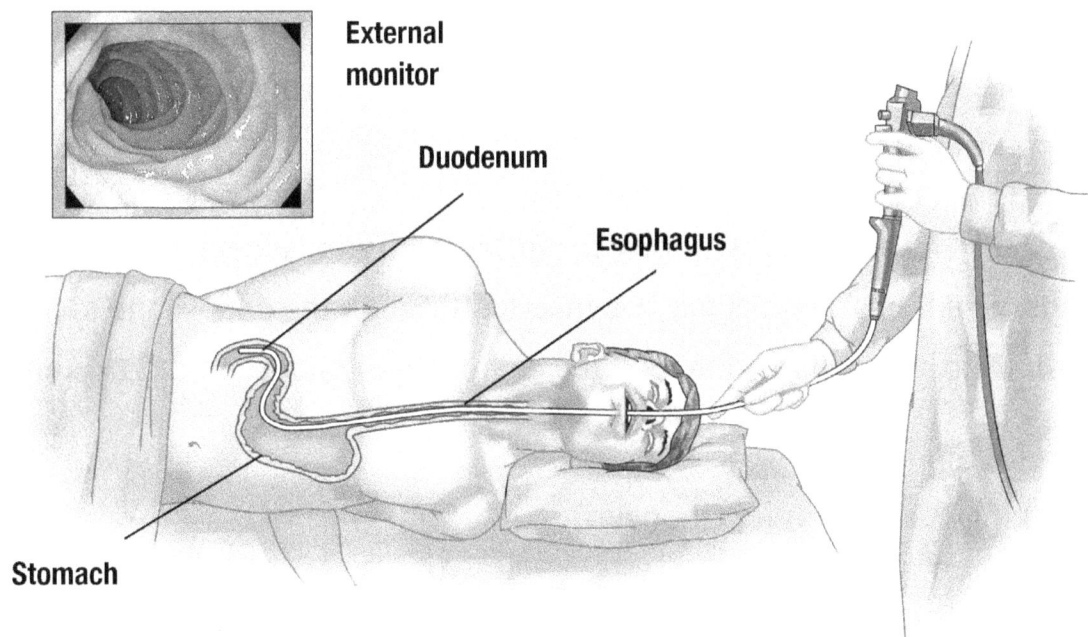

External monitor

Duodenum

Esophagus

Stomach

An endoscope exam provides a real-time image of your upper gastrointestinal tract, including the esophagus, stomach and duodenum. Images from the scope appear on an external monitor.

The tube is inserted via one of two routes. The first route is down through your mouth and esophagus to the stomach and upper small intestine (duodenum). The second route is up through your anus and into your rectum and all or part of your colon, even into the last part of the small intestine.

The instrument that your doctor uses to examine the gastrointestinal tract is called an endoscope. When it's used to examine the lower gastrointestinal tract, it's typically referred to as a colonoscope or, in a shorter version, a sigmoidoscope.

Upper endoscopy

A procedure called esophagogastroduodenoscopy (EGD) allows your doctor to look directly inside your food pipe (esophagus), stomach and the first part of the small intestine (duodenum). The images from this test help determine what might be causing signs and symptoms of the upper gastrointestinal tract such as difficulty swallowing, heartburn, nausea, vomiting, chest pain, bleeding or upper abdominal pain.

During an EGD, a doctor will look for inflamed tissue, ulcers and abnormal growths. Small instruments may be inserted through the endoscope to perform a variety of procedures. Some examples of endoscopic procedures include:

- Taking tissue samples (biopsies)
- Taking fluids samples
- Removing foreign objects or noncancerous growths (polyps)
- Stretching (dilating) your esophagus if it's narrowed by scar tissue
- Identifying and treating bleeding lesions

Your stomach needs to be empty for the test, so you can't eat or drink anything for at least six hours before the examination. Right before the procedure, you'll receive a sedating medication. You may also receive an anesthetic spray to numb your throat and help prevent you from gagging.

After the endoscope is placed in your mouth, you'll be asked to swallow to help pass the tube from your throat into your esophagus. The tube doesn't interfere with your breathing, but you may feel mild pressure or fullness as it slowly moves through your digestive tract. En route, the small camera transmits pictures, allowing your doctor to carefully examine the lining of your esophagus, stomach and upper small intestine for abnormalities.

Abnormalities that don't show up as well on an X-ray or CT image are more visible with endoscopy. This includes inflamed esophageal tissue from stomach reflux and abnormally dilated blood vessels (varices) in the esophagus. A doctor can also identify inflammation of the stomach lining, as well as small ulcers and tumors in the stomach and upper small intestine (duodenum).

For a better view of the stomach lining, air is used to inflate your stomach and stretch out its natural folds. The air may cause you to belch or pass gas afterward.

After the procedure, it takes an hour or more to recover from the sedative. You'll need someone to drive you home, since the sedative's effects can linger for 24 hours. During this time, don't drink alcohol, work with heavy machinery or make important decisions, even though you may feel fine. You may experience a mildly sore or irritated throat for a day or two.

Colonoscopy

Similar to upper endoscopy, a colonoscopy allows your doctor to visually examine your lower digestive tract. As the scope moves through your colon, your doctor examines the images being displayed.

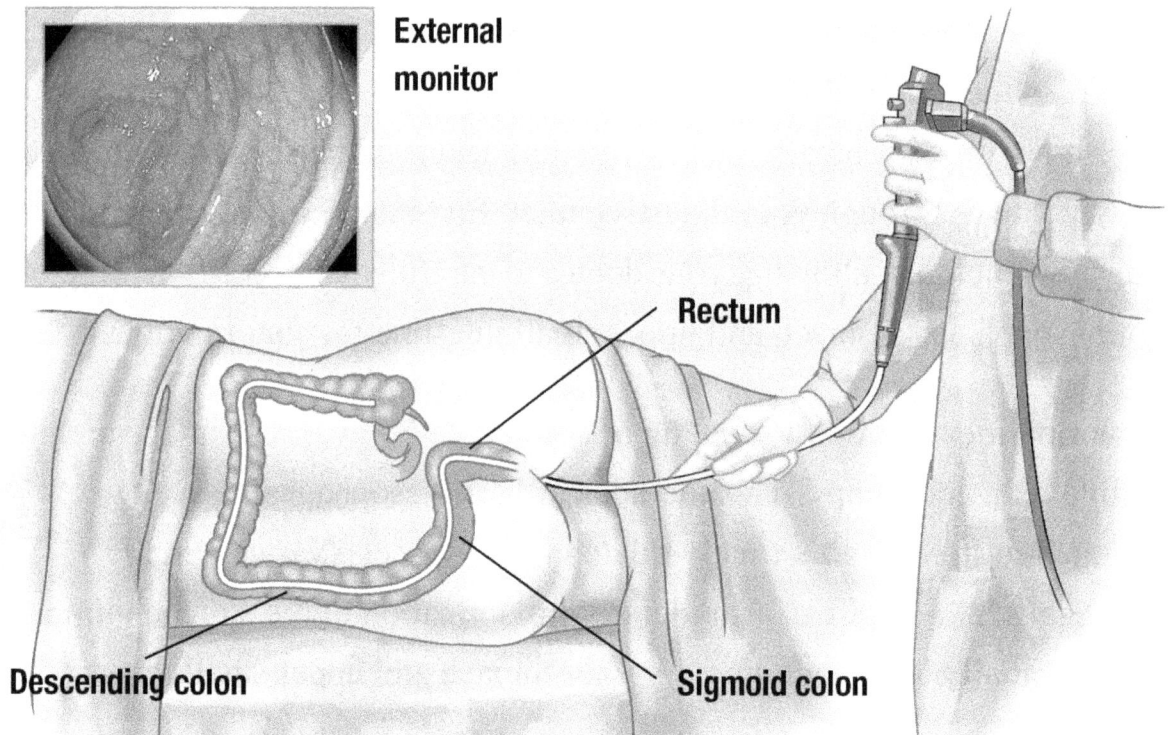

During a colonoscopy examination, a flexible tube is inserted into your rectum and threaded through the length of your colon. Images of your lower gastrointestinal tract appear on an external monitor.

During the procedure he or she can:

- Inspect for abnormalities such as bleeding, ulcers, inflammation, polyps, tumors, pouches (diverticula) and narrowed areas
- Take biopsy samples
- Remove polyps
- Treat bleeding lesions
- Stretch (dilate) narrowed areas

Your colon needs to be empty for this procedure so you'll want to follow a clear-liquid diet for one to two days beforehand. You'll also be given laxatives to take the night before and the morning of the procedure. Before the exam, a sedative is administered through a vein to help you relax. You may also be given a pain reliever.

During the exam, you lie on your left side. Air is pumped into your colon to inflate it for better views of the interior walls. You may feel some cramping or pressure during the exam. This should end when the scope is removed.

Once the exam is over, it takes an hour or more to recover from the sedative. You'll need someone to drive you home because it takes up to a day for the full effects of the sedative to wear off. You may experience some bloating and gas for a few hours afterward until you expel the injected air. This is not the best time for air travel because the gas may expand and become painful.

● ● ● ● ●

HOW TO MAKE COLONOSCOPY PREP EASIER

Many people will say that the prep work before a colonoscopy is the worst part of the procedure. A few tips can help make the process easier:

- *Two days beforehand.* Start eating a low-fiber diet. Avoid raw fruits and vegetables, whole grains, and nuts and seeds.
- *The day before.* Don't eat any solid food. Stick to clear liquids, broth soups, and popsicles and gelatin that aren't red or purple. The evening before your procedure, drink the first dose of your laxative preparation as directed.
- *The day of.* Drink clear liquids only and stop drinking all liquids two hours before your scheduled report time. Take the second dose of your laxative preparation at the time instructed.
- *Throughout.* Take your medications as directed. Drink

plenty of liquids to stay hydrated, except two hours prior to your test.

It's important that you drink all of the laxative preparation. If you find it difficult to do so because of the taste, try these tips:

- Refrigerate the solution and drink it cold.
- Suck on ice or a lemon or lime wedge.
- Chew gum right before you drink each glass of the solution.
- Drink the solution through a straw.

● ● ● ● ●

Sigmoidoscopy

For this procedure, a doctor examines just your rectum and sigmoid colon (and perhaps part of the descending colon) instead of the entire colon. You generally aren't sedated for sigmoidoscopy, and preparation for the test typically involves one or two enemas.

Your doctor may order a sigmoid exam to find the cause of diarrhea, abdominal pain or bleeding, or to look for signs of cancer. Sigmoidoscopy can be a part of cancer screening for people at average risk who are age 50 or older, often combined with a stool test to check for occult bleeding.

You may experience some bloating for a few hours afterward until you expel the injected air. If polyps are found during a sigmoid exam, the next step is generally a colonoscopy to remove the polyps and to examine the entire colon for additional polyps.

Capsule endoscopy

If endoscopic examinations of your upper and lower gastrointestinal tract are unable to identify the cause of digestive symptoms, your doctor may turn to capsule endoscopy. This test allows your doctor to see areas of your small intestine that aren't easily reached with the other procedures.

To start the exam, several adhesive patches are attached to your abdomen. Each patch contains an antenna with wires connected to a recorder that you wear on a belt around your waist. You then swallow a coated capsule about the size of a vitamin, which contains a minicamera. The camera takes pictures as it travels into your small intestine. The images are collected and stored on the recorder and then strung together to create a video.

The procedure is complete after about eight hours. During this time, you can perform most regular activities but there may be certain restrictions. You may need to avoid strenuous exercise or any activity that disrupts the recorder. When you see the capsule in the toilet after a bowel movement, it may be safely flushed down the toilet.

Capsule endoscopy is most often used to look for sources of gastrointestinal bleeding, such as ulcers or abnormal blood vessels. Sometimes, the procedure is used to diagnose inflammatory bowel disease, as well as polyps and tumors. The test can't be performed on individuals with bowel obstructions or narrow areas (strictures) in their intestinal tracts, which could cause the capsule to become stuck.

Studies are underway on the use of capsule endoscopy to examine the colon.

• • • • •

VIRTUAL COLONOSCOPY

Virtual colonoscopy, also called computerized tomography (CT) colonography, is an imaging technique that combines and digitally manipulates CT images of your abdominal organs to produce a detailed view of the inside of the colon and rectum. Unlike conventional colonoscopy, virtual colonoscopy doesn't require sedation or the insertion of a scope into the colon. Typically, it's used to screen people at average risk of colorectal cancer who are unable to tolerate traditional colonoscopy.

Before the scan, you're given laxatives to clear your colon of stool. To begin the exam, your colon is filled with air or carbon dioxide through a small catheter inserted inside the rectum. Images are then made of the entire colon and rectum with a CT scanner.

Virtual colonoscopy is usually faster than traditional colonoscopy. At times you may be asked to hold your breath to limit your abdominal movement and avoid distorting the images. In some cases, a contrast dye is administered intravenously to highlight polyps in the colon.

Studies comparing the results of virtual colonoscopy with those of traditional colonoscopy have found that virtual colonoscopy is often as sensitive in detecting most types of polyps as is traditional colonoscopy. Some polyps, including small ones, may be less likely to be detected with virtual colonoscopy. If suspect areas are found, traditional colonoscopy will be needed to get a better view of the area, perform biopsies and remove the polyps.

Virtual colonoscopy isn't the test of choice for individuals at high risk of precancerous polyps because it's highly likely that traditional colonoscopy will be required anyway.

● ● ● ● ●

Endoscopic ultrasound

As its name suggests, endoscopic ultrasound (EUS) combines an endoscopic examination with ultrasound technology. EUS creates images of internal organs using an endoscope that's equipped with both a video camera and an ultrasound probe.

● ● ● ● ●

COLON CANCER SCREENING TESTS

Following are the recommended tests to screen for colon cancer. Talk with your doctor about which test may be best for you. You can read more about each test in this chapter.

Colonoscopy During a colonoscopy exam, a long, flexible tube (colonoscope) is inserted through the anus into the rectum. A tiny video camera at the tip of the tube allows the doctor to detect changes or abnormalities inside the entire colon. Colon polyps that are identified during this examination are often removed using small surgical tools.

Stool DNA test The stool DNA test uses a sample of your stool to look for DNA changes in cells from your digestive tract that are present in stool. Such changes could indicate the possibility of colon cancer or precancerous conditions. The stool DNA test also checks for signs of blood in your stool.

Virtual colonoscopy (CT colonography) For this test, a computerized tomography (CT) scan produces cross-sectional images of the abdominal organs (see here for more information).

Flexible sigmoidoscopy During flexible sigmoidoscopy, a thin, flexible tube is inserted through the anus into the rectum. A tiny video camera at the tip of the tube allows the doctor to view the inside of the rectum and most of the lower part of the colon (sigmoid colon).

Occult blood test The idea behind this type of test is that blood vessels in larger colorectal polyps or cancers are fragile and easily damaged by the passage of stool. The damaged vessels usually bleed into the colon or rectum, but only rarely is there enough bleeding for blood to be seen in the stool. An occult blood test can detect small amounts of blood in stool.

● ● ● ● ●

First, an endoscope is positioned within your esophagus, stomach, duodenum, sigmoid colon or rectum. Then, ultrasound waves are emitted from the tip of the scope. The reflected signals are collected and projected on an external monitor, which allows your doctor to closely examine your gastrointestinal tract and nearby organs, such as the pancreas or liver. EUS also allows your doctor to take samples of abnormal tissue using ultrasound guidance to pass a fine needle through the stomach or intestinal wall.

As with other endoscopic tests, you'll be sedated for this test and need time to recover from sedation. This technology is particularly useful in viewing tumors and other abnormalities of the gastrointestinal tract and in getting an accurate assessment of tumor spread if the tumors are malignant.

AMBULATORY ACID (PH) PROBE TEST

This type of test is used to help determine if you have acid reflux, a condition in which stomach acid regurgitates into your esophagus and inflames esophageal tissue.

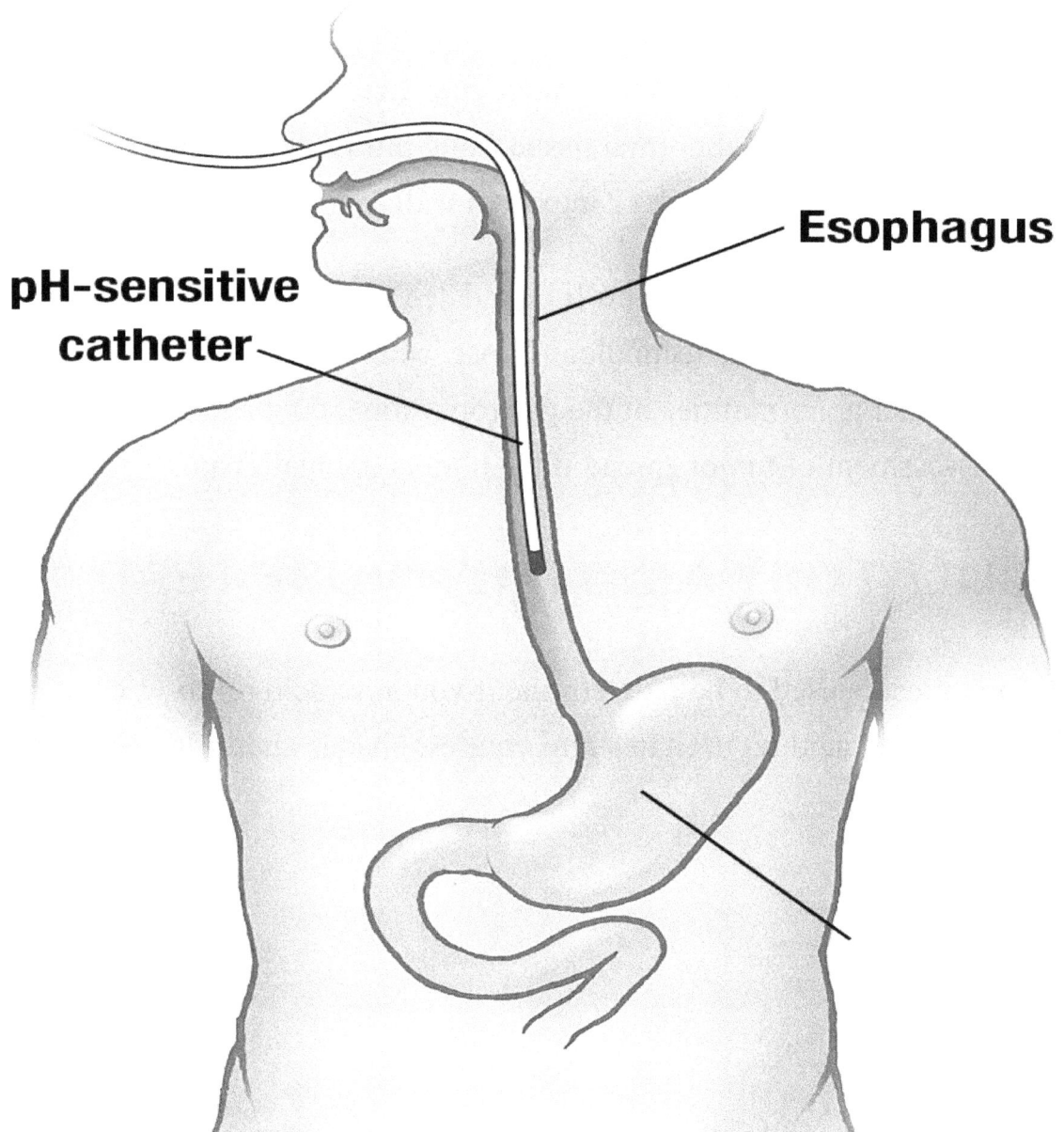

pH-sensitive catheter

Esophagus

Ambulatory acid (pH) probe test

An ambulatory acid probe test uses an acid-measuring (pH) probe (catheter) to identify when, and for how long, reflux takes place. Your doctor may give you medication to help relax you. A nurse or technician also may spray your throat with a numbing medication.

The doctor then inserts the catheter through a nasal passage (less frequently, your mouth) and into your esophagus. The catheter is positioned between your esophagus and stomach, just above the lower esophageal sphincter (LES). The device won't interfere with your breathing, and most people experience little or no discomfort during the procedure. Connected to the other end of the catheter is a small computer that records acid measurements. You wear the computer around your waist or with a strap over your shoulder. During the test, you may move around and go home.

While monitoring is taking place, you'll be instructed when to eat and drink, and you won't be allowed to bathe or go swimming. The following day you return to have the device removed.

Knowing how frequently and for how long periods of acid reflux take place helps your doctor determine how best to treat your problem. This test can also help determine if reflux may be causing other signs and symptoms, such as chest pain, coughing or wheezing, by correlating episodes of acid reflux with their onset. You may be asked to track these signs and symptoms.

An ambulatory acid (pH) probe test is sometimes used to determine if treatment to control acid reflux is working. In addition to probes in your upper and lower esophagus, a third probe may be placed in your stomach to measure the acid level there.

ESOPHAGEAL MUSCLE FUNCTION TEST

This test, also known as esophageal manometry, may be used if your doctor suspects that you have a swallowing problem (dysphagia) caused by esophageal muscles that aren't working properly. During the test, a tiny, pressure-sensitive catheter is inserted through your nose (less frequently, your mouth) and into your esophagus. There, it measures muscle pressures as you swallow water.

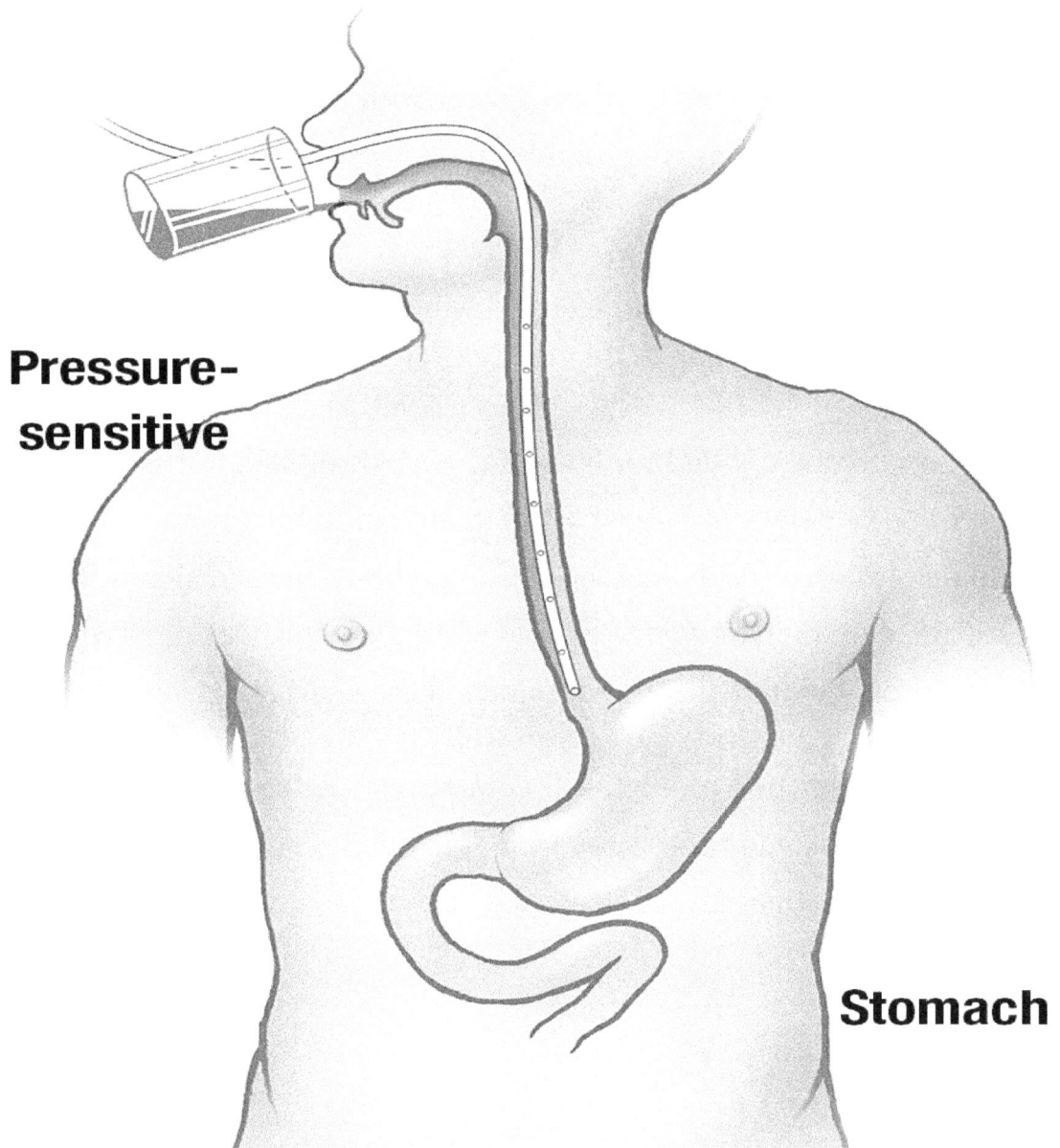

Pressure-sensitive

Stomach

Esophageal muscle function test

When you swallow, the muscles in your esophagus normally contract and relax in rolling waves (peristalsis) that propel food and liquid toward your stomach. In addition, muscular valves at the top and bottom of your esophagus (upper and lower esophageal sphincters) relax and open to let materials pass. They tighten again to protect the sensitive tissue lining the esophagus.

Malfunctions with the muscles in the walls of the esophagus or with the muscular valves (achalasia) can cause difficulty swallowing and lead to gastroesophageal reflux and chest pain. They can also cause pneumonia due to the aspiration of tiny bits of stomach contents into your lungs.

TRANSIT STUDIES

If other diagnostic tests can't determine a cause of persistent abdominal pain, nausea, vomiting, constipation or diarrhea, your doctor may order one of several transit studies. These tests measure how quickly food passes through your digestive tract, either in certain areas of the tract or in its entirety. If your digestive muscles or nerves aren't working properly, food may move through the tract too quickly or too slowly.

Gastric emptying

This test evaluates how quickly your stomach empties food into your small intestine. People with diabetes are at risk of a condition called gastroparesis in which the stomach empties too slowly. A doctor may also order this test for unexplained vomiting or in individuals who feel full after eating only a moderate amount of food.

You start the test with overnight fasting. At your doctor's office the following day, you eat breakfast that includes scrambled eggs. The eggs contain a few drops of a slightly radioactive tracer substance that's clear and tasteless.

After finishing breakfast, you stand or lie on your back while gamma cameras take pictures of the consumed eggs as they pass through your stomach. The pictures only show the radioactive tracer element in the eggs, not your internal organs.

The first pictures are taken right after you eat, followed by pictures at one, two and four hours. A four-hour test is more accurate than a two-hour test. Between picture sessions you can sit or walk around.

Your doctor is aware of the rate at which a normal stomach will empty and, by tracking the movement of the tracer element, he or she can compare the rate at which your stomach empties to the normal timeframe.

Gastric emptying and small bowel transit

This test is similar to the gastric emptying test, except that an additional series of pictures is taken at six hours. If your small intestine is moving food through it at the normal speed, most of the radioactive eggs will have passed through your small intestine by this time and be in your colon. The last set of pictures checks that the radioactive tracer has left the small intestine.

Whole-gut transit

A whole-gut transit test may be done if your doctor suspects that the digestive process isn't moving food normally, but he or she is uncertain of where in your gastrointestinal tract the problem is located.

You begin the exam by swallowing a capsule containing a radioactive tracer substance (see the image here). The capsule is designed to remain intact through the upper digestive tract until it reaches your colon. In the colon, it dissolves and releases the tracer into the lower digestive tract.

About one hour after consuming the capsule, you eat the same egg breakfast described in the other transit studies, followed by a similar schedule of pictures. This provides a record of how the upper gastrointestinal tract empties.

An important difference with this exam compared to other transit studies is that you come back for a picture session about 24 hours after taking the capsule. By this time, the capsule should have released the tracer, which should be mixed in with food residue in the middle or lower colon. If the tracer substance remains concentrated in the upper part of your colon, it may mean the colon isn't propelling food waste normally.

● ● ● ● ●

WHOLE-GUT TRANSIT STUDY

1. Capsule containing tracer is swallowed and egg breakfast is eaten.
2. Picture session shows tracer from egg moving through stomach and small intestine.

3. Capsule dissolves in colon, releasing tracer pellets.
4. Picture session reveals tracer from pellets mixed with food waste moving through colon.

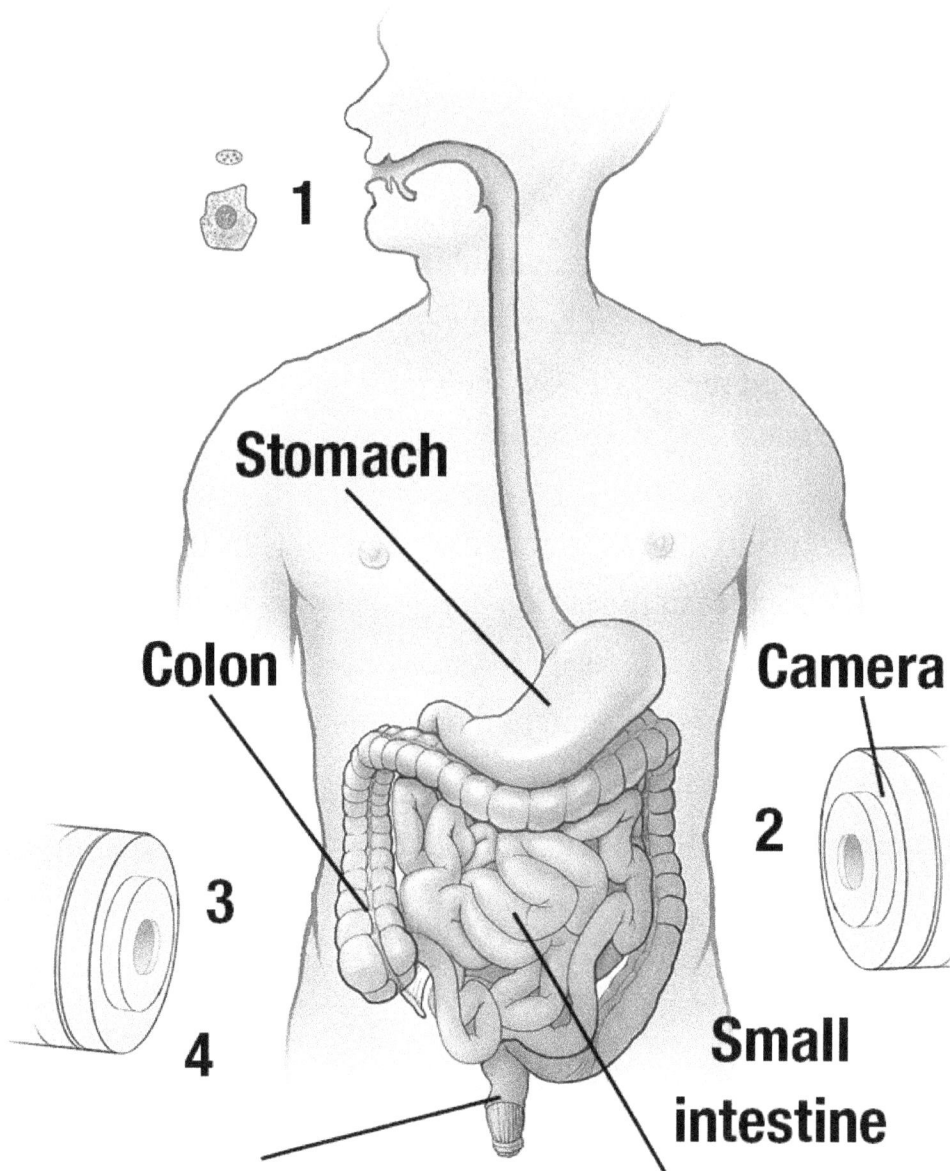

1

Stomach

Colon

Camera

2

3

4

Small intestine

Colonic transit

For people with severe, persistent constipation, a doctor may order a study that focuses on only the colon. You swallow the same capsule as that given in the whole-gut transit study but, in this case, you don't need to eat the specially prepared egg breakfast. Instead, a nurse or medical technician will instruct you on the times when you can eat meals throughout the day.

Pictures are taken as soon as you swallow the capsule, then four hours later. By the time of the four-hour picture, the capsule should have reached your upper colon. You'll need to return to the office 24 hours later for a picture session to see how far the tracer element has progressed within your colon. Sometimes the study is extended to 48 hours.

As in the whole-gut study, if the tracer element hasn't moved to your middle or lower colon, your colon isn't moving food fast enough. This would help explain your constipation.

MANOMETRY

Manometry tests are used to measure pressure and movement inside the gastrointestinal tract. A manometry test of the esophagus is also referred to as an esophageal muscle function test (see here).

Anorectal manometry

Anorectal manometry is typically performed in individuals with constipation or fecal incontinence. The test measures pressures inside your rectum and anal canal. A catheter is inserted into your rectum. It checks the strength of your anal sphincter muscles and their ability to relax and tighten at the proper times.

Two other tests are often performed in conjunction with anorectal manometry. These tests help evaluate if your rectum is functioning properly and its ability to sense stool.

Balloon expulsion exam The balloon expulsion exam tests your ability to push out (expel). As you lie on your side, a small catheter is inserted into your anus and rectum. The tube has a small, deflated balloon at one end. Once the tube is in place, the balloon is expanded and filled with water. You are asked to try to push it out.

The balloon senses the pressure inside your rectum, your internal anal sphincter and your external anal sphincter and then transmits the data to a computer. Abnormally low pressures may indicate a muscle strength or coordination problem.

Rectal sensation exam This test is used to check sensation in your rectum. The ability to sense stool in your rectum is critical to being able to know when you need to go to the bathroom. In addition, the test evaluates how well your rectum expands and contracts when stool enters.

DEFECATING PROCTOGRAM TEST (DEFECOGRAPHY)

This test is generally used in individuals having problems with fecal incontinence or constipation. It checks how the lower (sigmoid) colon and the rectum expel stool.

For the exam, your rectum is filled with a semisolid paste the consistency of soft stool. The paste contains barium, which is visible on an X-ray. Afterward, you sit on a toilet that's next to an X-ray machine. While on the toilet, you're asked to relax, then squeeze, then tense your abdomen and push out the paste.

X-rays and videos are taken during each phase of the exam. The X-ray film is analyzed to look for defects in the structure or function of your sigmoid colon and rectum. Results may reveal a prolapse or problems with muscle function and muscle coordination. A similar test may be performed using magnetic resonance imaging.

BREATH TESTS

For some gastrointestinal conditions, doctors may be able to determine if you have a condition by analyzing your breath. The two most common breath tests are those used to check for *Helicobacter pylori (H. pylori)* infection or sensitivity to the sugars lactose and fructose.

H. pylori breath test

H. pylori is a type of bacteria that can infect the stomach or upper small intestine (duodenum), causing inflammation or irritation of the stomach's inner layer and development of an ulcer.

For the breath test, you first blow into a balloonlike bag to provide a baseline sample of your normal breath. Then you drink or eat something that contains radioactive carbon, which *H. pylori* will break down in your stomach in the form of carbon dioxide. After a few minutes, you blow into a balloonlike bag again. If you're infected with *H. pylori*, your breath sample will show an increase in carbon dioxide.

Hydrogen breath test

The hydrogen breath test may be used to diagnose lactose or fructose intolerances. Lactose and fructose are forms of sugar. If you have an intolerance to either one, the sugar doesn't fully digest in the small intestine as it should, and it passes through to your colon where it produces hydrogen gas. This gas can be measured in your exhaled breath. A hydrogen breath test may also be used to help diagnose small intestine bacterial overgrowth, a condition in which excessive bacteria exist in your small intestine.

For the test, you first blow into a balloonlike bag to get a sample of your normal breath. Then you consume a specific form of sugar in liquid concentration and blow into balloonlike bags at timed intervals to see if hydrogen gas can be detected.

PART 2
Digestive diseases

CHAPTER 6
Obesity

If you struggle with being overweight, you're not alone. Almost 40 percent of American adults — more than 93 million people — meet the criteria for obesity. Obesity is defined as having an excess amount of body fat that increases your risk of health consequences. Individuals are usually diagnosed as being obese if they have a body mass index (BMI) of 30 or higher (see here). If you fall into the obese category, it means that your weight is at least 20 percent above what's considered ideal, or healthy.

Once considered a cosmetic issue, obesity is now classified as a chronic disease. It's also a complex disease in which a variety of factors appear to play roles in its development and progression.

Chances are, you're well aware that being overweight poses serious ramifications to your physical health. In addition to diabetes, cardiovascular disease and cancer, obesity increases your risk of a number of digestive problems, including gastroesophageal reflux disease (GERD), gallstones and nonalcoholic fatty liver disease.

Obesity also affects mental health. Many individuals who are overweight are targets of criticism and ridicule. They frequently experience discrimination, social bias, rejection and humiliation. These harsh behaviors can lead to problems with depression, anxiety and low self-esteem.

WHY AM I OVERWEIGHT?

The answer to why anyone is overweight often boils down to basic math. For most people, obesity results from consuming more calories each day than they burn through activities and exercise. But obesity is more complicated than a simple mathematical equation. A number of factors can play a role in the development of the condition.

Lifestyle factors

Eating high-calorie foods, eating large portions, working sedentary jobs, being less physically active, not exercising — all these factors increase your risk of obesity. And these are common reasons why many people today are overweight.

Our ancestors ate as much, if not more, than we do, yet they weighed less. Why is that? First off, they ate less fast food and fewer processed foods, which tend to be higher in fat and calories.

They were also always on the move. The automobile, television, modern technology and the changing nature of our work — switching from farm labor to computer desk jobs — have resulted in a dramatic drop in the number of calories humans burn each day.

Genetic factors

Evidence suggests that obesity tends to run in families, but the role that genes play is unclear. Scientists believe that obesity is more likely the result of a complex interaction between genes and environment. This means that although you may have a genetic predisposition to being overweight, it's not fate that you'll become obese. Ultimately, your weight is determined by dietary, physical activity and environmental influences.

• • • • •

GUT BACTERIA AND YOUR WEIGHT

As you read in Chapter 2, your gastrointestinal tract is home to a vast array of microorganisms, including more than 1,000 different species of bacteria.

Interestingly, researchers are discovering that obese individuals tend to have a different population of bacteria in their intestines than people who are lean. This has led to speculation that the makeup of your gut — the balance of "healthy" and "unhealthy" bacteria that reside there — may influence your weight by affecting how your body digests and metabolizes food.

Some scientists theorize that certain bacterial compositions may break down more food particles than others, supplying the body with more energy (more calories). In addition, certain bacteria may slow the secretion of hormones that signal the feeling of fullness, causing you to eat more than you need.

If you're wondering if probiotics might be the solution to your weight problem, the answer at this point is no. Studies haven't found probiotics to be an effective treatment for obesity. Probiotics, you'll recall, are beneficial microorganisms created through the fermentation process that promote the development of healthy bacteria (see here).

Clearly, there are more questions than there are answers and a lot left to learn. It will likely be several years before scientists have a better understanding of the relationship between gut bacteria and obesity. But don't let that become a reason not to seek help. No matter the cause of your obesity, treatments are available that can help you lose weight.

● ● ● ● ●

Psychological factors

People sometimes overeat to cope with life problems or deal with emotions such as boredom, sadness, stress or frustration.

Other factors

A variety of other factors can contribute to weight gain, but they generally aren't enough in and of themselves to cause you to become overweight.

- *Age.* With age, the amount of muscle in your body tends to decrease, lowering your metabolism. In addition, people tend to be less active as they get older. Both of these changes result in fewer calories burned.
- *Quitting smoking.* Many smokers gain weight after quitting smoking, usually because they turn to food as a coping mechanism while they

withdraw from tobacco use.

- ***Medication and illness.*** Some medications, such as corticosteroids, antidepressants and anticonvulsants, may cause weight gain. In some circumstances weight gain can be traced to a health disorder, such as low thyroid function or Cushing syndrome. Medical conditions such as arthritis, back problems or neuropathy can interfere with exercise, making weight gain more likely.

- ***Pregnancy.*** Some women gain more than the recommended amount of weight during pregnancy, and they have difficulty losing the weight after the baby is born.

WEIGHT-LOSS TREATMENTS

Despite recent discoveries, the formula for losing weight and maintaining a healthy weight still applies. Weight will come off only when you burn more calories than you consume.

Over the years you may be tempted by fad diets that promise fast and easy weight loss. The reality, however, is that there are no magic foods or quick fixes. While some people do lose weight on fad diets, most regain the weight when they stop the diet.

Your best chance at successful weight loss is with a multifaceted approach. Dietary changes, increased physical activity and behavior modifications are important first steps. To lose weight — and keep it off — you have to adopt healthy habits that you can maintain over time.

If you've tried to lose weight and you haven't been successful, or you lost weight but you weren't able to keep it off, seek help from an obesity expert.

Doctors have many tools to help you lose weight and to keep it off. These tools include prescription weight-loss medications, minimally invasive procedures and surgery.

DIET

So, what do you eat to lose weight? The first step is to eat less — more specifically, to consume fewer calories. Weight loss is the result of simple energy balance — fewer calories in and more calories out. Calories in come from the food you eat and calories out are dependent on how physically active you are.

To reduce the number of calories you consume, you want to follow a healthier diet. A healthy diet begins with plenty of vegetables and fruits. Studies show that individuals who eat the most vegetables and fruits daily tend to weigh less, and that people can lose weight by eating more plant-based foods.

Vegetables and fruits provide a lot of weight and volume (bulk) to help fill you up without adding a lot of calories. In addition, these foods are rich in fiber and nutrients and other healthy compounds.

At the same time, you want to limit sugar, fat and animal proteins such as red meat, as well as highly processed foods containing additives and artificial sweeteners.

Look for an eating plan that focuses on vegetables, fruits and whole grains and that limits saturated fats and sugars. The USDA's MyPlate is one example of such an approach. Another is the Mayo Clinic Diet, which is similar to MyPlate.

The Mayo Clinic Diet

The Mayo Clinic Diet is a lifestyle-based approach that focuses on getting rid of unhealthy eating habits and adopting healthier ones. It encourages weight loss based on a concept called energy density, or calorie density.

● ● ● ● ●

THE MAYO CLINIC HEALTHY WEIGHT PYRAMID AND DINING TABLE

Use the Mayo Clinic Healthy Weight Pyramid to help you make smart eating choices. To lose weight, you want to eat more from the food groups at the base of the pyramid and less from those at the top. The Mayo Clinic Healthy Dining Table graphic helps you visualize what your meals should look like on your plate.

Mayo Clinic Healthy Weight Pyramid

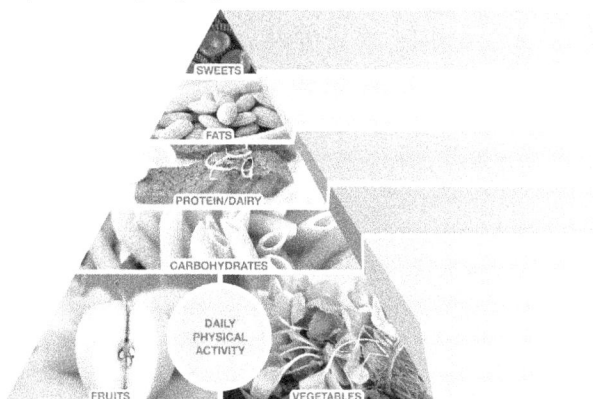

Mayo Clinic Healthy Dining Table

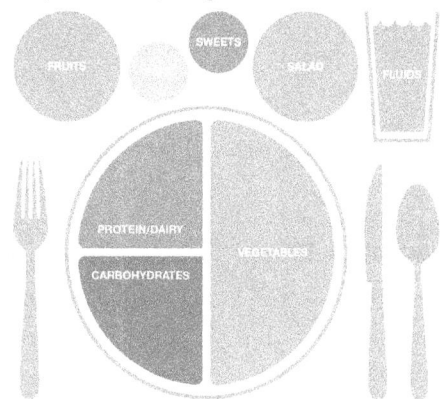

● ● ● ● ●

Some foods have a large number of calories in a small volume of food. Examples include baked goods containing butter and sugar. These foods are energy dense. In comparison, other foods have a small number of calories in a large volume of food — they aren't very energy dense. Vegetables and fruits are examples of bulky, low-calorie foods that are low in energy density.

By eating foods low in energy density, you can eat more food for fewer calories. Plus, foods low in energy density are more likely to fill you up, and they're rich in fiber and nutrients.

The Mayo Clinic Diet is based on the Mayo Clinic Healthy Weight Pyramid (see here). You'll see that vegetables and fruits form the foundation of the pyramid. These are the foods that you want to eat the most of because they're good for your health and they're low in energy density.

Moving up the pyramid, you come to the carbohydrates group. When eating carbohydrates, choose whole-grain products, which are healthier than their refined counterparts. Whole grains include whole-grain bread, whole-wheat pasta, oatmeal, brown rice and barley.

Your protein and dairy selections should be lean or low-fat. These include foods such as fish, lean poultry, beans and skim milk. For fats, choose foods that contain unsaturated fats, such as nuts and olive oil. Finally, an occasional sweet is OK, but it shouldn't be part of every meal.

The Mayo Clinic Healthy Dining Table that accompanies the pyramid illustrates how you can apply the pyramid to your meals. In general, more than half of the food on your plate should be vegetables. Including a salad and a bowl of fruit with your meals is an easy way to make sure you're getting enough vegetables and fruits.

Limit carbohydrates to a quarter of your plate — the same for protein and dairy. Eat fats and sweets sparingly; they may not be part of every meal. Nuts are a healthy fat, but you need to limit the amount you eat because they're high in calories, as are sweets. Some type of fluid (water is best!) rounds out the dining table.

Many individuals trying to lose weight underestimate the number of calories they consume each day in liquid form — be it nondiet soda, calorie-laden coffee drinks, fruit juices or alcohol. To lose weight and keep it off, pay attention to the number of calories in the beverages you drink and keep the calories to a minimum.

For additional information on the Mayo Clinic Diet and the best foods to eat, go to diet.MayoClinic.org.

● ● ● ● ●

BEFORE YOU GET STARTED

It's often a good idea to talk with your doctor before starting an exercise program. If you have a health problem or you're at risk of heart disease, you may need to take some precautions while you exercise. It's essential that you see your doctor if you:

- Are unsure of your health status
- Have experienced chest discomfort, shortness of breath or dizziness during or right after exercise or strenuous activity
- Are a male age 40 years or older or a woman age 50 years or older, and haven't had a recent physical exam

- Have a blood pressure of 140/90 millimeters of mercury (mm Hg) or higher
- Have diabetes, heart, lung or kidney disease, or are significantly overweight
- Have a family history of heart-related problems before age 55
- Are taking medication for diabetes, high blood pressure, heart problems or another medical condition
- Have bone or joint problems that could be made worse by some forms of physical activity

● ● ● ● ●

PHYSICAL ACTIVITY AND EXERCISE

Another key part of weight loss is getting enough physical activity and exercise. Physical activity is any movement that burns calories — whether it's gardening, a leisurely walk or stretching during a work break. Exercise is a structured repetitive form of physical activity that improves fitness — such as swimming laps, bicycling, brisk walking and lifting weights.

To prevent weight gain or maintain your weight loss, you want to move enough each day so that you take at least 10,000 steps. You can record your daily steps on your smartphone or with a tracking device (pedometer). Also, try to get at least 150 minutes of moderately intense physical activity each week. That equates to 30 minutes a day five days a week. If you've lost weight and you're trying to maintain the weight loss, you need to be even more active each day — up to 300 minutes a week of exercise.

You don't have to become an ultimate athlete, just find enjoyable ways to move more and sit less. If you aren't physically active, gradually increase the amount you exercise as your endurance and fitness improve. This table shows approximately how many calories you can burn from doing a variety of different activities.

One way to become more physically active is to take part in a fitness challenge or community wellness program. These events are often offered by employers or local medical clinics or sponsored by community agencies or organizations. In addition to improving your health, it's also a great way to meet people and socialize.

Keep in mind that you don't have to get all of your activity at one time. Walking for 15 minutes in the morning, spending 30 minutes in the afternoon mowing the lawn with a push mower, and enjoying a 15-minute bike ride in the evening all count toward your daily goal.

Becoming more physically active is important because it can improve your health in many ways — beyond just helping you lose weight. Physical activity improves your body's fat-to-muscle ratio. It can strengthen your heart, blood vessels and lungs — in addition to your muscles. Try not to think of physical activity as simply a tool to lose weight. Instead, view it as another component to a healthier lifestyle.

BEHAVIOR CHANGES

Everyone is different and has different obstacles to losing weight. For many individuals, excess weight is linked to unhealthy habits — regularly eating out, eating on the go, late-night snacking, eating to relieve stress or depression, skipping breakfast, not making time for exercise.

To be successful in your weight-loss efforts, you need to identify your unhealthy habits and find ways to change these troublesome behaviors. Behavior modification — also known as behavior therapy — is designed to help individuals lose weight by changing their behaviors. Options for changing behaviors include:

Working with a dietitian

A registered dietitian can help you develop an eating plan that fits your needs and circumstances. Your meal plan should be designed in such a way that you're likely to follow it. If your meal plan contains foods you don't like or won't eat, it doesn't do you much good.

Counseling

Meeting with well-trained professionals can help you address emotional and behavioral issues related to eating. Therapy can help you understand why you overeat and learn healthy ways to cope with anxiety or stress. You learn how to monitor your diet and activity, identify eating triggers and cope with food cravings.

Joining a support group

Many people enjoy the camaraderie of support groups made up of other individuals who share similar challenges. Talk to a member of your health care team about weight-loss support groups in your area.

Enrolling in a weight management program

Some medical centers offer multidisciplinary weight management programs focused on educating you about weight control and teaching you the steps you need to take to lose weight.

These programs often include cooking classes and one-on-one or small group training with a fitness instructor, as well as time spent with a counselor to address unhealthy behaviors.

There are also commercial weight management programs that focus on specific aspects of weight loss and often include regular support meetings. Weight Watchers is an example of this type of program. Before you join a commercial weight management program, talk with your doctor to make sure it's a good fit for you.

PRESCRIPTION MEDICATIONS

When lifestyle changes don't seem to be enough, medication may help. Anti-obesity medications are meant to be used in conjunction with diet, exercise and behavior changes, not in place of them. If you don't make other changes in your life, the medication is unlikely to be effective. In addition, anti-obesity drugs may have side effects, so make sure your doctor reviews the risks and benefits with you.

Anti-obesity medications should be tailored to other medications you take or preexisting health conditions. You'll need close medical monitoring while taking an anti-obesity medication, which often means checkups with your doctor every few months. Keep in mind that effects of the medication may wane over time, and when stopping the medication, many people regain the weight they lost.

Anti-obesity drugs available by prescription include orlistat (Xenical), liraglutide (Saxenda), lorcaserin (Belviq), phentermine and topiramate (Qsymia), and buproprion and naltrexone (Contrave). Orlistat also comes in a reduced strength and is sold over-the-counter under the brand name Alli. Other prescription medications may be prescribed for short-term use.

● ● ● ● ●

WHAT ABOUT WEIGHT-LOSS SUPPLEMENTS?

It may be tempting to purchase an over-the-counter product that promises to help you lose weight. But are you wasting your money? And is it safe?

There's minimal evidence that over-the-counter herbal products or other dietary supplements produce sustained weight loss. And there's relatively little research about most of these products, including their safety and effectiveness.

If you're considering nonprescription weight-loss products, be sure to talk with your doctor, especially if you have health problems, take prescription drugs, or are pregnant or breast-feeding. It's also important to get advice on possible interactions with your current use of medicine, vitamins or minerals.

Be aware that unlike prescription drugs, the makers of dietary supplements are responsible for ensuring the safety of their products and making honest claims about the possible benefits. These claims aren't subject to Food and Drug Administration (FDA) review or approval before marketing. Also, the type or quality of research used to support the claims can vary.

● ● ● ● ●

SURGERY AND ENDOSCOPIC PROCEDURES

A variety of procedures are available that are designed to promote weight loss. Similar to medication, these procedures by themselves — without a change in behavior — are unlikely to produce long-term benefits.

Surgery

Weight-loss surgery, also called bariatric surgery, offers the best chance of losing the most weight, but it doesn't come without serious risks. Surgery limits the amount of food you're able to comfortably eat or decreases the absorption of food and calories or both. Surgery may be considered when other means of losing weight haven't worked or produced the desired results. Weight-loss surgeries include:

Gastric bypass In Roux-en-Y gastric bypass, a surgeon creates a small pouch at the top of the stomach. The small intestine is then cut a short distance below the main stomach and connected to the new pouch. Food and liquid flow directly from the pouch into the small intestine, bypassing the main stomach. Gastric bypass surgery is the most effective treatment for severe obesity.

Gastric sleeve In this procedure, part of the stomach is removed, creating a narrow tube (reservoir) for food that looks similar to a sleeve. The new stomach is much smaller and it doesn't stretch when eating, helping you feel satisfied with less food. This surgery is less complicated than gastric bypass.

Biliopancreatic diversion with duodenal switch The surgeon removes a large part of the stomach, leaving the valve that releases food to the first part of the small intestine (duodenum). The surgeon then closes off the middle section of the intestine and attaches the last part directly to the duodenum. The separated section of the intestine is reattached to the end of the intestine to allow bile and digestive juices to flow into this part of the intestine.

Adjustable gastric banding Less commonly used today, in this procedure the stomach is separated into two pouches with an inflatable band. Pulling the band tight, like a belt, a surgeon creates a tiny channel between the two pouches. The band keeps the opening from expanding and is generally designed to stay in place permanently.

The decision about what type of procedure to have is important. Discuss your options with your surgeon, and make sure that he or she is experienced in weight-loss surgery.

Endoscopic procedures

A variety of minimally invasive procedures designed to promote weight loss are now available. Similar to medications, these procedures by themselves — without a change in behavior — are unlikely to produce long-term benefits. Also, because they're newer their long-term effectiveness is unknown.

Endoscopic procedures are performed without an open incision and generally without the need for hospitalization. Procedures that have been approved by the FDA include:

Gastric balloon A thin tube is threaded down the throat and into the stomach. A special balloon is released and placed in the stomach, where it remains for up to six months. The balloon occupies space normally available for food, thereby limiting how much can be eaten.

Aspiration therapy Recently approved by the Food and Drug Administration, this treatment is intended to reduce how many calories your body absorbs after a meal. A thin tube is placed in your stomach that connects the inside of the stomach to a small button (port) located on the outside of your abdomen. After each meal, the device enables you to empty (aspirate) up to 30 percent of your meal into a toilet via the abdominal port.

Endoscopic sleeve gastroplasty In this procedure, your stomach is sutured inside, creating a narrow tube (reservoir) for food to collect that looks similar to a sleeve. The new stomach is much smaller and it doesn't stretch when eating, helping you to feel satisfied with less food.

LOOKING AHEAD

Unfortunately, it's common to regain lost weight no matter what treatment methods you try. You can even regain weight after weight-loss surgery if you continue to overeat or overindulge in high-calorie foods.

One of the best ways to keep from regaining the weight you've lost is to exercise regularly. As you lose weight and gain better health, talk to your doctor about additional activities you might be able to do. Also keep in mind that other tools exist — medication, surgery and endoscopic procedures — to help you lose weight and keep if off.

Finally, don't be too hard on yourself. Take your weight loss and weight maintenance one day at a time and surround yourself with supportive resources to help ensure your success.

● ● ● ● ●

WHAT'S YOUR BMI?

To determine your BMI, find your height in the left column of the table below. Follow that row across to the weight nearest yours. Look at the top of that column for your approximate BMI. Or use this formula:

1. Multiply your height (in inches) by your height (in inches).
2. Divide your weight (in pounds) by the results of the first step.
3. Multiply that answer by 703. (For example, a 270-pound person, 68 inches tall, has a BMI of 41.)

Normal	Overweight	Obese

BMI	19	24	25	26	27	28	29	30	35	40	45	50
Height						**Weight in pounds**						
4'10"	91	115	119	124	129	134	138	143	167	191	215	239
4'11"	94	119	124	128	133	138	143	148	173	198	222	247
5'0"	97	123	128	133	138	143	148	153	179	204	230	255
5'1"	100	127	132	137	143	148	153	158	185	211	238	264
5'2"	104	131	136	142	147	153	158	164	191	218	246	273
5'3"	107	135	141	146	152	158	163	169	197	225	254	282
5'4"	110	140	145	151	157	163	169	174	204	232	262	291
5'5"	114	144	150	156	162	168	174	180	210	240	270	300
5'6"	118	148	155	161	167	173	179	186	216	247	278	309
5'7"	121	153	159	166	172	178	185	191	223	255	287	319
5'8"	125	158	164	171	177	184	190	197	230	262	295	328
5'9"	128	162	169	176	182	189	196	203	236	270	304	338
5'10"	132	167	174	181	188	195	202	209	243	278	313	348
5'11"	136	172	179	186	193	200	208	215	250	286	322	358
6'0"	140	177	184	191	199	206	213	221	258	294	331	368
6'1"	144	182	189	197	204	212	219	227	265	302	340	378
6'2"	148	186	194	202	210	218	225	233	272	311	350	389
6'3"	152	192	200	208	216	224	232	240	279	319	359	399
6'4"	156	197	205	213	221	230	238	246	287	328	369	410

Based on Circulation, 2014;129(suppl 2):S102; NHBLI Obesity Expert Panel, 2013.

Asians with a BMI of 23 or higher may have an increased risk of health problems.

● ● ● ● ●

● ● ● ● ●

APPROXIMATE CALORIES BURNED IN 1 HOUR

The number of calories burned in an hour of physical activity varies significantly depending on the type of activity, the intensity level and the individual.

Activity (1-hour duration)	Weight of person and calories burned		
	160 lbs.	200 lbs.	240 lbs.
Aerobics, low-impact	365	455	545
Aerobics, water	402	501	600
Bicycling, < 10 mph, leisure	292	364	436
Canoeing	256	319	382
Dancing, ballroom	219	273	327
Elliptical trainer, moderate effort	365	455	545
Golfing, carrying clubs	314	391	469
Hiking	438	546	654
Resistance (weight) training	365	455	545
Rowing, stationary	438	546	654
Running, 5 mph	606	755	905
Skiing, cross-country	496	619	741
Skiing, downhill	314	391	469
Stair treadmill	657	819	981
Swimming laps, light to moderate	423	528	632
Tai chi	219	273	327

Tennis, singles	584	728	872
Walking, 2 mph	204	255	305
Walking, 3.5 mph	314	391	469
Yoga, hatha	183	228	273

Based on Ainsworth BE, et al. 2011 Compendium of Physical Activities: A second update of codes and MET values. Medicine & Science in Sports & Exercise. 2011;43:1575.

● ● ● ● ●

CHAPTER 7

Constipation and fecal incontinence

Does it seem like you're spending too much of your life on the toilet? Has the bathroom become a battleground? If you're dealing with constipation, it can feel that way. You may be straining to pass stools that are hard and lumpy. Some days, it can feel as if you can't completely empty your bowels, no matter how hard you try.

Or maybe you're experiencing the opposite end of the spectrum. When you pass gas, do you also pass stool? Does stool leak onto your underwear without any warning? When you do feel the urge to move your bowels, are there times you can't make it to the bathroom on time? If you answered yes to any of these questions, you may have fecal incontinence.

Constipation and fecal incontinence can be bothersome conditions, but you shouldn't be embarrassed to get help. Neither problem is as uncommon as you might think, and there are steps you and your doctor can take to manage or treat the condition — whether your symptoms are simply annoying or severe enough to affect your daily life. You don't have to tough it out alone or suffer in silence. By working with your doctor and taking an active approach to your problem, you can feel better and live better.

CONSTIPATION

When your body digests food, the food passes from your stomach, through the small intestine and large intestine (colon), and finally through the rectum before it leaves your body. If you're having a hard time passing stool through your colon or rectum, you might have constipation.

Constipation is generally described as having fewer than three bowel movements a week, but the symptoms of constipation vary. You could have one bowel movement a week. Or you may have frequent, small bowel movements but not feel like you're ever able to empty your bowels. Generally speaking, anywhere from three bowel movements a day to three a week is considered normal. What matters more than how many bowel movements you have is how difficult it is for you to pass stool.

When the symptoms of constipation last for several weeks, it's considered chronic constipation. Chronic constipation is thought to affect up to 20 percent of adults in the United States, with more women reporting the problem than men. The condition becomes more common as you age, affecting up to one-third of people 65 or over. When the symptoms are severe and long lasting, they can impact your everyday life, from how productive you are at work to how much you want to socialize. Even so, only a minority of people talk to their doctors about their symptoms and seek help.

Rarely, constipation can be a sign of a serious problem. So, it's important to talk to your doctor if your symptoms don't get better with self-care, such as adding fiber to your diet or taking laxatives. In general, you should avoid taking laxatives or stool softeners for more than a week without consulting a doctor.

● ● ● ● ●

CONSTIPATION

Key signs and symptoms:

- Fewer bowel movements
- Lumpy or hard stools
- Straining during bowel movements
- Incomplete bowel movements

● ● ● ● ●

Symptoms

Doctors use guidelines known as Rome IV criteria to determine whether someone has chronic constipation. These guidelines, established by an international group of medical experts, outline common symptoms of chronic constipation.

You could have chronic constipation if you've experienced two or more of the following signs or symptoms for at least three months:

- Straining to have bowel movements
- Having lumpy or hard stools
- Feeling as if you can't completely empty the stool from your rectum
- Feeling as if there's a blockage in your rectum that prevents bowel movements
- Needing help to empty your rectum, such as using your hands to press on your abdomen and using a finger to remove stool from your rectum
- Passing fewer than three stools a week without the use of stool softeners or laxatives

Causes

There are many reasons why you could be experiencing constipation. Sometimes there may be a combination of causes, while in other cases an exact cause is unknown. Here are some common reasons why you might be constipated:

Diet or lifestyle imbalances If you don't eat enough fiber or get enough physical activity, you may develop constipation. Regularly ignoring the urge to have a bowel movement can also make you constipated.

Irritable bowel syndrome Irritable bowel syndrome (IBS) is a common disorder that affects the large intestine. Along with abdominal discomfort or pain, IBS can cause constipation or diarrhea. IBS with constipation is often called constipation-predominant IBS, and it can prevent you from having a bowel movement, even if you have the urge to go.

Pelvic floor dysfunction A normal bowel movement requires contraction of the diaphragm and relaxation of the pelvic floor muscles (puborectalis and anal sphincter). Pelvic floor dysfunction happens when these muscles aren't working together or relaxing properly.

Medications Pain medications such as opioids cause constipation. Some other medications linked to constipation include certain antihistamines, certain antidepressants, and some medications that lower blood pressure, prevent seizures or treat Parkinson's disease. Dietary supplements such as calcium and iron can also contribute to constipation.

Slow transit Sometimes stool takes longer to move through your intestines. Doctors call this problem slow transit. This may explain why stools become hard and difficult to pass.

Blockage or structural problems Rarely, problems in the anatomy of the colon or rectum may slow or stop the movement of your stool. These problems can include:

- Tears in the lining of the lower rectum (anal fissure)
- Bowel obstruction
- Cancers of the colon, rectum or abdomen
- Narrowing of the colon (bowel stricture)
- Rectum bulge through the back wall of the vagina (rectocele)
- Rectum slippage toward or outside the anus (rectal prolapse)

Other disorders Other conditions associated with constipation include metabolic disorders such as diabetes, hormonal disorders such as an underactive thyroid (hypothyroidism) and disorders of the nervous system, including Parkinson's disease and multiple sclerosis.

DIAGNOSING CONSTIPATION

If you've been struggling with constipation, your doctor will likely ask many questions about your signs and symptoms, your medical history, medications you take, and your lifestyle. These questions are important because they can help your doctor determine if you have constipation and what might be causing the problem.

Your doctor will likely also want to perform a physical examination of your rectum and abdomen. A physical exam can identify problems with the muscles involved in having a bowel movement. It can also help identify other issues, such as a blockage or structural problem.

During a digital rectal exam, your doctor will inspect your rectal area visually and physically by inserting a gloved, lubricated finger into your rectum (see the image below). If you feel pain during the rectal exam, tell your doctor. The exam may be uncomfortable, but it shouldn't be painful.

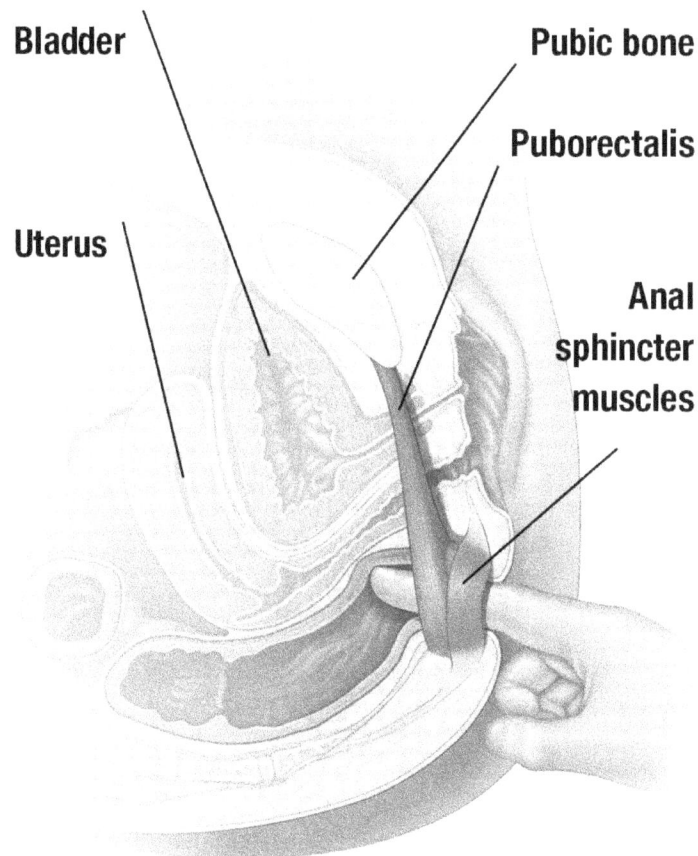

Bladder

Pubic bone

Puborectalis

Uterus

Anal sphincter muscles

During a digital rectal exam, a doctor inserts a gloved, lubricated finger into the rectum to evaluate the strength of the sphincter muscles or identify a mass of hard stool within the rectum.

After taking these steps, your doctor may perform one or more of the following tests to try to pinpoint the cause of your constipation. You can read more about the tests in Chapter 5.

- ***Blood tests.*** A sample of your blood is tested to check for systemic conditions such as low blood cell count or hypothyroidism.

- *Anorectal manometry.* This test measures the strength of your anal sphincter muscles and the ability of the muscles to relax and tighten at the proper times.
- *Balloon expulsion test.* Often used along with anorectal manometry, this test measures the amount of time it takes for you to push out a balloon that has been filled with water and placed in your rectum.
- *Defecography.* This procedure is often performed with the balloon expulsion test. A doctor inserts a soft paste or gel made of barium into your rectum that shows up on X-rays or magnetic resonance imaging (MRI). Movement of the barium mixture is analyzed as you pass the mixture through your rectum and anus as you would stool. This test helps detect structural abnormalities.
- *Colon transit study.* This test may be used to evaluate how well food moves through your colon. You swallow a capsule that contains either radiopaque markers or a wireless recording device. The progress of the markers through your colon is recorded over several days and seen on X-rays. In some cases, you may eat radiocarbon-activated food and a special camera will record its progress (scintigraphy).
- *Colonic manometry.* This procedure tests if the nerves and muscles involved in passing stool are working properly. You are sedated with a general anesthetic as your doctor performs a simple procedure to insert a motility tube into your colon. A motility tube is a flexible plastic tube slightly thicker than a straw. The tube is carefully taped into place on the thigh or buttock. The test allows your doctor to measure the strength of muscle contractions in your colon and to determine if the contractions are properly synchronized.
- *Others.* Other tests, such as a stool test or a colonoscopy, are less commonly used to diagnose constipation. Your doctor may suggest a

colonoscopy if you're experiencing blood in your stool, unexplained weight loss or fever.

TREATING AND MANAGING CONSTIPATION

You don't have to live with constipation. Many people get relief from simple changes to their diet and lifestyle, and that's a good place to start. For some people, however, those changes aren't enough. If that's the case for you, other options can help get your digestive system back on track.

Diet and lifestyle changes

Small changes can add up when it comes to constipation. To begin, your doctor might recommend trying some of the strategies that follow.

Increase your fiber intake Adding fiber to your diet increases the weight of your stool and speeds its passage through your intestines. Eat more fresh fruits and vegetables each day. Choose whole-grain breads and cereals. Make these changes to your diet slowly by increasing your fiber intake over a few weeks. (For more information on dietary fiber, see Chapter 3.)

Drink plenty of water Aim for 64 ounces of liquid a day, such as water or clear soups. If you're increasing how much fiber you eat, consuming more liquid may help the fiber work better.

Get regular exercise Regular physical activity may help improve your constipation symptoms. If you don't already exercise, talk to your doctor about whether you're healthy enough to start an exercise program.

Try bowel training Try to have a bowel movement at the same time each day. This can train your body to become more regular. Because eating activates your colon, you might try having a bowel movement 15 to 45 minutes after breakfast or another meal each day.

Don't ignore the urge to go If your body's telling you it's time to have a bowel movement, listen to it. Give yourself enough time to have a bowel movement, without distractions and without feeling rushed.

Medications

If changes to your diet and lifestyle don't relieve your constipation, your doctor may recommend medication. Many medications for constipation are sold over-the-counter, while others require a doctor's prescription.

Over-the-counter medications There are a variety of options for treating constipation. They include:

- ***Fiber supplements.*** Fiber supplements add bulk to your stool. They include psyllium (Metamucil), calcium polycarbophil (FiberCon), methylcellulose fiber (Citrucel) and wheat dexrin (Benefiber).
- ***Stimulant laxatives.*** Stimulants, including the medications bisacodyl (Dulcolax) and senna-sennosides oral (Senokot), cause your intestines to contract.
- ***Osmotic laxatives.*** Osmotic laxatives help fluids move through the colon. Examples include oral magnesium hydroxide (Phillips' Milk of Magnesia), magnesium citrate, lactulose (Kristalose) and polyethylene

glycol (Miralax).

- ***Stool softeners.*** Stool softeners sold over-the-counter under several names, including docusate sodium (Colace) and docusate calcium (Surfak), moisten stool by drawing water from the intestines.
- ***Enemas and suppositories.*** Sodium phosphate (Fleet), soapsuds or tap water enemas can help soften stool and produce a bowel movement. Glycerin or bisacodyl suppositories also can soften stool.

Prescription medications If over-the-counter medications don't help relieve your constipation, your doctor may recommend a prescription medication. Prescription medications work in different ways and include the drugs lubiprostone (Amitiza), linaclotide (Linzess) and plecanatide (Trulance). Polyethylene glycol, or PEG (Golytely, Nulytely), is a complete bowel preparation that's also used to clear the colon of stool in preparation for a colonoscopy or colon surgery.

Physical therapy

If your constipation is caused by pelvic floor dysfunction, your doctor may recommend pelvic floor retraining. For this therapy, you work with a health care provider to learn how to control and relax your pelvic floor muscles and change behaviors that may be contributing to your symptoms.

This type of therapy uses biofeedback, which gives you visual, audio and verbal feedback to help you retrain the muscles involved in having a bowel movement. During your physical therapy sessions, you'll also learn muscle relaxation techniques that you can use at home.

Ergonomics

When you're sitting on a toilet, you don't want your hips to be higher than your knees. That position, which occurs with taller, or "comfort height," toilets can make it more difficult to pass stool. If you have a taller toilet, your doctor might suggest that you use an angled toilet footrest. This type of footrest puts your body in a more ideal position that can help you relieve constipation.

Surgery

Depending on the cause of your constipation, surgery may be an option if other treatments haven't worked. Surgery may involve removing a blockage in the colon or rectum or removing part or all of the colon (colectomy).

● ● ● ● ●

THE TROUBLE WITH HIGH TOILETS

Tall toilets, sometimes called "comfort height" or "right height" toilets, are marketed as a more comfortable option than standard toilets. The increased height can make it easier to sit down on the toilet and stand up again, especially for older adults.

The problem is that this kind of toilet positions the hips well above the knees, which can make it more difficult to pass stool. If you recently purchased a taller toilet and developed constipation around the same time, be sure to mention it to your doctor. Your new toilet may be contributing to your bathroom woes.

● ● ● ● ●

COMPLICATIONS OF CONSTIPATION

Two common conditions that can result from constipation are hemorrhoids and anal fissures.

Hemorrhoids

Hemorrhoids are swollen veins in your anus and lower rectum, similar to varicose veins. Hemorrhoids have a number of causes, although often the cause is unknown. They may result from straining during bowel movements or from the increased pressure on the veins during pregnancy. Other causes of hemorrhoids include lifting heavy objects, sitting or standing for long periods, and obesity.

Internal hemorrhoid

External hemorrhoid

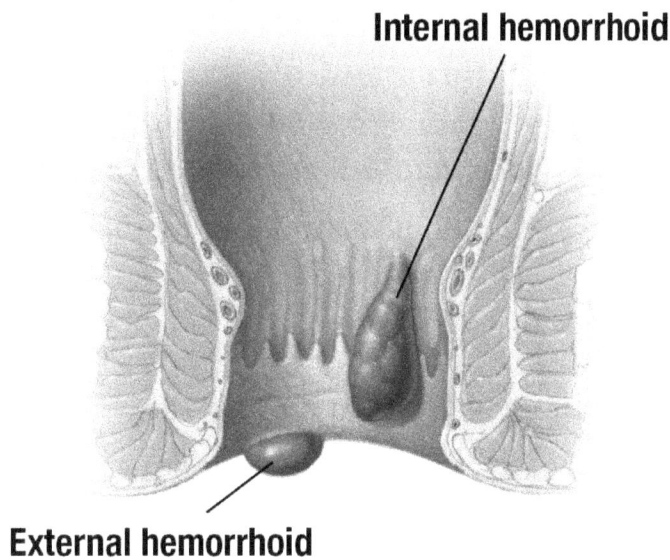

Hemorrhoids may be located inside the rectum (internal hemorrhoids), or they may develop under the skin around the anus (external hemorrhoids).

Hemorrhoids are very common. Nearly 3 out of 4 adults will have hemorrhoids from time to time. Sometimes they don't produce any signs or symptoms, but other times they cause itching, discomfort and bleeding.

Occasionally, a clot may form in a hemorrhoid (thrombosed hemorrhoid). A thrombosed hemorrhoid isn't dangerous, but it can be extremely painful and may need to be lanced and drained.

Treatment You can often relieve the mild pain, swelling and inflammation of hemorrhoids with home treatments.

- *Eat high-fiber foods.* Eat more fruits, vegetables and whole grains. Doing so softens stool and increases its bulk, which can help you avoid the straining that can worsen symptoms from hemorrhoids. Add fiber to your diet slowly to avoid problems with gas. A high-fiber diet also can help prevent hemorrhoids.

- *Use topical treatments.* Apply an over-the-counter hemorrhoid cream or suppository containing hydrocortisone, or use pads containing witch hazel or a numbing agent.
- *Soak regularly in a warm bath or sitz bath.* Soak your anal area in plain warm water for 10 to 15 minutes two to three times a day. A sitz bath fits over the toilet.
- *Keep the anal area clean.* Bathe (preferably) or shower daily to cleanse the skin around your anus gently with warm water. Avoid alcohol-based or perfumed wipes. Gently pat the area dry or use a hair dryer.
- *Don't use dry toilet paper.* To help keep the anal area clean after a bowel movement, use moist towelettes or wet toilet paper that doesn't contain perfume or alcohol.
- *Apply cold.* Apply ice packs or cold compresses on your anus to relieve swelling.
- *Take oral pain relievers.* You can use acetaminophen (Tylenol, others), aspirin or ibuprofen (Advil, Motrin IB, others) temporarily to help relieve your discomfort.

With these treatments, hemorrhoid symptoms often go away within a week. See your doctor if you don't get relief in a week, or sooner if you have severe pain or bleeding.

Medications If your hemorrhoids produce only mild discomfort, your doctor may suggest over-the-counter creams, ointments, suppositories or pads. These products contain ingredients, such as witch hazel, or hydrocortisone and lidocaine, that can relieve pain and itching, at least temporarily.

Don't use an over-the-counter steroid cream for more than a week unless directed by your doctor because it may cause your skin to thin.

External hemorrhoid thrombectomy If a painful blood clot (thrombosis) has formed within an external hemorrhoid, your doctor can remove the clot with a simple incision and drainage, which may provide prompt relief. This procedure is most effective if done within 72 hours of developing a clot.

Minimally invasive procedures For persistent bleeding or painful hemorrhoids, your doctor may recommend one of the other minimally invasive procedures available. These treatments can be done in your doctor's office or in another outpatient setting.

- ***Injection (sclerotherapy).*** In this procedure, a doctor injects a chemical solution into the hemorrhoid tissue to shrink it. While the injection causes little or no pain, it may be less effective than rubber band ligation, discussed below.
- ***Coagulation (infrared, laser or bipolar).*** Coagulation techniques use laser or infrared light or heat. They cause small, bleeding, internal hemorrhoids to harden and shrivel. While coagulation has few side effects and may cause little immediate discomfort, it's associated with a higher rate of hemorrhoids coming back (recurrence) than is the rubber band treatment.
- ***Rubber band ligation.*** A doctor places one or two tiny rubber bands around the base of an internal hemorrhoid to cut off its circulation. The hemorrhoid withers and falls off within a week. This procedure is effective for many people.

  Hemorrhoid banding can be uncomfortable, and it may cause bleeding, which might begin two to four days after the procedure. Rarely, however, is the bleeding severe. On occasion, more-serious complications can occur, but they are uncommon.

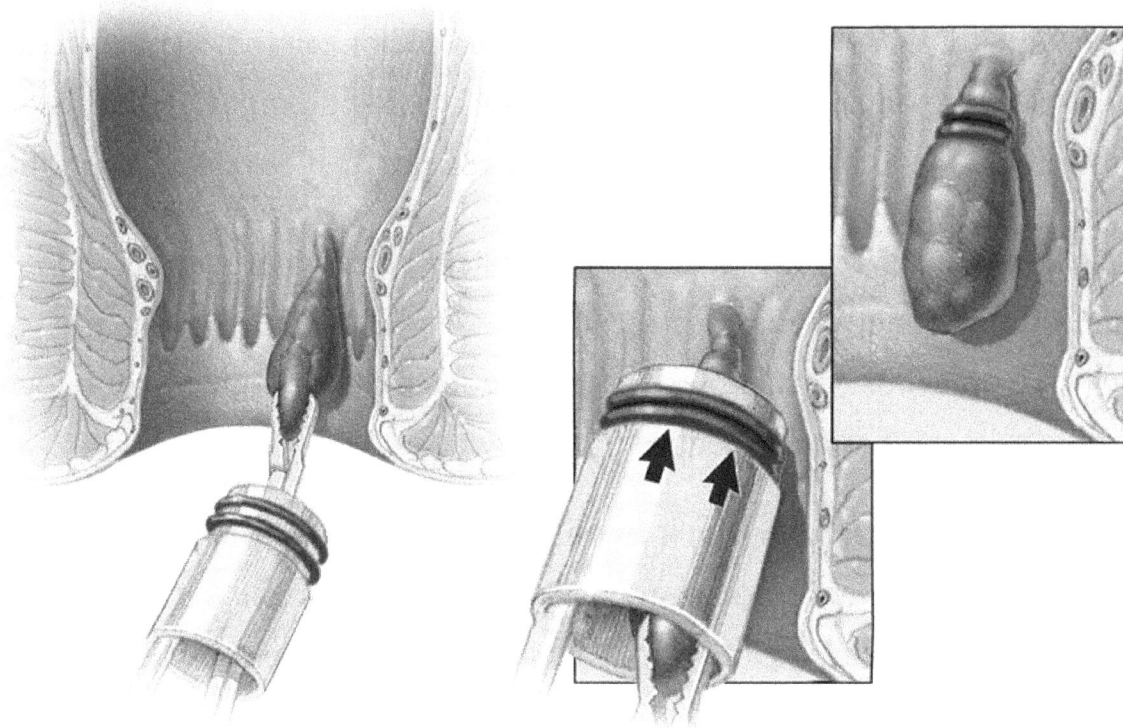

To remove an internal hemorrhoid with a rubber band, a doctor first attaches a special instrument (ligator) to the hemorrhoid and stretches it downward. A rubber band is then placed around the hemorrhoid to cut off its blood supply.

Surgical procedures If other procedures aren't successful or you have large hemorrhoids, your doctor may recommend a surgical procedure. Surgery may be done as an outpatient, or it may require an overnight hospital stay.

- ***Hemorrhoid removal.*** In this procedure, called hemorrhoidectomy, a surgeon removes excessive tissue that causes bleeding. Various techniques may be used. Hemorrhoidectomy is the most effective and complete way to treat severe or recurring hemorrhoids. Most people experience some pain after the procedure. Medications can relieve the pain. Soaking in a warm bath also may help.
- ***Hemorrhoid stapling.*** This procedure, called stapled hemorrhoidectomy or stapled hemorrhoidopexy, blocks blood flow to hemorrhoidal tissue.

It's typically used only for internal hemorrhoids. Stapling generally involves less pain than hemorrhoidectomy and allows for earlier return to regular activities. Compared with hemorrhoidectomy, however, stapling has been associated with a greater risk of recurrence and rectal prolapse, in which part of the rectum protrudes from the anus. Talk with your doctor about the best option for you.

Anal fissure

An anal fissure is a small tear in the thin, moist tissue (mucosa) that lines the anus. An anal fissure may result from constipation and straining during bowel movements or when you pass hard or large stools. Chronic diarrhea also can lead to small tears in the anus.

Anal fissures typically cause pain and bleeding with bowel movements. You also may experience spasms in the ring of muscle at the end of your anus (anal sphincter). Signs and symptoms generally include:

- Pain during bowel movements
- Pain after bowel movements that can last up to several hours
- Bright red blood on the stool or toilet paper after a bowel movement
- A visible crack in the skin around the anus
- A small lump or skin tag on the skin near the anal fissure

Treatment Anal fissures often heal within a few weeks if you take steps to keep your stool soft, such as increasing your intake of fiber and fluids. Soaking in warm water for 10 to 20 minutes several times a day, especially after bowel movements, can help relax the sphincter and promote healing.

If your symptoms persist, your doctor may recommend:

- ***Externally applied nitroglycerin (Rectiv).*** This medication helps increase blood flow to the fissure and promote healing and to relax the anal sphincter. Nitroglycerin is generally considered the medical treatment of choice when other conservative measures fail. Side effects may include headache, which can be severe.
- ***Topical anesthetic creams.*** The topical preparation lidocaine hydrochloride may be helpful for pain relief.
- ***Botulinum toxin type A (Botox) injection.*** An injection of Botox paralyzes the anal sphincter muscle and helps reduce spasms.
- ***Blood pressure medications.*** Medications such as oral nifedipine (Procardia) or diltiazem (Cardizem) can help relax the anal sphincter. These medications may be taken by mouth or applied externally and may be used when nitroglycerin is not effective or causes significant side effects.

For fissures that are resistant to treatment, surgery may be required. Doctors usually perform a procedure called lateral internal sphincterotomy, which involves cutting a small portion of the anal sphincter muscle to reduce spasm and pain, and promote healing.

Studies have found that for chronic fissure, surgery is much more effective than any medical treatment. However, surgery has a small risk of causing incontinence.

FECAL INCONTINENCE

Fecal incontinence isn't something you hear much about, but it can affect women, men and children. Fecal incontinence is the inability to control your bowel movements, causing stool (feces) to leak unexpectedly from your rectum. Also called bowel incontinence, fecal incontinence ranges from an occasional leakage of stool to a complete loss of bowel control. When you experience stool leakage because you don't sense the need to pass stool, it's called passive fecal incontinence. When you sense a bowel movement but aren't able to make it to the toilet in time, it's called urge fecal incontinence.

Fecal incontinence is more common in older people, but it can affect anyone, including children who are already toilet trained. It's difficult to determine how common the problem is, since many people are reluctant to see a doctor. According to the National Institute of Diabetes and Digestive and Kidney Diseases, between 7 and 15 percent of the general population may experience fecal incontinence. The condition becomes more common with age and frailty, affecting between 50 and 70 percent of older adults living in nursing homes.

Most people with fecal incontinence don't tell anyone about it, not even their doctor. Instead, they limit their activities and withdraw from friends and family. If your fecal incontinence is frequent or severe and is affecting your ability to enjoy life, talk to your doctor. Taking steps to deal with fecal incontinence will help ease the embarrassment, fear, anxiety and loneliness that often come with the physical problems. Fortunately, there are many effective ways to reduce or eliminate the symptoms of fecal incontinence.

• • • • •

FECAL INCONTINENCE

Key signs and symptoms:

- Leakage of stool
- Uncontrolled bowel movements

● ● ● ● ●

Symptoms

You've likely experienced a brief period of fecal incontinence during a bout of diarrhea. But if the problem's ongoing, it's called chronic fecal incontinence. Doctors use guidelines known as Rome IV criteria to determine whether someone has chronic fecal incontinence. These guidelines outline common symptoms of the condition.

According to the Rome IV criteria, you may have fecal incontinence if:

- You experience repeated episodes of uncontrolled bowel movements or stool leakage.
- The problem lasts for at least three months.

Causes

Bowel function is mainly controlled by the strength of your pelvic floor muscles (anal sphincter and puborectalis), the storage capacity of your rectum and your ability to sense stool. A problem in one or more of these areas can lead to fecal incontinence. These problems can arise for a variety of reasons.

Diarrhea Solid stool is easier to hold in than loose stool, so the loose stools of chronic diarrhea can cause or worsen fecal incontinence.

Overflow It's ironic, but a common cause of fecal incontinence is constipation. Chronic constipation may lead to a mass of stool in the rectum that's too large to pass (overflow). Overflow can cause the muscles of the rectum and intestines to stretch and eventually weaken, allowing watery stool from farther up the digestive tract to move around the impacted stool and leak out.

Loss of storage capacity in the rectum Normally, the rectum stretches to accommodate stool. If your rectum is scarred or your rectal walls have stiffened from surgery, radiation treatment or inflammatory bowel disease, the rectum can't stretch as much as it needs to and stool may leak out.

Muscle weakness Your anal sphincter and puborectalis muscles normally tighten to hold in stool. If either of these pelvic floor muscles are weak, it can be more difficult to hold in stool. The weakness is often caused by muscle damage. The damage can happen during childbirth, especially if you have an episiotomy or if forceps are used during delivery. Surgery to treat enlarged veins in the rectum or anus (hemorrhoids), as well as more complex operations involving the rectum and anus, also can lead to muscle weakness.

Loss of rectal sensation Normally, the nerves in the rectum sense when there's a need to pass stool. Damage to those nerves may lead to a loss of rectal sensation, which can result in fecal incontinence. The nerve damage can be caused by childbirth, constant straining during bowel movements, spinal cord injury or stroke. Some diseases, such as diabetes and multiple sclerosis, also can affect these nerves and cause damage that leads to fecal incontinence.

Anatomy problems of the colon or rectum Sometimes, problems with the anatomy of the colon or rectum may cause fecal incontinence. One problem is when the rectum drops down into the anus (rectal prolapse). In women, fecal incontinence can also occur if the rectum protrudes through the vagina (rectocele).

• • • • •

WHO'S AT RISK OF FECAL INCONTINENCE?

Fecal incontinence can affect men and women, young and old. But some factors increase your likelihood of incontinence. These risk factors include:

- ***Being older.*** Although it can occur at any age, fecal incontinence is more common in adults older than 65.
- ***Being female.*** Fecal incontinence can be a complication of childbirth.
- ***Having nerve damage.*** People who have long-standing diabetes or multiple sclerosis — conditions that damage the nerves that help control defecation — may be at risk of fecal incontinence.
- ***Having dementia.*** Fecal incontinence is often present in late-stage Alzheimer's disease and dementia.
- ***Having a physical disability.*** Being physically disabled may make it difficult to reach a toilet in time. An injury caused by a physical disability also may cause rectal nerve damage, leading to fecal incontinence.

• • • • •

DIAGNOSING FECAL INCONTINENCE

When you talk to your doctor about your fecal incontinence, he or she will likely ask many questions about your symptoms, medical history and lifestyle. The questions help determine whether you have true fecal incontinence and how severe it is.

Your doctor will likely want to perform a physical examination. A physical exam can help identify muscle weakness, injury or other problems in the anal and rectal area.

Your doctor may check for signs of neurological disease or nerve damage by checking your reflexes, walking gait and senses. Sensation in the area between your anus and genitals also may be checked.

The physical examination will most likely involve a rectal exam. During the rectal exam, your doctor will inspect your rectal area visually as well by inserting a gloved, lubricated finger into your rectum (digital rectal exam). If you feel pain during the rectal exam, tell your doctor. The exam may be uncomfortable, but it shouldn't be painful.

After taking these steps, your doctor may perform one or more tests to try to pinpoint the cause of the fecal incontinence. You can learn more about many of these tests in Chapter 5.

- *Anorectal manometry.* The test measures the strength of your anal sphincter muscles and nerve sensation in the rectum.

- *Balloon expulsion test.* A balloon expulsion test evaluates your ability to defecate. More precisely, it tests the ability of your puborectalis muscle to relax and the coordination of your abdominal, pelvic floor and anal sphincter muscles.
- *Defecography.* This test shows how much and how well your rectum can hold stool and how well your rectum works during defecation.
- *Anorectal ultrasound.* For this test, also called an anal endosonography, a narrow, wandlike instrument is inserted into the anus and rectum. The instrument produces video images that allow your doctor to evaluate the structure of your anal sphincter and to identify defects, scarring, thinning or other abnormalities in anal and rectal muscles.
- *Magnetic resonance imaging (MRI).* An MRI of the pelvis can provide clear pictures of the sphincter to determine if the muscles are intact or if there are structural problems, such as rectal prolapse and rectocele. A test called a dynamic MRI creates a real-time image of your pelvic floor as you contract the floor muscles and move your bowels, allowing the doctor to see any abnormalities that occur as you defecate.

TREATING AND MANAGING FECAL INCONTINENCE

A number of effective treatments are available for fecal incontinence. Treatment usually can help restore bowel control or at least substantially reduce the severity of your symptoms. The treatment you'll receive depends on the cause or causes of your incontinence and how severe the condition is.

Diet and lifestyle changes

To begin with, your doctor may recommend that you make small changes to your everyday habits. These changes may be enough to improve or eliminate your symptoms.

Alter your fiber intake The amount of fiber in your diet can affect the consistency of your stools. If diarrhea is contributing to your fecal incontinence, your doctor may recommend that you reduce the amount of fiber you consume. Or, your doctor may recommend high-fiber foods or fiber supplements to add bulk to your stools and make them less watery.

If constipation is causing the problem, fiber- rich foods or fiber supplements can make you less constipated and improve fecal incontinence. (For more information on fiber, see Chapter 3.)

Identify problem foods and beverages For people with fecal incontinence, certain foods or drinks may trigger diarrhea, which can make the problem worse. Make a list of what you eat for a week. You may discover a connection between certain foods and your bouts of incontinence. Once you've identified problem foods, stop eating them and see if your symptoms improve.

Common culprits are caffeine, dairy products containing lactose, and fructose found in foods and drinks such as fruit juice, honey and high-fructose corn syrup. Products that contain artificial sweeteners, such as sugar-free gum or diet sodas, also can act as laxatives.

Try bowel training Try to have a bowel movement at the same time each day, such as after a meal. Bowel training helps some people relearn how to control their bowels.

Physical therapy

Depending on the cause of fecal incontinence, physical therapy may reduce symptoms and improve your quality of life. Your doctor may recommend one or both of these treatments:

Kegel exercises If your fecal incontinence is caused by weak pelvic floor muscles, your doctor may suggest Kegel exercises. For these exercises, you contract and release the muscles that you would normally use to stop the flow of stool and urine. The exercises can strengthen your pelvic floor and rectal muscles. Before starting Kegel exercises, talk to your doctor and work with a physical therapist. In some people, the exercises can make fecal incontinence worse.

Biofeedback Kegel exercises are often used in combination with biofeedback treatment. Biofeedback gives you visual, audio and verbal feedback to help you retrain the muscles involved in having a bowel movement. This therapy can help strengthen and coordinate the muscles involved in holding in stool. It may also improve your ability to sense the presence of stool in your rectum.

Medications

There currently are no medications specifically approved for the treatment of fecal incontinence. These medications can help treat certain underlying causes of the condition:

Anti-diarrheal drugs If diarrhea is contributing to your symptoms, your doctor may recommend anti-diarrheal medications such as diphenoxylate and atropine sulfate (Lomotil) or loperamide hydrochloride (Imodium A-D).

Constipation medications If constipation has caused the problem of overflow, medications can help empty your bowels and improve your constipation symptoms. (For more information about medications to treat constipation, see here.)

● ● ● ● ●

CARING FOR YOUR SKIN

It can take time for fecal incontinence treatments to work, and sometimes the condition can't be completely corrected. Contact between watery stool and skin can cause pain or itching. Consider these tips to relieve anal discomfort:

- ***Wash with water.*** Gently wash the area with water after each bowel movement. Showering or soaking in a bath also may help. Soap can dry and irritate the skin. So can rubbing with dry toilet paper. Premoistened, alcohol-free, perfume-free towelettes or wipes may be a good alternative for cleaning the area.
- ***Dry thoroughly.*** Allow the area to air-dry, if possible. If you're short on time, you can gently pat the area dry with toilet paper or a clean washcloth.
- ***Apply a cream or powder.*** Moisture-barrier creams help keep irritated skin from having direct contact with stool. Be sure the area is clean and dry before you apply any cream. Nonmedicated talcum powder or cornstarch also may help

relieve anal discomfort.

- **Wear cotton underwear and loose clothing.** Tight clothing can restrict airflow, making skin problems worse. Change soiled underwear quickly.
- **Use self-care products.** When medical treatments can't completely eliminate incontinence, products such as absorbent pads and disposable underwear can help you manage the problem. If you use pads or adult diapers, be sure they have an absorbent wicking layer on top, to help keep moisture away from your skin.

• • • • •

Other nonsurgical treatments

Depending on the cause of your fecal incontinence, your doctor may recommend one of these procedures:

Injectable bulking agents Injections of materials such as dextranomer and sodium hyaluronate (Solesta) into the anal canal may help build tissue in the area around the anus. By growing, or "bulking," the surrounding tissue, the opening of the anus narrows, stopping or limiting leakage of stool.

Sacral nerve stimulation The sacral nerves run from your spinal cord to muscles in your pelvis. These nerves regulate the sensation and strength of your rectal and anal sphincter muscles. Implanting a device that sends small electrical impulses continuously to the nerves can strengthen muscles in the bowel.

Anal plug If other treatments haven't been successful, your doctor may suggest you try an anal plug. This small, cup-shaped device is made of foam. You insert it into your rectum to prevent stool leakage, and it can stay in place for up to 12 hours. Although this option works for some people, others find it too uncomfortable to use.

Surgery

Most people with fecal incontinence don't need surgery. But if other treatments aren't successful and the incontinence remains severe and disabling, surgery may be considered. Surgery may be helpful for people whose incontinence is caused by damage to the pelvic floor, anal canal or anal sphincter, perhaps from a tear during childbirth, a fracture or a past operation.

Various surgical procedures may be performed. They range from minor repair of damaged tissues to complex surgeries. Sometimes a combination of procedures may be used. Surgery isn't free of complications, but it's often effective.

CHAPTER 8
Irritable bowel syndrome and food intolerances

You're out with friends, and you've just finished a delicious meal when the familiar rumblings in your stomach begin. You excuse yourself and head for home, where you spend the next hour dealing with cramps and diarrhea. At other times, you may battle uncomfortable constipation. Either way, your quality of life suffers.

Irritable bowel syndrome (IBS) is a very common digestive problem that affects the intestines, mainly the large intestine (colon). It's estimated that 10 to 20 percent of the general population experiences symptoms of IBS. While the condition does occur in men, it most often affects women. The term *spastic colon* is sometimes used to describe IBS because spasms in the intestinal walls may be responsible for some symptoms, but spasms don't explain all symptoms of the disorder.

The walls of your intestines are lined with layers of nerves and muscles that contract and relax, helping to move food through your digestive tract. Normally, the muscles contract and relax in a coordinated rhythm. With IBS, the muscles may function abnormally. They may contract for a longer period of time, and with greater force than normal, causing pain. Food is forced through the intestines more quickly, producing gas, bloating and diarrhea.

Sometimes, the opposite may occur. Contractions may be weak, slowing the passage of food, which leads to hard, dry stools and constipation.

IBS can be disabling but it isn't life-threatening. If you have a mild form, the condition may be only a minor inconvenience — and most people have mild symptoms. Some people have moderate symptoms that are intermittent and can keep them from enjoying life events. A small fraction of people has severe symptoms that can produce unbearable pain, along with severe diarrhea or constipation.

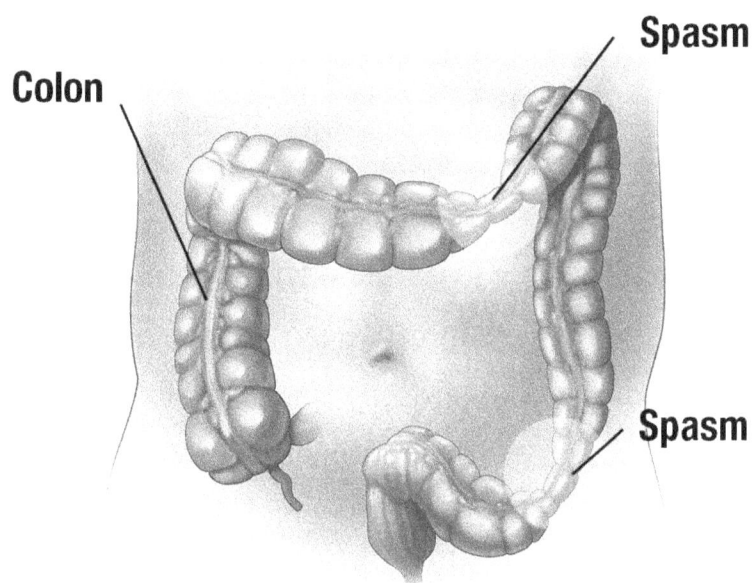

Spasm

Colon

Spasm

The highlighted areas represent severe muscle spasms that may occur in the large intestine (colon), causing pain. Spasms associated with irritable bowel syndrome can occur in one or more locations.

• • • • •

IRRITABLE BOWEL SYNDROME

Key signs and symptoms:

- Abdominal pain or discomfort
- Diarrhea
- Constipation

- Bloating or gas
- Mucus in stool

• • • • •

A FUNCTIONAL DISORDER

IBS is often referred to as a functional disorder, meaning that your intestines are not inflamed or infected — they look normal — but they function abnormally.

No one knows for certain what causes the dysfunction. The condition is likely related to nerves that control sensation. These nerves may be more sensitive than normal, causing you to react strongly to certain foods, physical activity, or the presence of air or gas in your intestines. Something that might not bother most people, such as a little gas, may cause pain or bloating if you have IBS.

It's well-known that stress and other psychological factors contribute to IBS. Many people find that their symptoms tend to be more severe or frequent during stressful events, such as variations to their daily routines, family troubles or a change of jobs.

For years, doctors attributed IBS to stress alone. But studies suggest both a functional (physiological) and an emotional (psychological) basis. Some people with IBS have a history of physical, sexual or emotional abuse, which may contribute to the symptoms. Food intolerances also are common in individuals with IBS, raising the possibility that in some people the disorder may be related to a sensitivity to certain food groups.

A number of foods are known to cause symptoms that mimic or aggravate IBS, including dairy products, beans and dried peas (legumes), and cruciferous vegetables such as broccoli, cauliflower, Brussels sprouts and cabbage. These foods increase intestinal gas, which can cause cramps.

Because women are twice as likely as men to have IBS, researchers speculate that hormonal changes may play a role. IBS may also result from another illness. Some people first experience IBS after a severe bout of diarrhea (post-infection IBS) caused by bacteria or a virus.

Studies suggest that IBS may result from an alteration in the types of bacteria in the gut — a shift from "good" to "bad" bacteria. You can read more about this possible association in Chapter 2.

IBS also runs in families, and researchers are investigating the genetic component of the condition. To date, scientists have identified a handful of variations in DNA that may be associated with IBS, but much about the genetics of the disorder is still unknown.

As for what IBS isn't: The disorder isn't the same as inflammatory bowel diseases such as Crohn's disease or ulcerative colitis. IBS also doesn't cause cancer or make you more likely to develop cancer. And while IBS is often long-lasting (chronic), it's not life- threatening.

RULING OUT OTHER CONDITIONS

There are no tests that can confirm, without a doubt, that you have IBS. Typically, the disorder is diagnosed after other conditions that produce similar symptoms, such as inflammatory bowel disease or celiac disease, have been ruled out. In some individuals suspected of having IBS, diagnostic tests may include blood, stool and breath tests, X-rays, endoscopic tests, and transit studies. See Chapter 5 for more about these tests.

Your doctor may also ask about your emotional health. Are you undergoing periods of stress? How well do you cope with stress? Do you often feel depressed or anxious?

Before a diagnosis of IBS is made, certain signs and symptoms — known as Rome criteria — must be present. The most important is abdominal pain or discomfort that has occurred at least one day a week for three months. The pain must be accompanied by at least two of the following symptoms:

- Bowel movements that provide temporary relief from the pain or discomfort
- A change in how frequently you have bowel movements — either more or less frequently
- A change in the consistency of your stool — softer or firmer, or both

As part of the diagnostic process, your doctor will consider your symptoms in determining the type of IBS you have. This information is important is deciding how to treat the disorder. There are three types, based on signs and symptoms:

- Constipation-predominant
- Diarrhea-predominant
- Mixed

TREATMENT

The focus of IBS treatment is on managing your signs and symptoms so that you can participate in normal activities and enjoy life more fully. Your success may depend on how well you achieve the following goals:

- Identify factors — foods, activities or situations — that trigger your signs and symptoms.
- Develop strategies to minimize your signs and symptoms.

A healthy diet and regular exercise are good starting points. They help keep your digestive system functioning more smoothly. Keep in mind, however, that your body may not respond immediately to the changes you make. Instead, look for signs of gradual improvement. Your goal is to find long-term, not temporary, solutions.

Constipation-predominant IBS

For individuals with constipation-predominant IBS, the following steps may help relieve constipation.

Drink plenty of liquids Liquids help relieve constipation and replenish body fluids that are absorbed by fiber during the digestive process. Make it your goal to drink at least eight 8-ounce glasses of fluid each day (see here).

Water is a good choice. Beverages containing alcohol cause you to urinate more — reducing rather than increasing body fluids. Avoid carbonated beverages because they can produce gas, which may add to the discomfort and bloating you already experience from IBS.

Experiment with fiber High-fiber foods soften stool and speed its passage through your colon, reducing constipation. The best approach is to increase the amount of fiber in your diet gradually over a period of weeks to prevent gas and cramping that can result from adding too much fiber to your diet too quickly.

For more information on how to increase the fiber in your diet, see here.

For additional information on constipation and steps you can take to help control symptoms, see Chapter 7.

Diarrhea-predominant IBS

For diarrhea-predominant IBS, the following steps can often help.

Limit high-fat foods Fat can stimulate abnormal muscle contractions in your colon, aggravating symptoms of IBS. It can also cause diarrhea. You don't need to avoid all fat in your diet, but if fat seems to worsen your pain and diarrhea, try limiting how much you eat.

The best way to reduce fat in your diet is to eat more plant-based foods. Plant-based foods — fruits, vegetables and foods made from whole grains — are naturally low in fat and contain many beneficial vitamins and minerals, as well as fiber. For more information on following a healthy diet, see Chapter 3.

Limit caffeine and alcohol Caffeine and alcohol may worsen diarrhea by stimulating or irritating your intestines. If you're bothered by gas and cramping, also try to avoid carbonated beverages, which can worsen symptoms.

All types

The following steps can improve all types of IBS — constipation predominant, diarrhea predominant and mixed.

Limit problem foods Many foods are only partially digested in the small intestine. When they reach the large intestine (colon) further digestion takes place, which can cause cramps and gas. Individuals bothered by gas and bloating may want to temporarily eliminate certain foods from their diets to see if their symptoms improve.

The most common gas-producing foods are legumes and cruciferous vegetables. Other potentially problem-causing foods include onions, celery, carrots, bananas, apricots, prunes and wheat.

Some individuals with IBS benefit from a more restrictive diet known as a low-FODMAP diet. FODMAPs are short-chain carbohydrates that ferment rapidly and are poorly digested, resulting in signs and symptoms such as pain and bloating. A low-FODMAP diet involves eliminating a large number of foods from your diet and then gradually reintroducing them to determine your tolerance for the food. A low-FODMAP diet should take place under the supervision of a trained dietitian. For more information on the diet, see here. For a list of foods containing FODMAPs, see here.

Eat at regular times It's best not to skip meals, and you want to try to eat at about the same times each day. Regularly scheduled meals help regulate your bowel function and lessen symptoms of constipation and diarrhea. That's because digestion involves stimulating the muscles in your gastrointestinal tract to contract and relax — the process necessary to move stool through your colon and into your rectum.

Some people find that eating frequent, smaller meals agrees with them better than eating three large meals a day. Either option is acceptable if it helps you manage your symptoms.

Get active Physical activity helps reduce feelings of stress. It also stimulates muscle contractions of your intestines, helping them to function normally. Physical activity can relieve constipation and may also alleviate symptoms of diarrhea. Exercise can also improve depression and make you feel better about yourself.

Aim for 30 to 60 minutes of moderate physical activity most days of the week. If you've been inactive, talk to your doctor before you start. Begin slowly and gradually increase the time you exercise. For information on setting up a fitness program, see here.

Manage stress Anyone can experience digestive upset from worry, anxiety or other stressful emotions. But among people with IBS, stress-related symptoms such as abdominal pain and diarrhea can occur more frequently and severely. A vicious cycle can develop — your signs and symptoms increase the level of stress, added stress causes your signs and symptoms to worsen, and so on.

An important strategy in controlling IBS is learning how to relax. There are many methods of relaxation. Some people relax while listening to or performing music, or surrounding themselves with soothing aromas (aromatherapy). Others benefit from massage, yoga, meditation or hypnosis.

Making certain changes to your day also may help reduce stress. These changes may include getting up earlier to give yourself more time to eat breakfast and get ready, simplifying your daily routine, following a schedule to avoid last-minute hassles, spending time with people who have a positive outlook and sense of humor, and getting enough sleep.

● ● ● ● ●

TOOLS FOR STRESS RELIEF

As you learn various relaxation therapies, here are two simple techniques you can use whenever you start to feel stressed.

Deep breathing

Stress typically causes rapid, shallow breathing from your chest. Deep, slow, relaxed breathing comes from your diaphragm. Deep breathing means your abdomen, not your chest, moves with each breath. You can use deep breathing as your only means of relaxation or as a warmup and cool-down method for other techniques.

Here's an exercise to help you practice deep, relaxed breathing. Rehearse it throughout the day until you can automatically apply it when you feel stressed:

1. Sit comfortably with your feet flat on the floor.
2. Loosen tight clothing around your abdomen and waist.

3. Place your hands on your lap or at your sides.

4. Close your eyes if it helps you to relax.

5. Take one hand and place it on your chest. (This helps you become aware of your breathing.)

6. Breathe in slowly through your nose while counting to four. Notice your abdomen expand as you breathe in.

7. Pause for a second and then exhale at a normal rate through your mouth.

8. Repeat until you feel more relaxed.

Progressive muscle relaxation

This technique involves relaxing various muscle groups one at a time. First, increase the tension level in one muscle group, such as a leg or an arm, by tightening the muscles. Then relax the muscles. Focus on slowly letting the tension subside. Then, move on to the next muscle group and do the same.

● ● ● ● ●

OVER-THE-COUNTER MEDICATIONS

Nonprescription medications may help relieve abdominal discomfort at the same time you're taking steps to change or improve your lifestyle. Most pharmacies, drugstores and grocery stores carry these over-the-counter products. The medications you use will depend on your signs and symptoms.

● ● ● ● ●

The following steps also may help relieve some signs and symptoms of IBS:

- Soak in a warm bath or lie down with a hot-water bottle or heating pad on your abdomen to decrease abdominal pain. Be careful not to burn your skin or to fall asleep.
- Wear comfortable, loosefitting clothing that doesn't put pressure on your abdomen.
- Go to the bathroom as soon as you feel the urge, but don't hurry yourself. Allow adequate time for a bowel movement without straining.
- Get a good night's sleep. Research suggests that sleep can help decrease the intensity of IBS symptoms.

● ● ● ● ●

Constipation-dominant IBS

Try one of the following products to see if it helps relieve your constipation.

Stool softeners Sold over-the-counter under several brand names, including docusate sodium (Colace) and docusate calcium (Surfak), stool softeners are the gentlest laxatives. Stool softeners increase the amount of water stool absorbs while it's in the gut, making the stool softer and easier to pass.

Some people take mineral oil to soften stool and relieve constipation. This isn't recommended. Mineral oil can block the absorption of key vitamins.

Never take mineral oil before lying down, as it could enter your lungs and cause pneumonia.

Fiber supplements Another way to relieve signs and symptoms of constipation is to use a natural fiber supplement such as Metamucil, Citrucel, FiberCon or Benefiber. Start by using a small amount, such as a teaspoon of supplement mixed in a glass of water or juice, and slowly increase your daily dose every one to two weeks. When taken regularly as directed, fiber supplements are generally safe and effective.

Because they're so absorbent, make sure to take fiber supplements with plenty of water. Otherwise, they can become constipating — the opposite of what you want.

Osmotic laxatives Osmotic laxatives work by drawing water into the large intestine from nearby tissue, thereby softening stool. They include products such as magnesium hydroxide (Phillips' Milk of Magnesia), magnesium citrate, lactulose (Kristalose) and polyethylene glycol (Miralax).

Stimulant laxatives These are the most powerful type of laxatives and should be used only when other measures don't induce a bowel movement. Stimulant laxatives promote the passage of stool by causing your intestines to contract. Over-the-counter brand names include Dulcolax and Senokot.

Avoid long-term, unsupervised use of these products, and talk with your doctor about the best approach for using any laxatives.

Diarrhea-predominant IBS

The following products sold over the counter can help relieve diarrhea.

Anti-diarrheals Relieving symptoms of diarrhea is an important concern in learning to manage IBS. Loperamide (Imodium A-D) slows the rate at which food leaves your intestines and increases water and sodium absorption, both of which help solidify stool. Other anti-diarrheals, such as bismuth subsalicylate (Pepto-Bismol), may ease the urgency of a bowel movement.

You need to be careful, however, not to use anti-diarrheal medications too often or for too long. Talk with your doctor about safe and effective use. One approach would be to take an anti-diarrheal after each loose bowel movement. Some people take an anti-diarrheal before they go out to eat, to serve as a safety net and to avoid embarrassment.

Oil of peppermint A specially coated tablet that slowly releases purified peppermint oil (enteric-coated peppermint oil) into the small intestine may help ease bloating, urgency and abdominal pain while passing stool. The product is sold under the brand names IBgard and Mentha-XL. Talk to your doctor before taking peppermint oil to make sure you are using it appropriately.

You might also experiment with peppermint tea (tea that contains peppermint oil). There's some evidence that it helps relieve diarrhea or gas accompanied by bloating. Be aware, however, that peppermint can aggravate heartburn.

PRESCRIPTION MEDICATIONS

When signs and symptoms of IBS are moderate to severe, more help than what lifestyle changes or over-the-counter medications can offer may be needed. Depending on your signs and symptoms, your doctor may recommend one of the following prescription medications. As a general rule, prescription medications are reserved for people whose signs and symptoms don't respond to more conservative treatment.

Constipation-predominant IBS

To treat more severe IBS that's dominated by constipation, one or more of the following medications may be prescribed.

Linaclotide Linaclotide (Linzess) works by increasing fluid secretion in the small intestine to help pass stool. The medication can cause diarrhea, but taking it 30 to 60 minutes before eating may help. Plecanatide (Trulance) is a similar drug that may be prescribed for individuals with constipation-predominant IBS.

Lubiprostone Lubiprostone (Amitiza) is a prescription laxative that stimulates the secretion of intestinal fluids, which helps move food through the intestines. It's approved for women who have constipation-dominant IBS and is generally prescribed only to women who have severe symptoms that haven't responded to other treatments. Headache and nausea may occur as side effects.

SSRI antidepressants In addition to treating depression, antidepressants may help relieve abdominal pain and constipation. Selective serotonin reuptake inhibitors (SSRIs), such as fluoxetine (Prozac, Sarafem) or paroxetine (Paxil), may help if you are depressed and have abdominal pain and constipation. In some people, SSRIs can cause nausea and cramping.

Antidepressants must be taken regularly to be effective. Because of this, these medications generally are prescribed only if you have chronic or recurring symptoms.

Diarrhea-predominant IBS

Among individuals with diarrhea-predominant IBS, the following medications may be prescribed.

Antispasmodic medications Antispasmodic (anticholinergic) drugs such as dicyclomine (Bentyl), block the nervous system's stimulation of the gastrointestinal tract, helping relax intestinal muscles and relieve muscle spasms. The medications are sometimes prescribed for people who have bouts of diarrhea. They tend to be most effective when taken preventively, before symptoms begin. Antispasmodic medications are generally safe but can cause constipation, dry mouth and blurred vision.

Tricyclic antidepressants The tricyclic agents imipramine (Tofranil), desipramine (Norpramine) and nortriptyline (Pamelor) can help relieve depression as well as inhibit the activity of neurons that control the intestines to help reduce pain. If you have diarrhea and abdominal pain without depression, your doctor may suggest a reduced dose. The medications need to be taken regularly to be effective.

Eluxadoline Eluxadoline (Viberzi) may ease diarrhea by reducing muscle contractions and fluid secretion in the intestine, and increasing muscle tone in the rectum. The medication can cause nausea, abdominal pain and mild constipation. It's also been associated with pancreatitis in certain individuals.

This medication should not be given to individuals who have had their gallbladders removed.

Bile acid binders In individuals who experience persistent diarrhea despite the use of other anti-diarrheal medications, sometimes a doctor might prescribe a bile acid binder, such as cholestyramine (Prevalite), colestipol (Colestid) or colesevelam (Welchol). These medications, however, can cause bloating and gas.

Alosetron Alosetron (Lotronex) is designed to relax the colon and slow movement of waste through the lower bowel. Alosetron can be prescribed only by doctors enrolled in a special program. It's intended for severe cases of diarrhea-predominant IBS in women who haven't responded to other treatments. It isn't approved for treatment in men. The medication has been linked to rare but serious side effects and should be considered only when other treatments aren't successful.

COUNSELING

Counseling is an important aspect of treatment if your condition is related to stress. A health care professional who specializes in behavioral medicine, such as a psychiatrist or psychologist, can help you reduce stress and anxiety by examining your responses to life events, and then helping you modify those responses.

You learn to identify stressful situations that cause bowel reactions and to develop strategies for controlling stress. For most people, counseling combined with medication works better than medication alone.

LACTOSE INTOLERANCE

Does this sound familiar? You love dairy products, but they don't love you. Shortly after a bowl of ice cream or a serving of cheesy lasagna, you experience cramps, bloating, gas and diarrhea. If your cramping and bloating occur mainly after eating dairy products, your signs and symptoms may be related to another condition called lactose intolerance.

Food intolerances or food sensitivities are terms used to describe signs and symptoms that develop when a person has difficulty digesting a particular food. This can lead to problems such as gas, abdominal pain or diarrhea — signs and symptoms similar to those of IBS. There are several types of food intolerances. One of the most common is lactose intolerance.

People with lactose intolerance have difficulty digesting the sugar (lactose) in dairy products because their bodies don't produce enough of the enzyme lactase — a substance normally found in the small intestine. Lactase breaks down lactose so it can be absorbed into your body. When lactose isn't absorbed, it travels to the colon where fermentation takes place. During fermentation, bacteria convert the lactose to gas and fluid, causing cramping, diarrhea, bloating and gas.

To digest lactose, you need the enzyme lactase. Babies are born with large amounts of lactase. As you grow older, your body often produces less of the enzyme. Adults whose intestines produce very little, if any, lactase have difficulty digesting foods containing lactose.

It's estimated that about one-third of Americans have difficulty absorbing lactose (lactose malabsorption). Lactose malabsorption can cause lactose intolerance, but not all people with lactose malabsorption have lactose intolerance.

Different types

There are three types of lactose intolerance. Different factors cause the lactase deficiency underlying each type.

Primary lactose intolerance This is the most common type of lactose intolerance. People with primary lactose intolerance begin life producing plenty of lactase — a necessity for infants who get all their nutrition from milk. As milk is gradually replaced with other foods, lactase production decreases, but remains high enough to digest the amount of dairy in a typical adult diet.

In primary lactose intolerance, lactase production falls off sharply by adulthood, making milk products difficult to digest. Primary lactose intolerance is genetically determined, occurring in a large proportion of people with African, Asian or Hispanic ancestry. The condition is also common among those of Mediterranean or Southern European descent.

Secondary lactose intolerance This form of lactose intolerance occurs when your small intestine decreases lactase production after an illness, injury or surgery involving your small intestine. Among the diseases associated with secondary lactose intolerance are celiac disease, bacterial overgrowth and Crohn's disease. Treatment of the underlying disorder may restore lactase levels and improve signs and symptoms, though it can take time.

Congenital or developmental lactose intolerance In rare cases a baby is born with lactose intolerance caused by a complete absence of lactase activity. This disorder is passed from generation to generation in a pattern of inheritance called autosomal recessive, meaning that both the mother and the father must pass on the same gene variant for a child to be affected. Premature infants also may have lactose intolerance because of an insufficient lactase level.

Diagnosing the disorder

Tolerance to lactose varies. Most people can handle the amount of lactose in half a cup of milk, and don't have a problem consuming small amounts of dairy products. Signs and symptoms occur when they consume several dairy products at once, or they eat a large portion of a product containing lactose. People with a more severe intolerance aren't able to eat any dairy products without experiencing distressing symptoms.

Your doctor may suspect lactose intolerance based on your symptoms and your response to reducing the amount of dairy foods in your diet. A blood test or breath test that gauges your body's reaction to high levels of lactose can confirm the diagnosis.

Managing lactose intolerance

There's no way to boost your body's production of lactase but you can usually avoid the discomfort of lactose intolerance with the following steps:

Keep it small Avoid large servings of milk and other dairy products. The smaller the serving the less likely it is to cause problems. If you're cutting back on dairy products, make sure you are getting your calcium from other sources.

Experiment Not all dairy products have the same amount of lactose. For example, hard cheeses, such as Swiss or cheddar, have small amounts of lactose and generally cause no symptoms. Other foods that are lower in lactose include butter, margarine and sherbet. Nondairy creamers are lactose-free.

You may be able to tolerate cultured milk products, such as yogurt, because the bacteria used in the culturing process naturally produce the enzyme that breaks down lactose. Look for yogurt with active yeast cultures. The highest concentrations of lactose per serving are in milk and ice cream.

Look for alternatives Eat or drink lactose-reduced or lactose-free milk or milk products. You can find these products in most supermarkets in the refrigerated dairy section.

Use lactose enzyme products Prior to consuming dairy foods, use over-the-counter products that break down lactose. Tablets or drops containing the lactase enzyme (Dairy Ease, Lactaid, others) may help you digest dairy products. The tablets can be taken just before a meal or snack. Or you can add the drops to a carton of milk. Some milk sold in grocery stores also contains lactase. Not everyone with lactose intolerance is helped by these products, however.

With some trial and error, you may be able to predict your body's response to different foods containing lactose and figure out how much you can eat or drink without discomfort. Fortunately, few people have such severe lactose intolerance that they have to cut out all milk products.

• • • • •

WATCH OUT FOR THESE FOODS

To reduce signs and symptoms of lactose intolerance, avoid these high-lactose foods or eat them in small amounts.

- Cheese spreads
- Chip dip or potato topping
- Cottage cheese
- Dry milk
- Evaporated milk
- Half-and-half
- Ice cream or ice milk
- Milk
- Ricotta cheese
- Sour cream
- Sweetened condensed milk
- White sauce

• • • • •

OTHER INTOLERANCES

Lactose intolerance is just one example of a food intolerance. There are a variety of ingredients in food to which some people are sensitive.

Because the signs and symptoms of a food intolerance are often similar to those of IBS, it's not uncommon for IBS to actually be related to a particular food or food ingredient. That's why it's important to pay attention to when your signs and symptoms occur and if they seem to develop after eating a particular food.

A food intolerance may be related to a deficiency in the enzymes needed to digest certain foods, such as a deficiency in lactase. Some people have problems processing certain chemicals, such as artificial sweeteners. Or it may be that an individual is sensitive to particular additives in foods, such as dyes or preservatives.

For people with a food sensitivity, symptoms usually begin within a few hours of eating the food to which they're sensitive. You can be sensitive to a variety of foods or food ingredients.

Gluten

Some people with IBS report an improvement in diarrhea symptoms if they stop eating gluten, which is found in wheat, barley and rye. A sensitivity to these grains is different from celiac disease, a serious condition stemming from an autoimmune reaction to gluten. See Chapter 9 for more information on celiac disease.

Nonceliac gluten sensitivity is basically a milder form of celiac disease that doesn't damage the intestinal tract but that can produce digestive discomfort.

Sensitivity varies from person to person, and ranges from mild to more severe.

Yeast

Similar to gluten, yeast fungi used in breads and baked goods can cause digestive discomfort in some people.

Histamine

Histamine is a chemical found in aged foods, such as wine, cheese and preserved meats. It can cause digestive symptoms in some people.

Caffeine

The chemical caffeine can trigger digestive troubles for some individuals. In addition to coffee, caffeine is found in a wide variety of beverages, as well as chocolate and even some medications.

FODMAPs

Individuals with IBS may have a sensitivity to certain dietary sugars, called FODMAPs, that are poorly absorbed in the small intestine. As these dietary sugars (carbohydrates) travel into the large intestine, they are broken down (ferment) by bacteria, causing gas and bloating. Some people also experience diarrhea.

There generally is no treatment for a food intolerance. The best way to manage the problem is to avoid the offending foods. Individuals whose IBS symptoms are related to a food intolerance typically see an improvement in symptoms when certain foods are eliminated from their diets.

LOW-FODMAP DIET

If you have irritable bowel syndrome or suspect that you may be sensitive to particular foods, you might benefit from a diet known as a low-FODMAP diet. But don't start this diet without first talking with your doctor or a registered dietitian.

Researchers studying a group of naturally occurring dietary sugars known as FODMAPs have found that these sugars don't always digest well, and for some people this can lead to gas, bloating and diarrhea. FODMAPs stands for fermentable oligosaccharides, disaccharides, monosaccharides and polyols.

Foods that contain FODMAPs include wheat products, garlic, onions, and dried peas and beans (legumes). Dairy products contain FODMAPs, and so do honey, certain fruits and foods made with high-fructose corn syrup. Low-calorie sweeteners such as sorbitol and mannitol are made from polyols.

FODMAPs don't absorb well in the small intestine and can pull water into the intestine, causing abdominal pain and diarrhea in some individuals. When they reach the bowel, undigested FODMAPs serve as a source of "food" for bacteria living in the digestive tract. The bacteria ferment the FODMAPs. This can cause abdominal bloating and pain and excess gas, especially among individuals with a more sensitive gastrointestinal tract. Some people experience both diarrhea and constipation.

A low-FODMAP diet is designed to relieve gastrointestinal symptoms by restricting foods that are high in FODMAPs. The diet is generally recommended for individuals with irritable bowel syndrome (IBS) or those who feel that their gastrointestinal tracts may be sensitive to something in the food they eat.

The diet works by eliminating all foods that contain FODMAPs and gradually adding them back until you're able to determine which carbohydrates are triggering your pain, discomfort and stool problems.

Different people are sensitive to different FODMAPs, so it's important to identify which ones are the culprits. Most people need to avoid only a few foods long-term. Because most FODMAPs are good sources of prebiotics, you want to be able to eat as many of them as you can.

For more information on the diet and to learn which foods contain FODMAPs, see here.

CHAPTER 9
Celiac disease

You notice the symptoms start after you eat a cracker or a slice of pizza. Or maybe you're not sure what you ate that could be making you feel so ill. But the warning signs are there — diarrhea, bloating and gas that often seem to follow certain meals. These signs and symptoms are typical of celiac disease, a condition that arises from not being able to digest gluten, a dietary protein. However, not all individuals with celiac disease experience such symptoms. Some have none at all.

Gluten is found in all food made of wheat, barley, rye and some oats. Avoiding gluten is critical if you have celiac disease. Eating food containing gluten damages the interior of the small intestine and interferes with its ability to absorb certain nutrients from food.

But avoiding gluten can be a challenge because the protein is found in common grain products that are prepared and eaten every day, including bread, pasta, pizza crust, cookies, cakes and pastries. (Products made with corn or rice flour don't contain gluten and are safe to eat if you have celiac disease.)

Celiac disease — also known as celiac sprue, nontropical sprue and gluten sensitive enteropathy — is one of many different malabsorption disorders. After a period of dramatic increase in the number of celiac disease cases diagnosed, research shows that rates in the United States have stabilized over the past several years, with a little more than 1 percent of the population affected.

Interestingly, recent years have also brought an increase in the number of people following gluten-free diets who haven't been diagnosed with celiac disease. The potential long-term health risks or benefits of a gluten-free diet among people who don't have celiac disease or a related condition isn't known.

• • • • •

CELIAC DISEASE

Key signs and symptoms:

- Diarrhea
- Gas
- Bloating
- Abdominal pain
- Fatigue
- Weight loss
- Stunted growth (in children)
- Bone loss
- Anemia
- Balance problems
- Numbness in legs and hands

• • • • •

HOW GLUTEN CAUSES HARM

Celiac disease is an immune system disorder — a condition in which your own immune system is harming you. If you have celiac disease and you eat food that contains gluten, your immune system responds to the gluten the same as it would a foreign invader such as a virus or bacterium — it tries to attack and destroy it. This reaction inflames and damages the inner lining of your small intestine.

The inflammation causes tiny hairlike projections (villi) in the small intestine to shrink and even disappear (see this image).

Normally, your small intestine is lined with millions of villi, resembling the deep pile of a plush carpet on a microscopic scale. The villi work to absorb nutrients from the food you eat.

When celiac disease damages villi, the inner surface of your small intestine becomes less like a plush carpet and more like a tile floor. Your body is unable to absorb many essential nutrients necessary for good health. Instead, fat, protein, vitamins and minerals are eliminated from your body via your stool.

Over time, poor absorption (malabsorption) affects your brain, nerves, bones, liver and other organs. The result is often malnutrition and may lead to other illnesses. No treatment can cure celiac disease, but you can effectively manage the disease through diet, allowing the small intestine to heal so villi can regrow.

The cause of celiac disease is unknown but it may be inherited. If someone in your immediate family has it, there's an increased chance you may as well. Celiac disease can occur at any age, and it tends to be more common in people of European descent, those with Down syndrome or Turner syndrome, those diagnosed with microscopic colitis, and people with other autoimmune disorders, such as lupus erythematosus, type 1 diabetes, Addison's disease, rheumatoid arthritis or autoimmune thyroid disease.

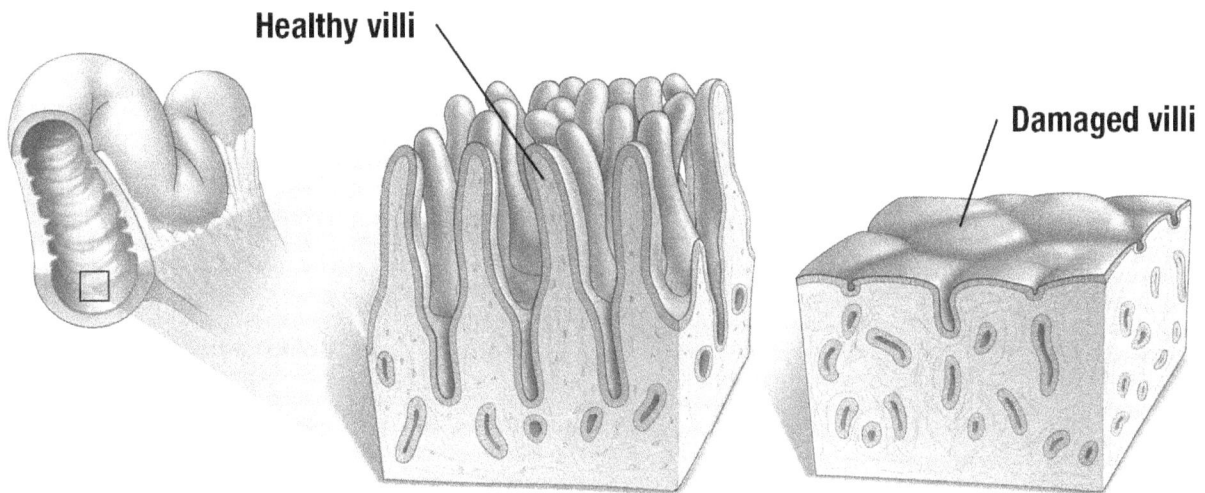

Healthy villi

Damaged villi

The inner surface of a healthy small intestine is lined with millions of villi (left). Celiac disease damages the villi, causing them to shrink and disappear (right). This affects your body's ability to absorb nutrients from the food you eat, leading to malnutrition and other illnesses.

SIGNS AND SYMPTOMS

Celiac disease dates back thousands of years, but only in the past 60 years or so have researchers gained a better understanding of the condition and how to treat it.

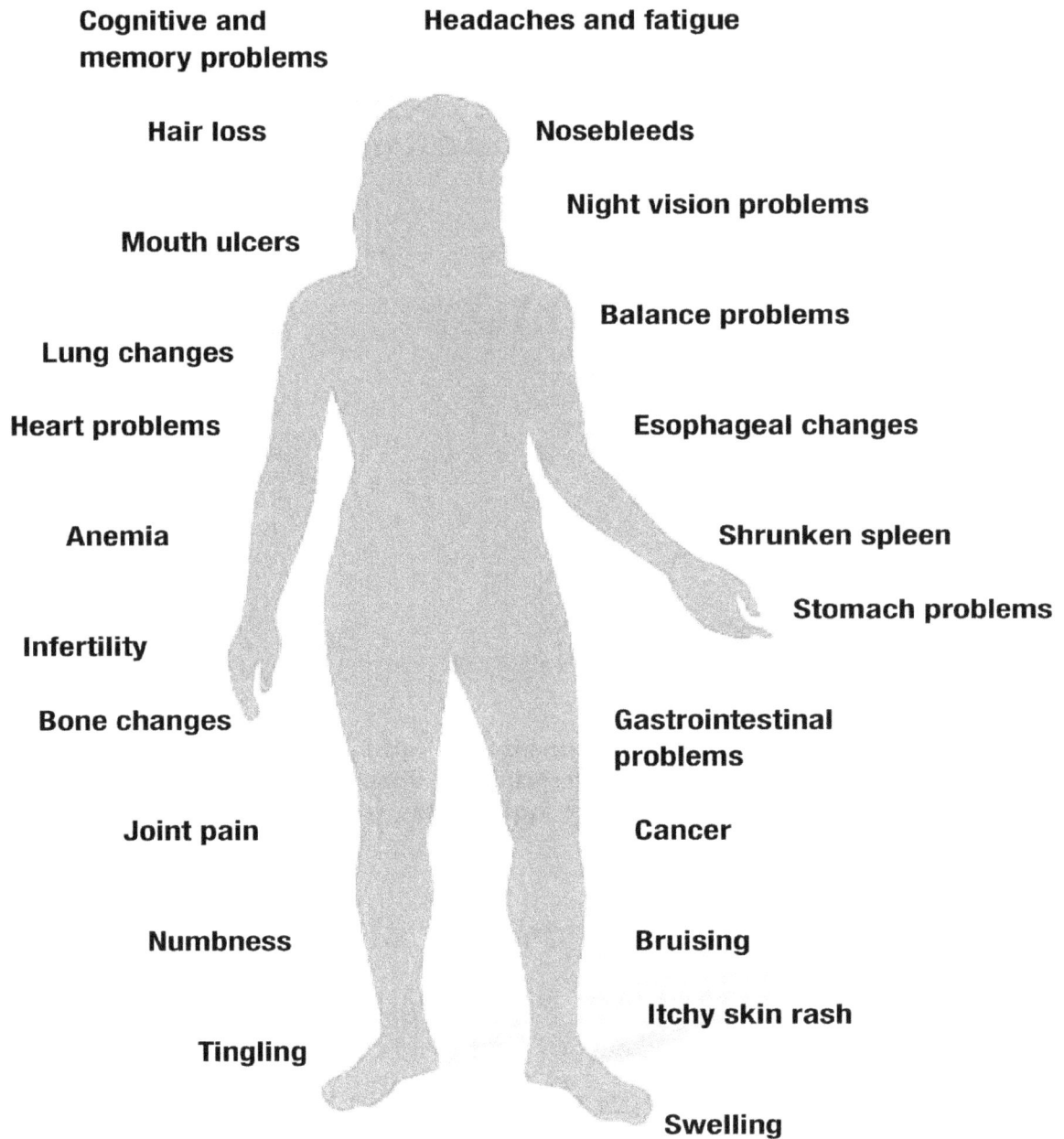

Cognitive and memory problems

Headaches and fatigue

Hair loss

Nosebleeds

Night vision problems

Mouth ulcers

Balance problems

Lung changes

Heart problems

Esophageal changes

Anemia

Shrunken spleen

Stomach problems

Infertility

Bone changes

Gastrointestinal problems

Joint pain

Cancer

Numbness

Bruising

Itchy skin rash

Tingling

Swelling

Almost all parts of the body may be affected by celiac disease. The disease presents itself in many different ways. This is why celiac disease can be difficult to diagnose.

There is no typical form of the disease. Some people have few or no signs and symptoms and may live with celiac disease for years before it's diagnosed later in life when they're adults. Some people first notice the signs and symptoms as children.

Many times, for reasons that aren't clear, the disease emerges after some form of trauma, such as an infection, physical injury, the strain of pregnancy, severe stress or surgery. How or why these conditions trigger the onset of celiac disease is unknown. For other people, the signs and symptoms vary and may include fatigue, abdominal pain, intermittent diarrhea, bloating, nausea, weight loss and excessive passing of gas.

Fatigue can result from a sharp reduction of red blood cells in your bloodstream (anemia) or from not being able to absorb calories from the foods you eat, which supply energy. Other indications of poor absorption (malabsorption) are weight loss and lighter colored, foul-smelling stools.

Celiac disease may also present itself in less obvious ways, including changes in behavior such as irritability or depression, joint pain, muscle cramps, skin rash, mouth sores, dental and bone disorders, infertility, tingling in the legs, and delayed growth in children.

Dermatitis herpetiformis is a chronic skin condition caused by a reaction to gluten consumption. The vast majority of people with dermatitis herpetiformis also have celiac disease. Extremely itchy bumps or blisters appear on both sides of the body, most often on the forearms near the elbows, as well as on the knees and the buttocks, and along the hairline. The condition affects about 5 to 10 percent of people with celiac disease and is treated with a gluten-free diet, in addition to medication to control the rash.

DIAGNOSING CELIAC DISEASE

People with celiac disease who eat gluten usually have higher than normal levels of certain proteins (antibodies) called tissue transglutaminase antibodies circulating in their bloodstreams. In addition, their immune systems produce antibodies against some of their body's own proteins (auto-antibodies).

Several diagnostic tests are available, but the most reliable and commonly used tests for detecting celiac disease look for elevated levels of different antibodies in your blood, indicating an immune reaction to gluten.

If your signs and symptoms and blood test results suggest celiac disease, your doctor will likely remove a small tissue sample (biopsy) from your small intestine and examine it under a microscope for damaged villi. The sample is obtained by threading a thin, flexible tube (endoscope) through your upper gastrointestinal tract and into the small intestine.

It's important to confirm celiac disease through diagnostic testing before you eliminate gluten from your diet. You shouldn't go on a gluten-free diet without first consulting your doctor. Doing so may create false-negatives. The results of blood tests and biopsies appear normal when the disease is actually present.

● ● ● ● ●

NON-CELIAC GLUTEN SENSITIVITY

The term *non-celiac gluten sensitivity* describes individuals who cannot tolerate gluten and who experience signs and symptoms similar to those of celiac disease — such as bloating, diarrhea and mental fog — within hours or days of eating food containing gluten. Similar to celiac disease, symptoms of non-celiac gluten sensitivity resolve when gluten is removed from the diet. But when tested, these individuals don't have the same blood antibodies and intestinal damage that's seen in celiac disease. They also don't test positive for wheat allergy, an allergic reaction to wheat whose symptoms can sometimes resemble celiac disease.

Some studies have suggested that non-celiac gluten sensitivity may be just as common or even more common than celiac disease.

Despite the name, research hasn't been able to definitively prove that gluten is, in fact, the culprit. More study is needed to determine potential triggers and if a strict, gluten-free diet is the best course of treatment.

● ● ● ● ●

Similar but different

Testing is important because some people who think they have celiac disease actually don't. Other conditions can mimic celiac disease, causing many of the same symptoms such as gas, bloating, abdominal discomfort and loose stools. A few conditions commonly mistaken for celiac disease are lactose intolerance, wheat intolerance and non-celiac gluten sensitivity (see the box above).

Wheat intolerance is similar to other food intolerances, such as lactose intolerance in which people are intolerant to the sugar (lactose) in dairy products (see here). With wheat intolerance, a carbohydrate in wheat (fructan) isn't completely digested in the small intestine and is passed into the colon, where bacteria ferment it, producing gas and loose stools. This is different from celiac disease, which involves a reaction to gluten, a protein found in wheat and certain other grains.

Several other conditions also may cause problems or damage to the small intestine, producing signs and symptoms that can resemble celiac disease. They include tropical sprue, Whipple's disease, giardiasis infection, medication-related injury, bacterial overgrowth, immunoglobulin deficiency, Crohn's disease, ulcerative colitis, irritable bowel syndrome and pancreatic disorders. A doctor often can identify special features on blood tests that distinguish these conditions from celiac disease. In addition, the conditions don't respond to a gluten-free diet.

People who take a class of drugs called angiotensin II receptor blockers to treat high blood pressure, including the medication olmesartan (Benicar), may experience a condition called drug-induced villous atrophy, which results when the medication damages villi in the small intestine. The villi become flattened and produce symptoms similar to celiac disease, such as diarrhea and weight loss, but celiac disease isn't the cause.

●　●　●　●　●

FOODS THAT CONTAIN GLUTEN

Foods made from the grains wheat, barley and rye contain gluten. Avoid the foods listed below unless they're made with corn or rice or labeled as gluten-free.

- Breads
- Cereals
- Crackers
- Pasta
- Pizza crust
- Cookies
- Cakes and pies
- Gravies
- Sauces

● ● ● ● ●

● ● ● ● ●

FOOD INGREDIENTS THAT CONTAIN GLUTEN

Gluten may be present in foods that you didn't expect. Avoid all food products that list any of the following as ingredients.

- Wheat (wheat flour, white flour, wheat bran, wheat germ, farina, wheat starch, graham flour, semolina, durum)
- Barley
- Malt, a derivative of barley
- Rye
- Bulgur
- Kasha
- Kamut
- Matzo meal

- Oats, unless labeled gluten-free
- Spelt
- Triticale

For years, there's been some difference of opinion whether individuals with celiac disease can eat oats and oat products — such as oat flour, oat brain and oatmeal. Based on research, a statement from the North American Society for the Study of Celiac Disease says that oats uncontaminated by wheat, barley or rye are safe for people with celiac disease to consume, and oats provide multiple nutritional benefits.

But here's the problem: While oats don't naturally contain gluten and reaction to them is rare, oats that you find in the store may be shipped or processed in containers or facilities containing wheat, barley and rye. This can contaminate the oats and trigger an inflammatory response. In addition, a small percentage of people with celiac disease react even to pure oats.

If you want to introduce oats into your diet, make sure to check with your doctor or dietitian before adding oats to meals. Look for oats that are certified as pure or gluten-free and incorporate them slowly. New products containing oats appear on the market periodically. Avoid these products until you can verify their safety from a reliable source, such as a dietitian.

• • • • •

A NEW WAY OF EATING

Celiac disease is a lifelong condition, and there are no medications or medical procedures such as surgery that can cure it. The focus of treatment is on healing the small intestine and relieving signs and symptoms while allowing you to maintain a varied, balanced and nutritious diet.

Managing the disease and preventing its complications will require you to change the types of food you eat. It's essential that you avoid gluten. That means avoiding all foods or food ingredients made from the grains wheat, barley and rye, as well as being on the lookout for gluten in more unexpected places, such as candies, salad dressings and processed lunchmeats. A dietitian can help educate you on how to scrutinize food labels and what to look for.

● ● ● ● ●

SURPRISING SOURCES OF GLUTEN

You may ingest gluten in ways that you would never expect. Examples are through cross-contamination, when gluten-free foods come in contact with foods containing gluten. This may happen if you share a knife for spreading butter that has bread crumbs on it, use the same toaster as others, or eat deep-fried foods that are cooked in the same oil used for breaded foods.

Some common products also may contain gluten, including:

- Certain prescription or over-the-counter medications, which may use gluten as a binding agent or other inactive ingredient
- Vitamin supplements

- Lipstick
- Communion wafers
- Toothpaste

Your best bet is to contact the manufacturers of these products to find out if the products contain gluten. Allow a pharmacist to inspect the containers of each medication you take.

● ● ● ● ●

COMPLICATIONS OF CELIAC DISEASE

If you accidentally eat a food product that contains gluten, you may or may not experience signs and symptoms such as abdominal pain, headaches, fatigue and diarrhea. Trace amounts of gluten in your diet can be damaging to the villi in your intestinal tract even if you don't develop symptoms. That's why you shouldn't rely on your symptoms to determine if a food contains gluten.

Over time, these small amounts of gluten may increase your risk of many serious complications. If not diagnosed and treated promptly, celiac disease can cause:

- *Malnutrition.* The damage to your small intestine means it can't absorb enough nutrients, leading to vitamin deficiencies, anemia and weight loss. In children, this may cause slow growth and reduced height.
- *Bone conditions.* Malabsorption of calcium and vitamin D may lead to a softening of the bone (osteomalacia or rickets) in children and a loss of bone density (osteoporosis) in adults.

- *Infertility and miscarriage.* Malabsorption can contribute to reproductive problems.
- *Lactose intolerance.* Damage to your small intestine may cause you to experience abdominal pain, bloating and diarrhea after eating lactose-containing dairy products, even though they don't contain gluten ([see here](#)).
- *Cancer.* People with celiac disease who don't maintain a gluten-free diet have a greater risk of developing several forms of cancer, including intestinal lymphoma and small bowel cancer.
- *Neurological problems.* Some people with celiac disease may develop neurological problems such as seizures; damage to the nerves leading to the hands and feet (peripheral neuropathy); or ataxia, a condition that causes balance problems, seizures and cognitive impairment.

In children, celiac disease can also lead to growth failure, delayed puberty, weight loss, irritability, dental enamel defects, anemia, arthritis, and epilepsy.

When celiac disease is first diagnosed and you begin making dietary changes, you may also need to take vitamin and mineral supplements recommended by your doctor or dietitian to help correct nutritional deficiencies. Common deficiencies include calcium, vitamin D, vitamin B-12, iron, folate and zinc. As your symptoms subside and your ability to absorb nutrients improves, the need for supplements may diminish. If you have osteoporosis, you may need to continue taking calcium and vitamin D supplements long term.

Within just a few weeks of removing gluten from your diet, the inflammation in your small intestine will likely begin to subside. But it can take from several months to two to three years for your intestine to heal completely.

Getting used to your new diet can be difficult. It may take months to sort out which foods you can or can't eat. You may crave certain foods that you're no longer allowed to eat. But don't get discouraged and give up. With time, most people learn to adjust to a gluten-free diet, and it becomes a normal part of daily life.

• • • • •

SOURCES OF SUPPORT

Many professionals can help you adjust to a gluten-free diet. A registered dietitian is first on the list. Also check to see if a support group for people with celiac disease exists in your community. A support group is a great way to learn about eating gluten-free from others who live with celiac disease.

If there's not a support group in your area, you may be able to find one online. Several national organizations, such as the Celiac Disease Foundation, also provide support services, including diet information.

• • • • •

A gluten-free diet

When you first learn that you have to follow a gluten-free diet the rest of your life, you may feel as if your food choices have been severely restricted and eating will no longer be fun. Take heart that there's a wide variety of nutritious, tasty foods that don't contain gluten. With time and patience, mixed with a little creativity and a willingness to explore new options, you can find many common foods to enjoy.

You'll want to base your diet on a foundation of fresh vegetables and fruits, which are naturally gluten-free, and plain meat that's not breaded. Eating becomes more challenging whenever you buy packaged foods at the grocery store, order at a restaurant, or are invited to social events and parties.

A gluten-free diet can include foods such as:

- Plain meats, poultry and fish
- Fruits
- Vegetables
- Pasta made from corn, rice and other gluten-free grains
- Legumes
- Quinoa
- Rice, including cereal and crackers made from rice
- Potatoes and potato flour
- Most dairy products
- Tapioca
- Amaranth
- Buckwheat
- Millet

There are many gluten-free flours and baking mixes to choose from to make your own breads, cakes and other foods. Be aware, however, that naturally gluten-free grains can be contaminated with grains that contain gluten. This can happen accidentally during harvesting, transporting or processing. Check that the label indicates the flour is gluten-free or that the manufacturer ensures that it is.

If you don't enjoy cooking, you can purchase ready-made gluten-free products. A registered dietitian can help you locate them. You may find such products in large supermarkets or food coops, or you can order them online.

Some celiac disease support groups also have published lists of commercially produced or packaged items that don't contain gluten, to help you with shopping.

● ● ● ● ●

CELIAC DISEASE AND LACTOSE INTOLERANCE

When your small intestine becomes damaged from gluten, foods that don't contain gluten also may cause abdominal pain, bloating and diarrhea. For example, some people with celiac disease aren't able to digest the sugar (lactose) found in dairy products — a condition known as lactose intolerance. In addition to avoiding gluten, these people also must limit products containing lactose.

After your small intestine has healed, you may be able to tolerate dairy products once again, or small amounts of dairy. Dairy products contain varying amounts of lactose. Many people can tolerate lower amounts of lactose, such as the small amount in aged cheese. Sometimes, though, lactose intolerance may continue despite successful management of celiac disease. If that's the case for you, you'll need to limit or avoid most dairy products the rest of your life.

A dietitian can help you plan a diet that's low in lactose as well as gluten-free. If you can no longer eat dairy products, it's important that you find other sources of calcium.

● ● ● ● ●

Reading food labels

Food labels are important tools for making safe food choices when you have celiac disease. Always read the food label before purchasing any product. Some foods that seem acceptable, such as rice or corn cereals, may actually contain small amounts of gluten. If you can't tell by the label if a food includes gluten, don't eat it.

Also, be aware that manufacturers may change a product's ingredients at any time without announcing it. A food that was once gluten-free may no longer be. Unless you read the label every time you shop, you won't know. If it's unclear if the product contains gluten, contact the manufacturer.

Eating in and dining out

Preparing your own meals is the best way to ensure your diet is gluten-free, and you don't have to be a chef to make delicious gluten-free meals.

If you're just starting out on your gluten-free journey, you'll want to make sure your kitchen is free of all gluten remains — anywhere crumbs can lurk such as cabinets, cupboards, countertops, utensil drawers, knife block, or the refrigerator, microwave or oven. Use a clean sponge or dishrag to thoroughly clean your kitchen.

You'll need to replace hard-to-clean appliances and utensils, such as the toaster, cutting boards, strainers, flour sifters, wooden utensils and any kitchen items that are scratched or made of porous materials. If you're uncertain if an item or appliance contains gluten residue, it's best just to replace it.

You'll also want to have a good stockpile of gluten-free foods on hand. Take a careful inventory of what is safe to eat, such as rice, beans, fresh fruit and vegetables, and meats, and make sure you have those items.

If members of your household will be eating foods containing gluten, you'll need to devise a way to keep your foods separate. Label all foods to avoid confusion. Consider keeping your food items on the top shelf and your family's gluten-containing foods on the bottom shelf, where they're less likely to contaminate your food. The important thing is to find a system that works for your household.

If you're feeling overwhelmed by the idea of cooking and preparing new foods, go slow. Start with gluten-free foods you already know how to make, such as a chicken breast and salad, then move on to meals that require simple substitutions to make them gluten-free, such as gluten-free macaroni and cheese.

When you feel more comfortable cooking gluten-free, you can start experimenting with more-challenging recipes. There are many gluten-free cookbooks available and you can also find recipes online.

Of course, you may not always feel like eating at home. Consider these guidelines to ensure you have a safe dining experience when eating out:

- Select a restaurant that specializes in the kinds of foods you can eat. You may call the restaurant in advance to discuss its menu options.
- Visit the same restaurants so that you become familiar with their menus and so the staff get to know your needs. Let them know you have celiac disease and you're not eating gluten-free by choice.
- If you have a phone app that lists gluten-free meals at restaurants, still verify with the server that the meal is made without gluten.
- Ask members of your support group for suggestions of restaurants that serve gluten-free food.
- Follow the same practices you do at home. Select simply prepared or fresh foods and avoid all breaded or batter-coated foods. Other foods that may contain gluten include soups, sauces, foods fried in the same oil as batter-fried foods (such as french fries) and combination dishes.

A recent study suggests that gluten is present in more than 30 percent of restaurant food labeled as gluten-free. So, don't be afraid to ask questions about how a restaurant prepares its food, what ingredients are in a particular dish and if the kitchen is set up to accommodate your needs. Many people ask a lot of questions and make specific requests — even if they don't have a medical condition — so the restaurant staff is likely used to it.

If you find it easier, consider printing out gluten-free dining-out cards, which contain a clear description of the foods and preparation methods that are allowed and not allowed when following a gluten-free diet. You may find free versions of this card on the internet.

WHEN DIET ISN'T ENOUGH

Most people with celiac disease who follow a gluten-free diet start to feel better within a few weeks and return to normal health within several months. A small percentage don't improve with a gluten-free diet. This is known as nonresponsive celiac disease.

Nonresponsive celiac disease can often be traced back to contamination of your diet with gluten. In other words, even though you don't think you are, you're still consuming gluten. This underscores the importance of working closely with a doctor and dietitian to ensure that you're eliminating all gluten from your diet.

If you continue to experience signs and symptoms despite following a gluten-free diet for six months to one year, your doctor may recommend further testing and look for other explanations for your symptoms.

If you didn't undergo complete testing, it could be that you don't actually have celiac disease and your symptoms are associated with another disease or disorder. Other conditions can cause signs and symptoms you may think are due to celiac disease. They include poor pancreas function, irritable bowel syndrome, and an intolerance to lactose or fructose. An excessive number of bacteria in the small intestine (small intestine bacterial overgrowth) or an inflammation of the large intestine (microscopic colitis) also can produce similar symptoms.

In rare instances, the intestinal injury of celiac disease persists and leads to substantial malabsorption, even though you're following a strict gluten-free diet. This combination is known as refractory celiac disease. Treatment for refractory celiac disease often includes medications such as steroids to control intestinal inflammation and other conditions resulting from malabsorption.

Because celiac disease is a lifelong condition, it's important to see your doctor regularly to monitor your health.

CHAPTER 10

GERD and other esophageal diseases

You're getting ready for bed after an enjoyable evening having dinner with friends. Suddenly, you have a burning feeling in the middle of your chest.

Nearly everyone has experienced heartburn, that hot, burning sensation in your chest, and sometimes in your throat, caused by stomach acid washing back into your esophagus. It may be because you ate too much at dinner. Or perhaps you didn't let a bedtime snack digest before you went to sleep.

Heartburn is common, and an occasional episode is generally nothing to worry about. Many people, however, battle heartburn regularly. More than 60 million Americans experience heartburn at least once a month, and some people have heartburn every day.

Frequent or constant heartburn can be a serious problem and it deserves medical attention. Most often, it's a symptom of gastroesophageal reflux disease (GERD).

WHAT'S GERD?

After you chew and swallow, a soft, rounded mass of food (bolus) travels down your esophagus to the muscular valve called the lower esophageal sphincter (LES) that separates your esophagus from your stomach. This valve opens to allow food to pass into your stomach and then it closes tightly again.

Sometimes, the muscles in the LES can weaken. When this happens, the valve doesn't seal off the lower esophagus from the stomach as it should. Stomach acid washes back into the esophagus through the opening. The flowing back of stomach acid into the esophagus is known as reflux. Reflux can cause frequent heartburn both day and night. Stomach acid also may regurgitate higher to your upper esophagus, leaving a sour taste in your mouth. Rarely, reflux can cause additional symptoms such as a cough.

When reflux occurs frequently, the problem is called gastroesophageal reflux disease (GERD). GERD is a common problem with potentially serious consequences if left untreated.

Constant backwash of stomach acid can irritate the lining of the esophagus, causing inflammation (esophagitis). Over time, inflammation may erode the lining of the esophagus, causing an open sore to form (esophageal ulcer) that may bleed and cause pain. Damage to the lining can also lead to the formation of scar tissue, which narrows the esophagus and makes swallowing food difficult. Changes in the color and composition of the esophageal lining from reflux (a condition called Barrett's esophagus) are associated with a higher risk of esophageal cancer.

Anyone can have GERD — even children and infants. Many infants are born with an immature sphincter valve, which is why they often spit up milk or food. By age 1, the valve is more fully developed and reflux of stomach acid into the esophagus becomes much less common. Among adults, the opposite tends to be true. Signs and symptoms may become more severe with age.

●　●　●　●　●

Key signs and symptoms:

- Heartburn
- Acid reflux
- Difficulty swallowing
- Upper abdominal pain
- Chest pain
- Persistent coughing
- Hoarseness

• • • • •

VARIED SIGNS AND SYMPTOMS

Acid reflux and heartburn are two problems that most people with GERD will share. The condition may also be accompanied by a variety of other signs and symptoms:

Difficulty swallowing

Swallowing problems may indicate a narrowing (stricture) or an inflammation of the esophagus that limits its ability to propel food toward the stomach. In severe cases, you may choke or feel as if food is lodged behind your breastbone.

Chest pain

The pain is often worse after a heavy meal or at night. Because GERD and heart disease can coexist, have any chest pain evaluated to make sure it's not associated with a heart condition.

Bleeding

Inflammation and erosion of the esophageal lining or the formation of an esophageal ulcer can produce bleeding. The blood may be bright red or darker in color (even black) and appear in vomit or mixed in with stool.

Throat problems

Uncommonly, acid reflux and inflammation of esophageal tissue may produce symptoms such as hoarseness or the need to keep clearing your throat.

Coughing and wheezing

Some people experience a chronic cough with GERD. Stomach juices that back up into your throat may be composed of acid, digestive juices, bile from the liver or all three. Any of these juices may irritate your throat, resulting in a chronic cough.

● ● ● ● ●

GERD is the most common cause of an inflamed esophagus (esophagitis), but esophagitis can have other causes. A fungus or virus can inflame esophageal tissue, especially in people with weakened immune systems, such as individuals with diabetes or who are taking corticosteroid medication.

Certain pills also may irritate throat tissue during swallowing (pill esophagitis), especially if they're taken without adequate liquid or while lying down. These pills include the antibiotics erythromycin and tetracycline, the osteoporosis medication alendronate (Fosamax), vitamin C, iron and potassium tablets among others.

● ● ● ● ●

WHAT PUTS YOU AT RISK?

It isn't always easy to pinpoint the cause of GERD. Some people with the disease lack common risk factors that often trigger the condition. Risk factors associated with GERD include the following:

Being overweight

Many, but not all, people with GERD are overweight. Excess weight is a problem because it puts extra pressure on your stomach and diaphragm — the large muscle that separates your chest and abdomen. This extra pressure can force open the lower esophageal sphincter. Eating very large meals or meals that contain a lot of fat can have similar effects.

Hiatal hernia

Hiatal hernia is the name for a condition that occurs when part of your stomach protrudes upward into your lower chest and your diaphragm. As a result, the diaphragm is no longer able to support the lower esophageal sphincter, causing the valve to weaken and stomach acid to reflux into the esophagus (see here for more information).

● ● ● ● ●

WHAT'S A HIATAL HERNIA?

If the upper portion of your stomach protrudes into your lower chest cavity, it forms a pocket known as a hiatal hernia. A hiatal hernia was once thought to be the most common cause of gastroesophageal reflux disease (GERD), but doctors now take a different view. Only moderate to large hiatal hernias seem to play a role.

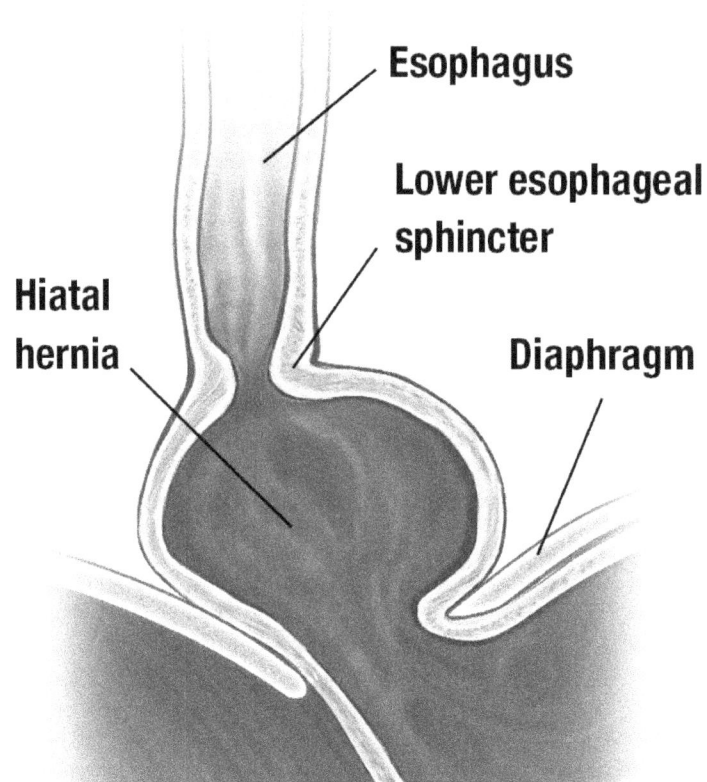

With a hiatal hernia, the upper stomach protrudes above the diaphragm.

Your chest cavity and abdomen are separated by a large, dome-shaped muscle called the diaphragm. A small opening (hiatus) in the diaphragm allows the esophagus to pass through to the stomach. A hiatal hernia forms when the upper stomach pushes upward through the hiatus into the cavity above the diaphragm.

A small hiatal hernia isn't likely to cause problems. In fact, most hiatal hernias cause no signs and symptoms at all. Moderate or large hernias can contribute to heartburn in one of two ways. Normally, your diaphragm is aligned with your lower esophageal sphincter, supporting and providing pressure on the sphincter to keep it closed. A hiatal hernia displaces the sphincter into the chest cavity, reducing pressure on the valve and allowing it to open. A hiatal hernia can also cause heartburn if it becomes a reservoir for stomach acid, which can travel up the esophagus.

Pain, bloating, difficulty swallowing or an obstruction may occur if the portion of the stomach that protrudes into the chest cavity becomes twisted. In rare cases, blood flow to the stomach may be restricted. Large hiatal hernias that pose these kinds of problems are generally treated with surgery to fix the problem and restore pressure on the sphincter to keep it closed.

● ● ● ● ●

Certain foods

Certain foods such as chocolate, fatty foods and foods containing mint may contribute to or aggravate GERD. Chemicals in these food ingredients can cause the lower esophageal sphincter to relax and open. Caffeine products can increase stomach acid production, which may worsen GERD.

● ● ● ● ●

FOODS TO BE AWARE OF

Limit or stop eating foods that bring on GERD symptoms or make your symptoms worse. Some foods that can cause or worsen GERD are listed below. You don't need to stop eating or cut back on all of these foods, only those that seem to be a problem for you.

- Fatty foods, including cream sauces, butter, margarine and shortening
- Fatty meat, including high-fat hamburgers, bacon and sausage
- Chocolate, especially high-fat milk chocolate
- Spearmint and peppermint
- Tomatoes and tomato-based products
- Citrus fruit and juice
- Beverages containing caffeine
- Carbonated drinks, especially soda with caffeine
- Fried foods, such as french fries and onion rings
- High-fat dairy products including whole milk
- Peanut butter and high-fat nuts
- Hot sauces and peppers
- Garlic
- Onion
- Apples
- Cucumbers and pickles
- Spicy food

● ● ● ● ●

Smoking and excessive alcohol

Smoking may increase the production of stomach acid, aggravating reflux. Alcohol reduces pressure on the lower esophageal sphincter, allowing it to relax and open. Alcohol may also irritate the lining of the esophagus. A combination of smoking and alcohol use can create even worse problems.

Family history

Mayo Clinic researchers believe that a genetic link may predispose some people to GERD. If your parents or siblings have or had the condition, your chances of also developing GERD are increased.

ASSOCIATED CONDITIONS

Other conditions or diseases can aggravate or trigger symptoms of GERD. However, unlike the risk factors just discussed, these conditions generally aren't considered a cause of GERD.

Pregnancy

GERD is more common during pregnancy because of increased production of the hormone progesterone. Progesterone relaxes many muscles in the body, including the lower esophageal sphincter. GERD can also develop during pregnancy because of increased pressure on the stomach as the fetus grows and the uterus expands.

Asthma

Asthma and acid reflux often occur together. It isn't clear why or whether one causes the other. But it is known that acid reflux, which causes heartburn, can worsen asthma and asthma can worsen acid reflux — especially severe acid reflux associated with GERD.

Connective tissue disorders

Diseases that cause muscular tissue to thicken and swell, such as scleroderma, can prevent digestive muscles from relaxing and contracting normally, causing acid reflux.

Zollinger-Ellison syndrome

One complication of this rare disorder is that your stomach produces large amounts of stomach acid, increasing your risk of reflux and GERD.

COMPLICATIONS OF GERD

If persistent acid reflux is left untreated, it can lead to one or more of these common complications.

Esophagitis

Esophagitis is an inflammation of the lining of the esophagus, the muscular tube that delivers food from your mouth to your stomach. Left untreated, the condition can become painful and lead to difficulty swallowing, scarring of the esophagus and the development of ulcers.

Treatment of esophagitis depends on the underlying cause and the severity of the tissue damage. Medications are often the first line of treatment. In some situations, surgery or minimally invasive procedures may be used.

Esophageal narrowing

Some people with GERD will develop esophageal narrowing (stricture). Exposure to stomach acid damages the cells lining the inner surface of the lower esophagus, resulting in the formation of scar tissue. The scar tissue narrows the opening through which food must pass to reach the stomach, obstructing the passage of food and interfering with swallowing.

Treatment for esophageal narrowing often consists of a procedure that stretches and widens the esophageal passage, as well as acid-suppressing medication to help prevent the passage from re-narrowing.

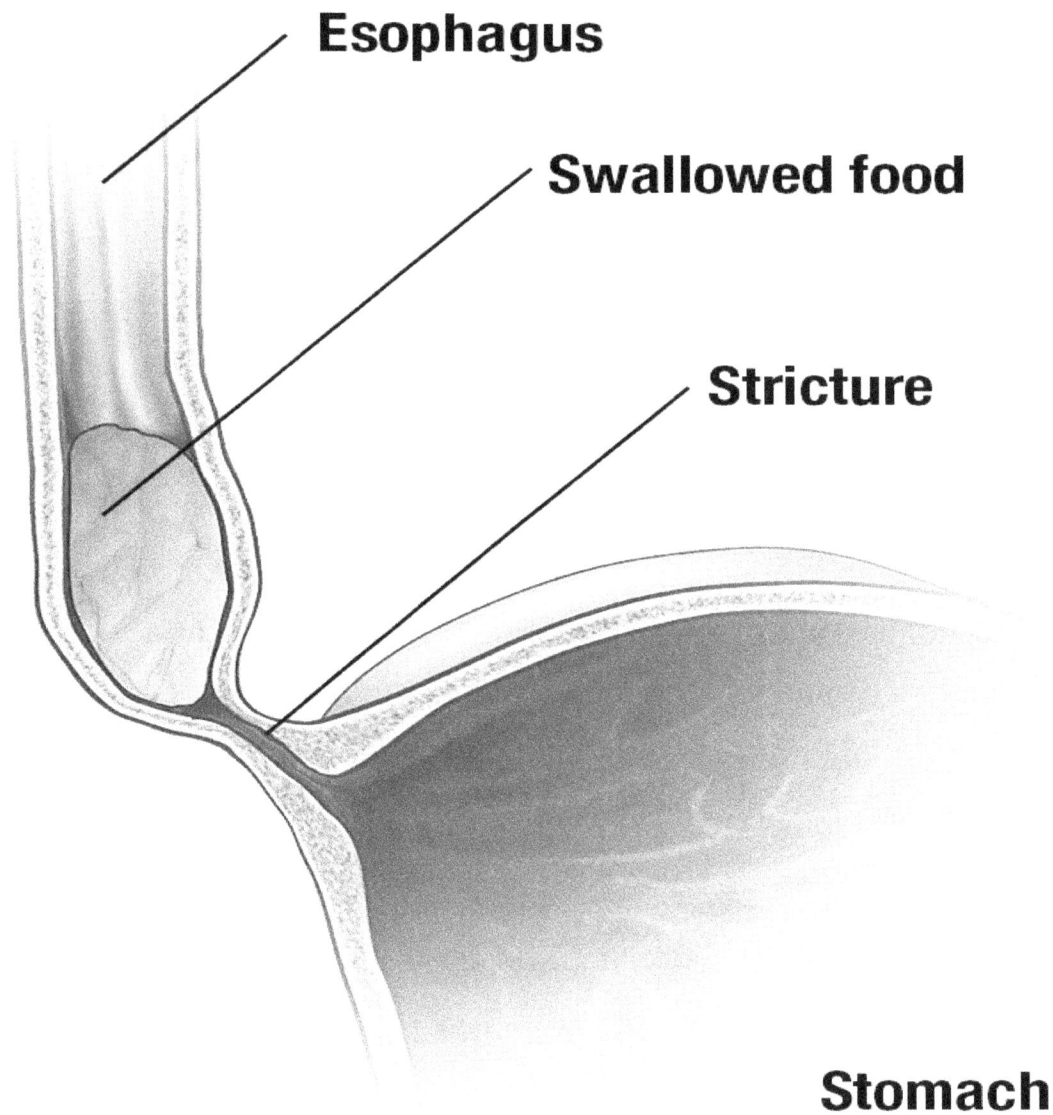

Esophagus

Swallowed food

Stricture

Stomach

A stricture of the esophagus often prevents swallowed food from reaching the stomach.

Esophageal ulcer

An open sore may form where stomach acid severely erodes tissue in the esophageal walls. The ulcer may be painful, bleed and make swallowing difficult. Medications and lifestyle changes to control stomach acid reflux generally are needed to give damaged tissue time to heal and help cure the ulcer.

Barrett's esophagus

Barrett's esophagus is a potential complication of GERD. In this condition, normal tissue lining the esophagus changes to tissue that resembles that of the small intestine. Changes in the color and composition of the tissue signal the development of Barrett's esophagus.

Instead of being pink, the tissue turns a salmon color. When looking at the tissue under a microscope, instead of flat, tile-shaped cells (similar to skin cells), the tissue contains tall cells that resemble the surface of a shag carpet (similar to cells lining the inner surface of the small intestine). This cellular change is called metaplasia — the abnormal replacement of one type of cell for another type.

Metaplasia is brought on by repeated and long-term exposure to stomach acid, and the tissue change is associated with a higher risk of getting esophageal cancer. It's estimated that .5 to 2 percent of the American population has Barrett's esophagus, but many cases go unrecognized.

If you have Barrett's esophagus, your chances of developing esophageal cancer are higher than those of the general population. However, most people with Barrett's esophagus don't develop cancer. The risk of esophageal cancer in someone with GERD remains low.

Endoscopy is the most common procedure for identifying Barrett's esophagus (see Chapter 5). A thin, flexible tube that contains a tiny camera (endoscope) allows a doctor to directly examine the esophagus for tissue damage. If tissue changes are present and your doctor suspects Barrett's esophagus, he or she may remove small pieces of tissue (biopsies) from the lower esophagus and have them examined in a laboratory. In addition to confirming the development of Barrett's esophagus, the biopsies are examined for evidence of precancerous cellular changes (dysplasia).

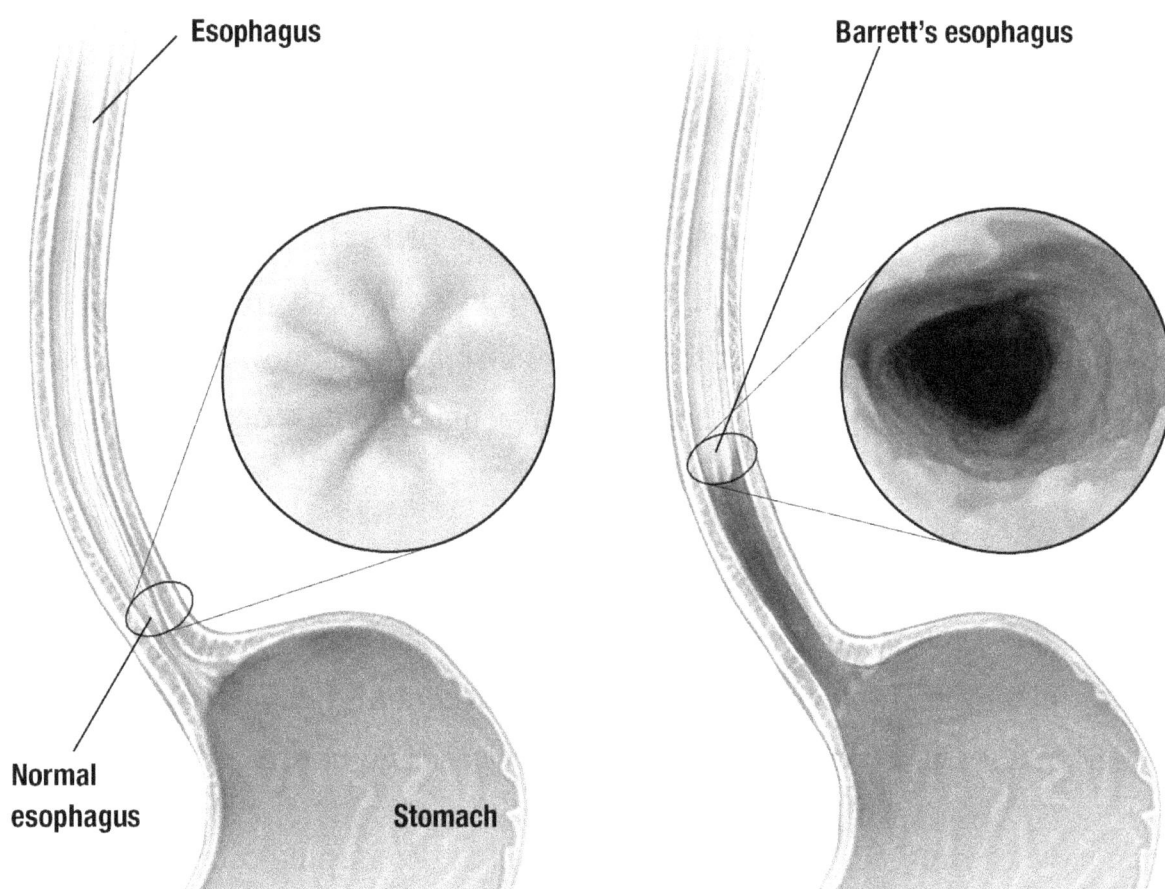

Esophagus

Barrett's esophagus

Normal esophagus

Stomach

The image at left shows the color and composition of tissue in a normal esophagus. With Barrett's esophagus, in the image at right, a change has taken place in the size, shape and composition of cells lining the esophagus, possibly caused by long-term exposure to acid reflux.

The degree of precancerous change in Barrett's esophagus ranges from none, to small but noticeable changes (low-grade dysplasia), to extensive changes (high-grade dysplasia), and finally, to invasive cancer. The more extensive the change, the greater the risk that cancer is present or that it will develop.

Treatment for Barrett's esophagus typically involves steps to control GERD by way of dietary and lifestyle changes, in addition to use of medications to control acid reflux. Your doctor may recommend periodic endoscopic examinations to monitor tissue changes.

If you have high-grade dysplasia, a potential precursor to esophageal cancer, treatment often includes a procedure to burn away the damaged tissue with high-frequency electrical current (radiofrequency ablation).

Who should be screened? The American College of Gastroenterology recommends consideration of screening for Barrett's esophagus among men who experience GERD symptoms at least weekly, who don't respond to treatment with proton pump inhibitor medication, and who have at least two additional risk factors, including:

- Older than age 50
- White
- Excessive abdominal fat
- Current or past smoker
- Family history of Barrett's esophagus or esophageal cancer

SEE YOUR DOCTOR

If you experience heartburn at least twice a week for several weeks, or your symptoms seem to be getting worse, you should see your doctor to discuss your symptoms.

At the initial visit, your doctor may ask about your general health and about the signs and symptoms you're experiencing. Questions may include the following: When did your signs and symptoms start? How often do they occur? Are they becoming more severe? Do certain factors, such as a type of activity or food, seem to make your signs and symptoms better or worse?

Your doctor may also ask questions about your lifestyle. Do you smoke? What are your eating habits? Have you gained weight recently? How much alcohol do you drink?

If you have the typical signs and symptoms of GERD — heartburn and acid reflux — but you don't have additional problems, you may not need any diagnostic tests. However, if your heartburn is severe or you have additional signs and symptoms including unexplained weight loss or difficulty with swallowing (dysphagia), you'll probably need some testing before your doctor can make a diagnosis.

To diagnose GERD and identify any complications, your doctor may recommend that you undergo one or more of the following tests. You can read more about these tests in Chapter 5.

Upper endoscopy

Endoscopy is a common test for diagnosing GERD because the procedure allows your doctor to examine the lining of your esophagus and stomach directly. During the examination, your doctor may also take tissue samples (biopsies) for laboratory analysis.

Upper gastrointestinal X-ray

It can detect abnormalities or obstructions in your upper gastrointestinal tract. Before the test, you drink a barium solution that coats your digestive tract, making your esophagus and stomach more visible on X-ray film.

Ambulatory acid (pH) probe test

This test is used to measure the amount of time, day or night, that stomach acid is present in your esophagus. The test involves placement of a catheter via a nasal passage (transnasal catheter) that measures acid reflux over a 24-hour period. Close analysis of the test results can help determine the frequency and duration of acid reflux.

Bravo test

The Bravo test is a catheter-free pH monitoring system. For this test, a miniature pH capsule, about the size of a small gelcap, is temporarily attached to the wall of your esophagus. The capsule measures the pH level in the esophagus and transmits the information wirelessly to a portable receiver you wear on your waistband. You're also given a diary to record the times you experience reflux symptoms. The study lasts approximately 48 hours.

Esophageal manometry

Esophageal manometry measures the rhythmic muscle contractions in your esophagus when you swallow. It also measures the coordination and force exerted by the muscles of the esophagus.

TREATMENT STARTS WITH SELF-CARE

Regardless of the severity of your signs and symptoms, the first step in managing GERD is to assess your behaviors and lifestyle. To control mild signs and symptoms, some small changes to your daily routine may be all that's needed to manage the disease. For more-severe signs and symptoms, profound lifestyle changes and medication may make your condition easier to control.

- *Stop smoking.* Smoking decreases the lower esophageal sphincter's ability to function properly. It also increases acid reflux and it can dry up saliva. Saliva helps protect your esophagus from stomach acid.
- *Lose excess weight.* Heartburn and acid reflux are more likely to occur when there's added pressure on your stomach from excess weight.
- *Eat smaller meals.* Smaller portions reduce the pressure on your lower esophageal sphincter. Too much pressure can force the valve open, allowing acid reflux.
- *Allow time to digest.* Wait at least three hours before lying down to sleep or nap. By then, most of the food in your stomach will have emptied into the small intestine. Don't exercise immediately after a meal. Wait two to three hours before engaging in strenuous physical activity.
- *Avoid tightfitting clothes.* A tight or constricting fit can put more pressure on your stomach.
- *Limit fatty foods.* Fatty foods relax the esophageal sphincter, permitting stomach acid to flow into the esophagus. Fat also slows stomach emptying, increasing the time acid can regurgitate into the esophagus.

- *Avoid problem foods.* Foods and beverages such as onions, spicy foods, chocolate, mint and caffeinated drinks tend to increase stomach acid. Chocolate and mint may relax the lower esophageal sphincter. Acidic foods, such as citrus fruits and tomato-based products, can irritate an inflamed esophagus, worsening symptoms in some people.
- *Limit or avoid alcohol.* Alcohol relaxes the lower esophageal sphincter and may irritate the esophageal lining, worsening symptoms.
- *Raise the head of your bed.* Raising the head of your bed 3 to 6 inches provides a gradual decline from your head to your feet and helps prevent stomach acid from flowing back into your esophagus while you sleep. The best way to do this is by placing blocks of wood or other sturdy materials under the legs at the head of your bed. Using bigger (or more) pillows to raise your head may worsen acid reflux or cause neck pain.
- *Take time to relax.* Stress can slow digestion and worsen GERD symptoms. Relaxation techniques, such as meditation, guided imagery or progressive muscle relaxation, may improve GERD by reducing stress.

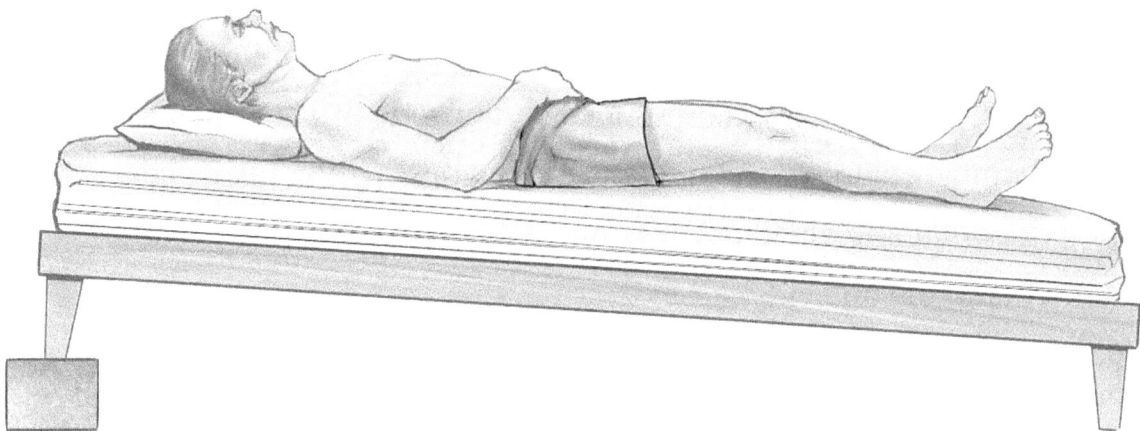

Raising the head slightly above the foot of your bed 3 to 6 inches helps prevent acid reflux.

MEDICATIONS TO TREAT GERD

Perhaps you've already tried a number of things to improve your symptoms. You've cut back on fatty foods, you're eating smaller meals and you've even lost some weight. Yet your reflux continues to bother you or has improved very little. When lifestyle changes aren't effective, the next step may be medication.

Antacids

Over-the-counter antacids are best suited for occasional or mild heartburn. They neutralize stomach acid for quick relief. Products have different neutralizing agents. For example, Tums and Rolaids are chewable tablets that contain calcium carbonate. Mylanta and Maalox come in liquid or tablet form and contain magnesium. Liquids generally work faster than do tablets, but some people find them less convenient.

Antacids can relieve signs and symptoms, but they won't cure the cause of acid reflux or heal an inflamed esophagus. The products are generally safe, but if taken frequently they can produce certain side effects, such as diarrhea (especially magnesium-containing antacids), constipation (especially aluminum-containing antacids) or congestive heart failure (especially sodium-containing antacids).

Some antacids may also interact with other medications, including medications for kidney or heart disease. Constant use of products containing magnesium may cause a magnesium buildup, which can aggravate or result in kidney disease, especially if you have diabetes. Too much calcium can result in kidney stones. If you take an antacid regularly, discuss these concerns with your doctor.

• • • • •

DRUGS AND SUPPLEMENTS TO BE AWARE OF

Certain medications and dietary supplements can irritate the lining of your esophagus, causing heartburn pain (pill esophagitis), while others can increase the severity of gastroesophageal reflux disease.

Medications and dietary supplements that can irritate your esophagus and cause heartburn pain include:

- Antibiotics, such as tetracycline
- Bisphosphonates taken orally, such as alendronate (Fosamax), ibandronate (Boniva) and risedronate (Actonel)
- Iron supplements
- Quinidine
- Pain relievers, such as ibuprofen (Advil, Motrin IB, others) and aspirin
- Potassium supplements

Medications and dietary supplements that can increase acid reflux and worsen GERD include:

- Anticholinergics, such as oxybutynin (Ditropan XL), prescribed for overactive bladder and irritable bowel syndrome
- Tricyclic antidepressants (amitriptyline, doxepin, others)

- Calcium channel blockers and nitrates used for high blood pressure and heart disease
- Narcotics (opioids), such as codeine, and those containing hydrocodone and acetaminophen
- Progesterone
- Quinidine
- Sedatives or tranquilizers, including benzodiazepines such as diazepam (Valium) and temazepam (Restoril)
- Theophylline (Elixophyllin, Theochron)

If you take any of these medications, make sure to take them with plenty of water and don't lie down for at least 30 minutes after taking them. Talk to your doctor if you think medications you take may be contributing to your reflux symptoms.

● ● ● ● ●

Acid blockers

Also known as histamine (H-2) blockers, these medications are available over-the-counter and by prescription. Instead of neutralizing gastric acid, they reduce the amount of acid produced in your stomach.

Acid blockers differ from antacids in that they don't act as quickly. However, they can prevent acid reflux and heartburn, not just relieve it. They're also longer acting, relieving heartburn for up to 12 hours, rather than four hours or less for antacids.

Acid blockers include the medications cimetidine (Tagamet HB), famotidine (Pepcid), nizatidine (Axid AR) and ranitidine (Zantac). Prescription versions of these drugs contain stronger versions of the medication than do over-the-counter varieties.

It's best to take acid blockers before any meal that may give you heartburn. You can take them after the symptoms occur, but it may take about 30 minutes before they start to work.

Acid blockers help heal inflammation (esophagitis) and ulcers by reducing the exposure of esophageal tissues to stomach acid. Your doctor may recommend that you take an acid blocker for several months, or longer, if it helps to keep your symptoms at bay.

The medications are generally safe but infrequently can cause side effects, including diarrhea, constipation, dry mouth, dizziness and drowsiness. Some acid blockers, especially cimetidine, carry the risk of dangerous interactions with other medications. Check with your doctor or pharmacist about possible drug interactions.

Proton pump inhibitors

Proton pump inhibitors (PPIs) are the most effective treatment for GERD. Dexlansoprazole (Dexilant), esomeprazole (Nexium), lansoprazole (Prevacid), omeprazole (Prilosec, Zegerid), pantoprazole (Protonix) and rabeprazole (Aciphex) are available by prescription. Omeprazole (Prilosec OTC, Zegerid OTC), lansoprazole (Prevacid 24HR) and esomeprazole (Nexium 24HR) are available over-the-counter.

PPIs block the production of gastric acid and allow time for damaged esophageal tissue to heal. PPIs are convenient to use because you generally take them only once, sometimes twice, a day. However, the drugs may be more expensive than other GERD medications.

PPIs are generally safe and well-tolerated for long-term treatment of GERD. In trials, PPIs have been found safe to use for up to at least 10 years. If your GERD is severe, your doctor may recommend PPIs for indefinite use to keep your symptoms under control.

Although generally well-tolerated these medications can cause some side effects, including stomach or abdominal pain, diarrhea, constipation, headache, or lightheadedness. Research suggests that long-term use may be associated with an increased risk of *Clostridium difficile* (*C. diff.*) infection, osteoporosis, pneumonia, vitamin deficiency and kidney disease. However, a direct cause-and-effect relationship between PPIs and these potential side effects hasn't been established and the associations are relatively weak.

The current recommendation at Mayo Clinic is that PPIs should be used when needed and at the lowest dose possible to treat symptoms of GERD, and they shouldn't be used longer than required. Calcium and vitamin D supplementation also may be considered but isn't universally recommended.

It's important to take your PPI about 15 to 30 minutes before a meal. Your stomach makes acid after food enters it. The medications need to be in your system before the acid is made. The drugs are far less effective if taken while you're fasting.

SURGERY TO TREAT GERD

Because of the effectiveness of medications, surgery to treat GERD is uncommon. However, surgery may become an option if you can't tolerate the medications, if the medications are ineffective or if you can't afford the cost of drugs long term. Your doctor may also recommend surgery if you have any of the following complications:

- Large hiatal hernia (see "What's a hiatal hernia?")
- Severe esophagitis, especially with bleeding
- In rare instances, severe pulmonary problems, such as bronchitis or pneumonia, due to acid reflux

Nissen fundoplication

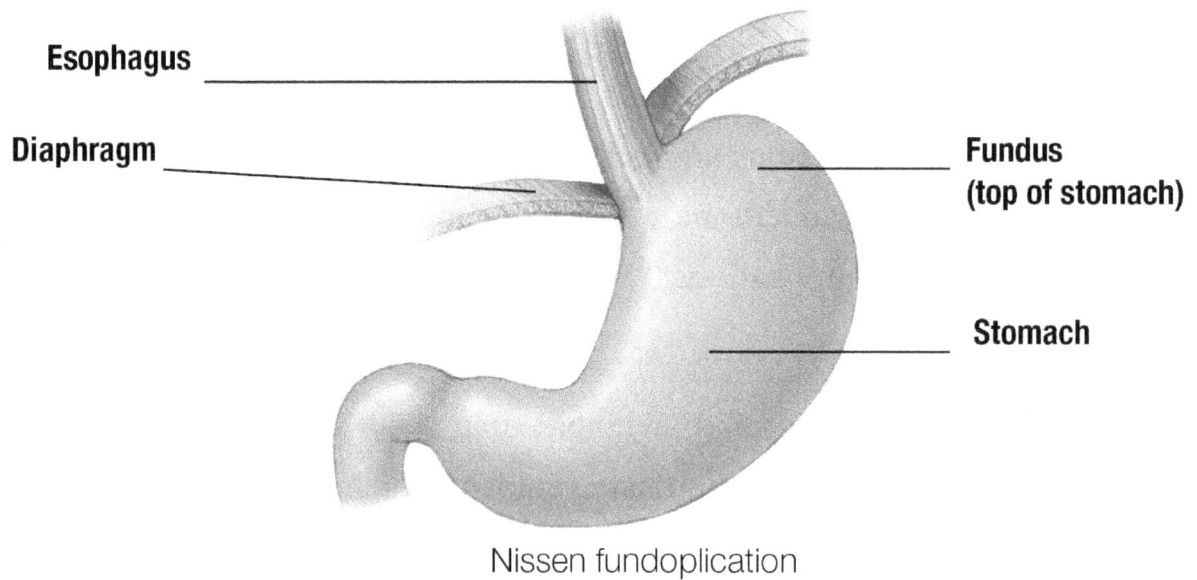

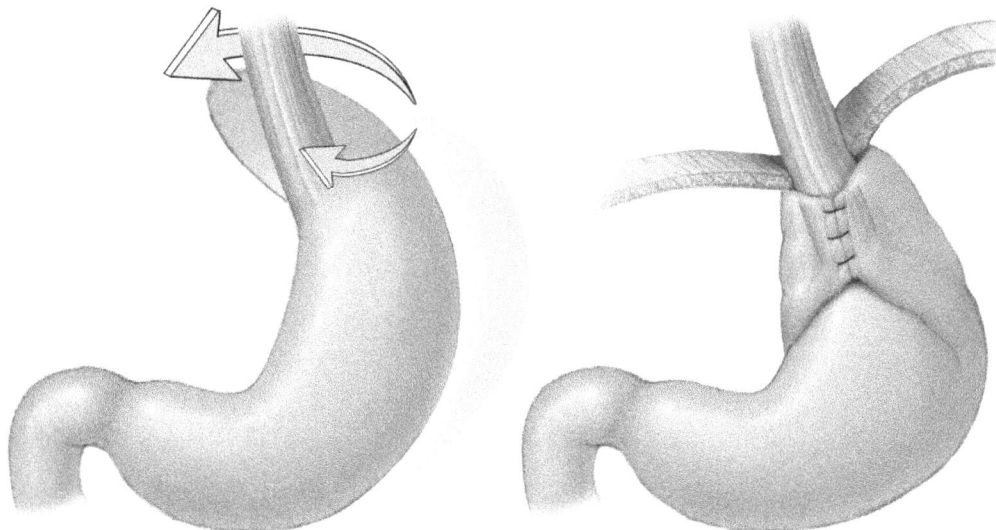

A. (left) Fundus wrapped around backside of esophagus
B. (right) Wrap secured with sutures to anchor lower esophagus below diaphragm

Fundoplication

The surgery of choice to treat GERD is a procedure called fundoplication. In this procedure, a surgeon wraps the upper part of the stomach (fundus) around the lower esophageal sphincter (LES), to tighten the sphincter muscle and prevent reflux.

Fundoplication is usually done as a minimally invasive (laparoscopic) procedure. Three to four tiny incisions are made in your abdomen through which the surgeon can insert small instruments, including an endoscope equipped with a tiny camera to see the procedure. To provide more space for the surgeon to work, your abdomen is inflated with carbon dioxide.

Sometimes, as part of fundoplication surgery, the surgeon needs to lengthen the esophagus. This is because prolonged reflux can shorten the esophagus. The lengthening procedure also helps prevent a hiatal hernia from redeveloping after surgery due to the tension a shortened esophagus can cause.

Linx device

In this procedure, a ring of tiny magnetic beads is wrapped around the lower esophageal sphincter. The magnetic attraction between the beads is strong enough to keep the muscle closed to prevent refluxing acid, but weak enough to allow food to pass through. The Linx device is implanted using minimally invasive (laparoscopic) surgery.

Endoscopic procedures

The following treatments are performed without any incisions. Instead, surgical tools are threaded down through the esophagus to the lower esophageal sphincter. These are newer procedures that lack long-term data to evaluate their effectiveness.

Transoral incisionless fundoplication (TIF). During this procedure, a portion of the stomach is folded up and around the lower esophageal sphincter and anchored with polypropylene fasteners. Similar to minimally invasive surgery, the stomach is used to reinforce the sphincter muscle.

Medigus Ultrasonic Surgical Endostapler (MUSE). It uses five titanium surgical staples to attach the stomach to the wall of the esophagus, helping to enforce the esophageal muscle.

Complications from any of the surgical procedures to treat GERD may include difficulty swallowing, bloating, diarrhea and a sense of feeling full after eating only a moderate amount — a sensation known as early satiety.

CANCER OF THE ESOPHAGUS

Cancer of the esophagus affects more than 17,000 Americans each year, and it's more common among men than women. Researchers aren't certain what causes esophageal cancer, but your risk is increased if you smoke tobacco or drink excessive amounts of alcohol. Barrett's esophagus, a complication of gastroesophageal reflux disease (GERD), is another risk factor (see here).

Unfortunately, the small tumors that develop in your esophagus in the early stages of the disease usually don't produce signs and symptoms. Often, the first indication of a tumor may be difficulty swallowing, when the tumor has grown to fill about half the opening of the esophagus.

As the cancer develops, other signs and symptoms may occur. You may experience weight loss, chest pain, and blood in vomit or stool.

There are two types of esophageal cancer, based on the cells involved:

- **_Squamous cell carcinoma._** This cancer forms in flat, scaly (squamous) cells that line the entire length of your esophagus. Tobacco and excessive alcohol use increase your risk of this type of cancer.
- **_Adenocarcinoma._** This cancer develops in glandular tissue in your lower esophagus. People with severe acid reflux disease and Barrett's esophagus are at greater risk of this type of cancer.

● ● ● ● ●

ESOPHAGEAL CANCER

Key signs and symptoms:

- Difficulty swallowing
- Blood in vomit or stool
- Weight loss
- Chest pain

● ● ● ● ●

Diagnosis

If you're experiencing signs and symptoms, your doctor may examine your esophagus for tumors or suspicious tissue. This is often done with a procedure called endoscopy, in which a thin, flexible tube with an attached camera (endoscope) is inserted down your throat. The endoscope may also collect a sample of tissue (biopsy) to be examined in a laboratory.

If cancer is identified, the next step is to determine how far the disease has spread. For this, you may undergo other tests including blood tests, a computerized tomography (CT) scan or endoscopic ultrasound. All of these tests are described in greater detail in Chapter 5.

There are no recommended tests to screen for cancer of the esophagus in individuals at low risk. However, periodic endoscopy examinations may be recommended for some people with Barrett's esophagus.

Treatment

Different types of treatment may be recommended depending on the type of cells involved, the severity and location of the cancer, your overall health, and your personal preferences.

Surgery Surgery is the most common treatment for esophageal cancer. If the cancer is small and confined to the inner layers of the esophagus, your doctor may recommend endoscopic removal of the cancer along with a margin of healthy tissue that surrounds it. With this type of surgery, an endoscope is passed down the throat and into the esophagus, and the cancer is removed by way of tools attached to the endoscope.

In most cases, a large portion of the esophagus is removed during surgery. A portion of the upper stomach also may be removed, as well as nearby lymph nodes. The surgeon then pulls the stomach up to meet the remaining esophagus. Rarely, a surgeon may form a new passageway from the throat to the stomach using intestinal tissue, often a part of the colon.

Surgery may be performed as an open procedure involving a large incision or laparoscopically, using special surgical tools that are inserted through several small incisions in your skin. The type of surgery you have, open or laparoscopic, will depend on your individual situation and your surgeon's particular approach to managing the disease.

Radiation Radiation therapy is most often combined with chemotherapy in the treatment of esophageal cancer. It is typically used before surgery, and sometimes afterward. Radiation therapy may also be used to relieve complications of advanced esophageal cancer, such as when a tumor grows large enough to stop food from passing to your stomach.

Chemotherapy Chemotherapy uses drugs to destroy cancer cells. In the treatment of esophageal cancer, it's often recommended prior to surgery, in conjunction with radiation. Sometimes chemotherapy, with or without radiation, is the primary treatment for advanced esophageal cancer.

Future treatments Targeted therapies that use drugs or other substances to identify and attack specific cancer cells are being studied as potential treatments for esophageal cancer. Monoclonal antibody therapy is one type of targeted therapy under investigation. With this therapy, specific immune system proteins (antibodies) are made in a laboratory and infused into the body. Once in the body, their goal is to identify and attack substances that help cancer cells grow.

Nutrition therapy Your doctor may recommend a feeding tube if you're having trouble swallowing or if you're having surgery. A feeding tube allows nutrition to be delivered directly to your stomach or small intestine, giving your esophagus time to heal after cancer treatment.

CHAPTER 11

Ulcers and stomach pain

Too much stress, too much spicy food, and you could be headed for an ulcer. Is this really true? Not long ago, the common belief was that ulcers were a direct result of how you lived your life. That burning pain in your chest was the outcome of an intense job or eating too much of the wrong foods.

A great deal has changed. Doctors now know that most ulcers are the result of a bacterial infection and certain medications. Smoking and alcohol also may increase your risk when accompanied by other risk factors. As a result, how ulcers are treated is very different now than from years past.

But stress management and a healthy diet still play a role in ulcer treatment. If you have an ulcer, anxiety or spicy or acidic foods, along with alcohol and tobacco, can worsen your symptoms and may delay healing.

AN OPEN SORE

Ulcer is the medical term for an open sore on your body. There are several types of ulcers. A pressure ulcer (decubitus ulcer), also called a bedsore, can occur on your back or buttocks from lying too long in one position. A stasis ulcer on an ankle generally develops from obstructed blood flow.

The most common type of ulcer — and the type that people generally associate with the term *ulcer* — is a peptic ulcer. Peptic ulcers are open sores in the upper part of the digestive tract — stomach and upper small intestine — that form when acid erodes the lining of the digestive tract or when the protective layer of mucus on the lining breaks down, making tissues more susceptible to damage. According to the Centers for Disease Control and Prevention (CDC), about 25 million Americans experience an ulcer at some point during their lifetimes.

A peptic ulcer that occurs in your stomach is called a gastric ulcer. If an ulcer develops in your small intestine, it's named for the section of the intestine where it's located. The most common is a duodenal ulcer. This type of ulcer develops in the first, or uppermost, part of the small intestine (duodenum).

Left untreated, a peptic ulcer may cause internal bleeding and create a hole in the wall of your stomach or small intestine, putting you at risk of infection or serious inflammation in your abdominal cavity (peritonitis). Peptic ulcers may also cause scar tissue to develop, which can obstruct the passage of food through the digestive tract.

● ● ● ● ●

ULCER

Key signs and symptoms:

- Gnawing pain in stomach or upper abdomen
- Feeling of fullness, bloating or belching
- Blood in vomit
- Blood in stool
- Nausea
- Heartburn
- Pain in the midback

Ulcer pain

Many people with peptic ulcers don't experience any symptoms. Among those who do, the most common symptom is a gnawing pain in the upper abdomen between the navel and breastbone (sternum). This pain, caused by stomach acid washing over the open sore, may linger for just a few minutes, or it may last for hours.

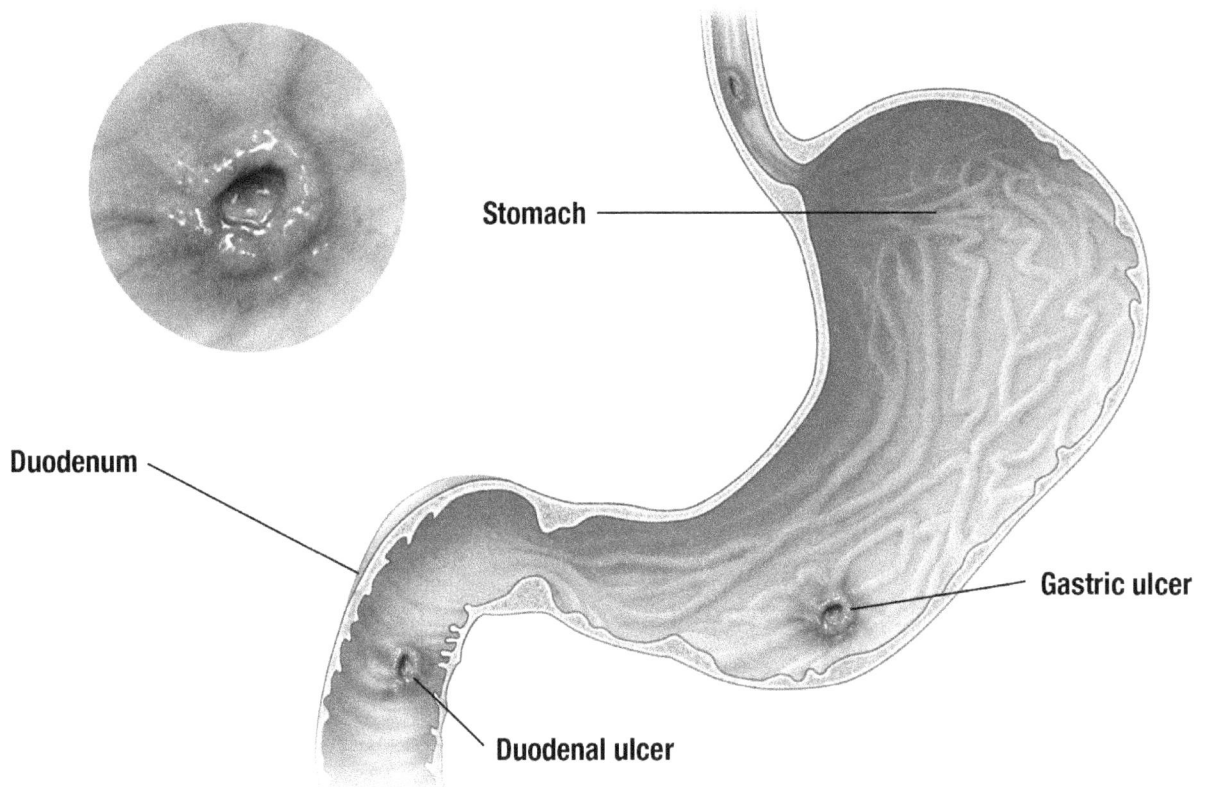

A peptic ulcer is a sore in the lining of your stomach or small intestine. A peptic ulcer located in your stomach is called a gastric ulcer. A peptic ulcer in the small intestine most often occurs in the uppermost part (duodenum), and is called a duodenal ulcer.

Pain from an ulcer is often worse when your stomach is empty. Therefore, the pain tends to flare at night. In contrast, food helps buffer stomach acid. That's why eating often temporarily relieves the pain. Some people with ulcers experience weight gain because their pain leads them to eat more often.

Other signs and symptoms of peptic ulcers include vomiting bright red or black blood, which may look similar in appearance to coffee grounds. Your stools may also contain dark-colored blood. Sometimes an ulcer can produce pain in the midback region.

BACTERIA A COMMON CULPRIT

A major breakthrough in the understanding and treatment of peptic ulcers occurred in 1983 when two Australian researchers noticed corkscrew-shaped bacteria in the biopsy specimens of people who had ulcers (see this image) and persistent stomach inflammation (gastritis).

The bacteria discovered by the researchers is called *Helicobacter pylori*. *H. pylori* bacteria commonly live in the mucous layer that covers and protects tissues that line the stomach and small intestine. Often, *H. pylori* causes no problems. But sometimes it can increase gastric acid and erode digestive tissues, producing an ulcer. The majority of peptic ulcers are caused by *H. pylori* infection.

Although it's not clear how the bacteria spread, they appear to be transmitted from person to person by direct contact with saliva or fecal matter. Children sharing beds, poor food handling and substandard sanitation practices are thought to be common routes of transmission. Because scientists have found

H. pylori in water samples, they suspect the infection may also be transmitted by drinking contaminated water.

Your stomach and the acid inside it make a hostile environment for many bacteria, but *H. pylori* is well-adapted for survival in the stomach. The bacteria produce an enzyme that creates a buffer zone to resist stomach acid, creating an alkaline microenvironment that enables *H. pylori* to survive.

Risk factors

The risk of developing a peptic ulcer due to *H. pylori* is greater if a person:

- Is born in a developing country
- Has a lower socioeconomic standard of living
- Lives with a large family or in crowded conditions
- Is exposed to the vomit of an infected individual

It's likely that genetics also play a role in ulcer development, as studies have shown that having a family member with a peptic ulcer increases your risk.

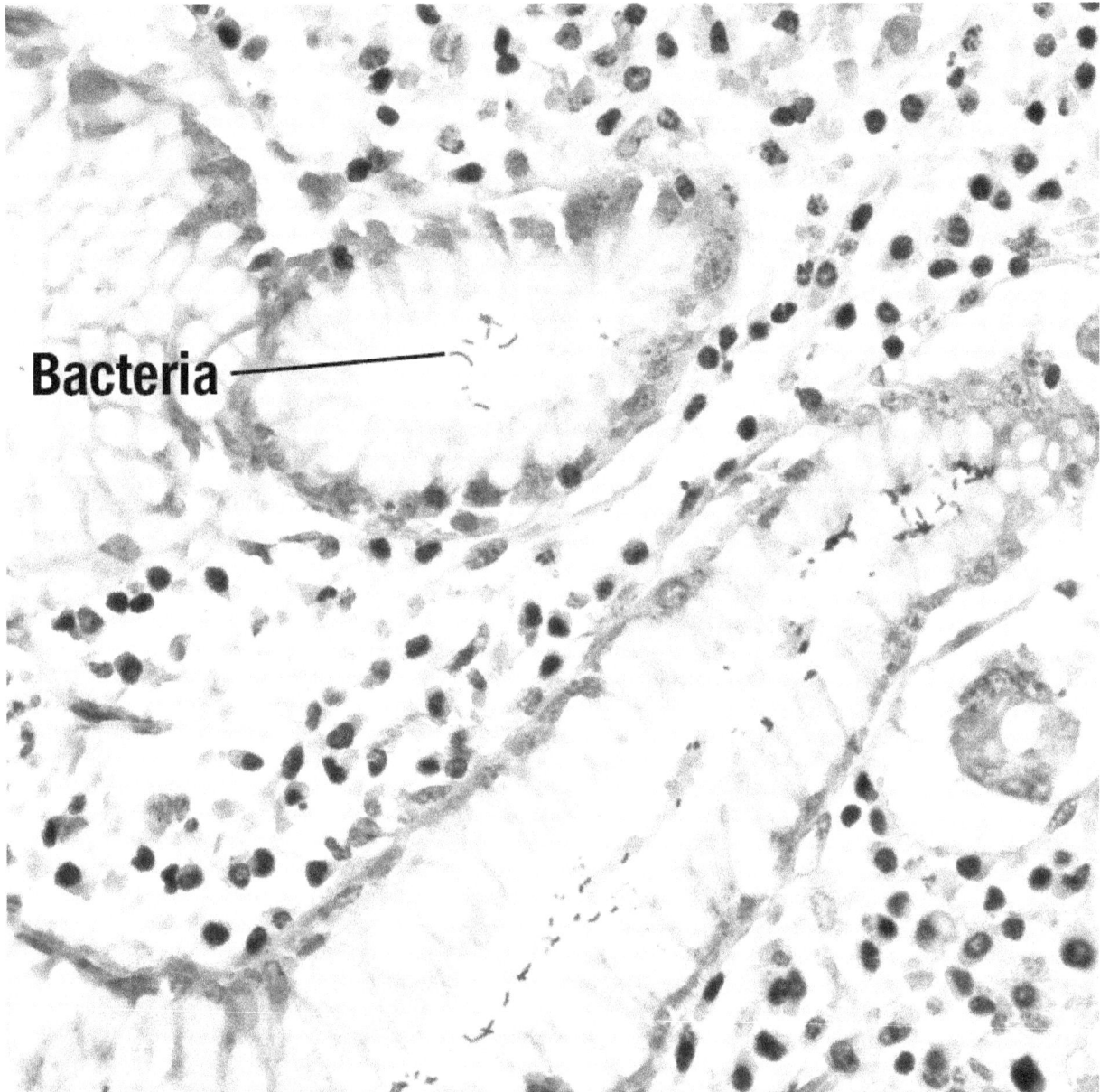

This biopsy sample reveals _H. pylori_ bacteria in the mucous layer overlying stomach tissue.

The good news is that the rate of new infections from _H. pylori_ seems to be dropping in the United States. American children raised in the 1920s to the 1940s were much more likely to have been infected by _H. pylori_ than are today's children.

Factors that may have contributed to the decrease in _H. pylori_ infection include improvements in socioeconomic status and in public hygiene and sanitation.

Another factor is the widespread use of antibiotics in children. Treatment of ear infections and other common childhood illnesses with antibiotics may have resulted in prevention and treatment of *H. pylori* infection early in life.

Other causes

While *H. pylori* is the most common cause of peptic ulcers, it's not the only one.

Aspirin and nonsteroidal anti-inflammatory drugs (NSAIDs) can irritate or inflame the lining of your stomach and small intestine. Approximately 10 percent of peptic ulcers result from regular use of aspirin and NSAIDs, which include the medications ibuprofen (Advil, Motrin IB, others), and naproxen sodium (Aleve).

These drugs inhibit the production of an enzyme that produces prostaglandins — hormonelike substances that protect your stomach lining. Without this protection, stomach acid can erode the lining, causing bleeding and ulcers. Among individuals already infected with *H. pylori* bacteria, frequent NSAIDs use increases their ulcer risk.

Older adults who take pain relievers frequently or who take other medications along with aspirin and NSAIDs — such as steroids, anticoagulants, selective serotonin reuptake inhibitors (SSRIs), alendronate (Fosamax) and risedronate (Actonel) — are more likely to experience ulcers.

You may also be at increased risk of an ulcer if you smoke or drink alcohol frequently. Smoking or alcohol alone don't cause ulcers, but they can contribute to ulcer development when other factors are present, such as *H. pylori* bacteria or use of nonprescription pain relievers. Nicotine, the primary active ingredient in tobacco, increases the volume and concentration of gastric acid in your stomach. Alcohol can irritate and erode the mucous lining of your stomach and intestines, causing inflammation and bleeding.

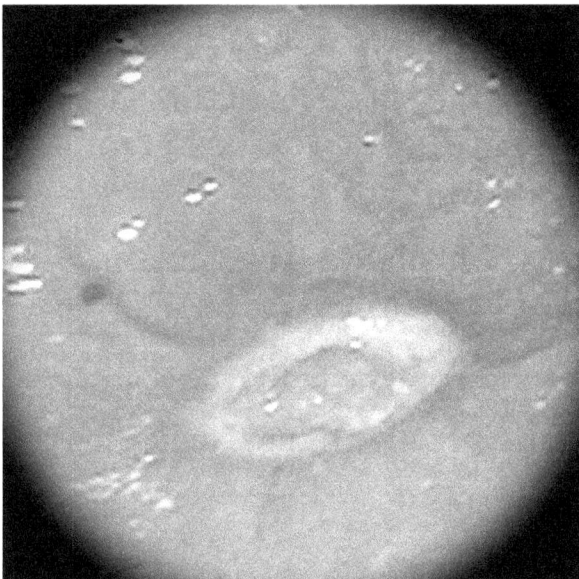

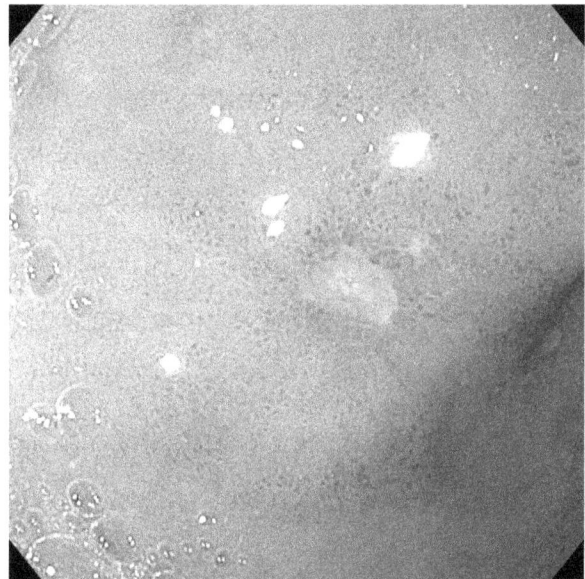

The endoscopic image on the left reveals a large gastric ulcer. Surrounding the open sore is a white ring consisting of dead tissue and debris. The endoscopic image on the right shows a duodenal ulcer. The red color surrounding the sore indicates inflammation of the intestinal lining.

DIAGNOSING ULCERS

To diagnose an ulcer, your doctor may first take a medical history and perform a physical examination. You then may need to undergo diagnostic tests, such as:

Laboratory tests

Your doctor may recommend tests to determine whether *H. pylori bacteria* are present in your body. He or she may check for *H. pylori* using a breath or stool test. Both breath and stool tests accurately indicate the presence of *H. pylori*. Blood tests are not routinely used because they can't accurately distinguish an active infection from a past infection.

For the breath test, you drink or eat something that contains radioactive carbon. *H. pylori* breaks down the substance in your stomach. Later, you blow into a bag, which is then sealed. If you're infected with *H. pylori*, your breath sample will contain the radioactive carbon in the form of carbon dioxide. You can read more about this test in Chapter 5.

If you're taking an antacid, an antibiotic or a bismuth-based medication, make sure to let your doctor know before testing for *H. pylori*. Certain medications need to be discontinued for a period of time before tests are performed. The medications can produce false-negative results, indicating you don't have *H. pylori* infection when you really do.

If your ulcer is caused by *H. pylori*, about four weeks after starting your medication your doctor may want to have you tested again to determine that the infection is gone. This is generally done with either a breath test or stool test.

● ● ● ● ●

DANGERS OF UNDIAGNOSED ULCERS

It's important that peptic ulcers be identified and treated, even if you aren't experiencing any symptoms. Left untreated, ulcers can result in:

- *Internal bleeding.* Bleeding can occur as slow blood loss that leads to anemia or as severe blood loss that may require hospitalization or a blood transfusion. Severe blood loss may cause black or bloody vomit or black or bloody stools.
- *Infection.* Peptic ulcers can eat a hole through (perforate) the wall of your stomach or small intestine, putting you at risk of infection of your abdominal cavity.
- *Obstruction.* Peptic ulcers can block passage of food through the digestive tract, causing you to become full easily, to vomit, and to lose weight through either swelling from inflammation or scarring.

● ● ● ● ●

Endoscopy

Your doctor may want to examine your upper digestive system with a small device called an endoscope. During a procedure called endoscopy, a doctor passes a hollow tube equipped with a light and a lens down the throat and into the esophagus, stomach and small intestine. With the aid of the endoscope, he or she looks for ulcers or other abnormalities.

If your doctor detects an ulcer, small tissue samples (biopsy) may be removed for examination in a laboratory. In addition to identifying the presence of *H.*

pylori bacteria, a biopsy can rule out other causes of the abnormality, such as cancer.

A doctor is more likely to recommend endoscopy among individuals who are older, have signs of bleeding, or have experienced recent weight loss or difficulty eating and swallowing. If the endoscopy identifies an ulcer, a follow-up exam should be performed after completion of drug treatment to confirm the ulcer has healed.

Upper gastrointestinal series

Also known as a barium swallow, this test involves a series of X-rays of your upper digestive system. During the procedure, you stand or sit in front of an X-ray machine and drink barium, a chalky liquid that coats your digestive tract and makes an ulcer more visible. X-rays are then taken, creating images of your esophagus, stomach and small intestine.

TREATMENT WITH MEDICATION

Over-the-counter antacids and acid blockers may help relieve the gnawing pain of an ulcer, but your relief will be short-lived. A peptic ulcer isn't something you should attempt to treat solely on your own.

With a doctor's help, you can find prompt relief from ulcer pain as well as a lifelong cure from the disease. Because most ulcers stem from *H. pylori* bacteria, doctors use a two-pronged approach to treatment:

- Eradicate *H. pylori* bacteria
- Reduce the amount of acid in your digestive tract to help relieve pain

and encourage healing

Accomplishing these two steps generally requires use of a combination of the following medications:

Antibiotics

A combination of antibiotics is often used to kill the *H. pylori* bacteria. Those most commonly prescribed for treatment of *H. pylori* include amoxicillin (Amoxil), clarithromycin (Biaxin XL), metronidazole (Flagyl), tinidazole (Tindamax), tetracycline and levofloxacin (Levaquin). However, the medications used in initial treatments are changing as *H. pylori* bacteria become increasingly resistant to a number of anti-biotics.

You'll likely need antibiotics for two weeks, as well as additional medications to reduce stomach acid, including a proton pump inhibitor and possibly bismuth subsalicylate (Pepto-Bismol). Other medications you may be prescribed are taken for a longer period of time.

Some pharmaceutical companies package a combination of two antibiotics together, with an acid suppressor or cytoprotective agent specifically developed for treatment of *H. pylori* infection.

Proton pump inhibitors

Proton pump inhibitors (PPIs) reduce stomach acid by blocking the action of tiny pumps at work within acid-secreting cells. PPIs include prescription and over-the-counter medications such as dexlansoprazole (Dexilant), esomeprazole (Nexium), lansoprazole (Prevacid), omeprazole (Prilosec), pantoprazole (Protonix) and rabeprazole (AcipHex).

PPIs are generally safe and well-tolerated. In trials, they have been found safe to use for at least 10 years. However, the medications may cause some side effects, including stomach or abdominal pain, diarrhea, constipation, headache, or lightheadedness.

Among older adults, research suggests that long-term use may be associated with an increased risk of *Clostridium difficile* (*C. diff.*) infection, pneumonia, vitamin B-12 deficiency and kidney disease. Therefore, older adults who regularly take PPIs should be periodically evaluated for potential side effects.

The current recommendation at Mayo Clinic is that PPIs should be used when needed and at the lowest dose possible. They shouldn't be used longer than required.

Acid blockers

Acid blockers — also called histamine (H-2) blockers — reduce the amount of stomach acid released into your digestive tract, which relieves ulcer pain and encourages healing. Available by prescription or over- the-counter, acid blockers include the medications cimetidine (Tagamet HB), famotidine (Pepcid), nizatidine (Axid AR) and ranitidine (Zantac).

Antacids

Your doctor may recommend an antacid (Maalox, Rolaids, Tums, others) as part of your drug regimen to neutralize stomach acid and help provide pain relief. Side effects can include constipation or diarrhea, depending on the main ingredients.

Cytoprotective agents

Cytoprotective agents help the tissues that line the stomach and small intestine. They include the prescription medications sucralfate (Carafate) and misoprostol (Cytotec). Sucralfate may cause constipation. Misoprostol can cause diarrhea and bleeding. Misoprostol shouldn't be taken by women who are pregnant or planning to become pregnant because it can cause miscarriage. Another cytoprotective agent is bismuth subsalicylate (Pepto-Bismol).

SELF-CARE STEPS TO PROMOTE HEALING

Before the discovery of *H. pylori*, people with ulcers were often placed on restricted diets and told to reduce stress in their lives. We now know that food and stress don't cause ulcers. However, while an ulcer is healing, it's still advisable to watch what you eat and try to manage worry and anxiety. Stress slows digestion, allowing food and digestive juices to remain in your stomach and intestines for longer periods of time.

The following steps may help to relieve your pain:

- *Eat healthy.* Follow a diet rich in fruits, vegetables and whole grains. Vitamin- rich foods, especially those containing vitamins A and C, help promote healing. Limit or avoid spicy or acidic foods until your ulcer has healed because these foods can worsen ulcer pain.

- ***Consider switching pain relievers.*** If you take NSAIDs regularly, ask your doctor whether acetaminophen (Tylenol, others) may be an option for you.
- ***Control stress.*** Stress may worsen the signs and symptoms of a peptic ulcer. Consider the sources of your stress and do what you can to address the causes. Some stress is unavoidable, but you can learn to cope with stress with exercise, relaxation techniques, spending time with friends or writing in a journal.
- ***Don't smoke.*** Smoking may interfere with the protective lining of the stomach, making your stomach more susceptible to the development of an ulcer. Smoking also increases stomach acid.
- ***Limit or avoid alcohol.*** Excessive use of alcohol can irritate and erode the mucous lining in your stomach and intestines, causing inflammation and bleeding.
- ***Get enough sleep.*** Sleep boosts the health of your immune system. A good night's rest also helps counter stress.

● ● ● ● ●

ULCERS THAT FAIL TO HEAL

Most peptic ulcers treated with medication heal within 12 weeks; some heal within just a couple of weeks. Unfortunately, a few ulcers don't heal. They are called refractory ulcers.

There are many reasons why an ulcer may fail to heal. Not taking medications according to directions is one reason. Another is that some types of *H. pylori* are resistant to antibiotic medications. Other factors that can interfere with the healing process include regular use of tobacco, alcohol, aspirin, ibuprofen (Advil, Motrin IB, others) or naproxen sodium (Aleve). Sometimes, the problem is accidental — people are unaware that a medication they're taking contains aspirin or an NSAID.

In rare cases, refractory ulcers may be a result of extreme overproduction of stomach acid, an infection other than *H. pylori*, or the development of other digestive diseases, including Crohn's disease or cancer. Some people develop ulcers without any known reason for getting them.

Treatment for refractory ulcers generally involves eliminating certain factors that may interfere with healing, along with prescribing different antibiotics or stronger doses of ulcer-healing medications. Sometimes, new medications may be added to the initial combination. Surgery to help heal an ulcer is rare and generally limited to serious complications such as acute bleeding or a stomach or intestinal perforation.

● ● ● ● ●

FUNCTIONAL DYSPEPSIA

Frequently, people will see their doctors for what they think are signs and symptoms of an ulcer, but diagnostic tests don't reveal a digestive problem — all results come back normal. Instead of an ulcer, these individuals may have a condition called functional dyspepsia, also known as nonulcer dyspepsia or nonulcer stomach pain.

In this condition, symptoms often mimic those of an ulcer. Functional dyspepsia commonly causes pain or discomfort in your upper abdomen near your ribs that's often accompanied by bloating, belching and nausea. Other signs and symptoms may include gas or feeling full after eating only a small amount of food.

Functional dyspepsia is common and can be long lasting. Signs and symptoms may disappear for a period of time and then return. Women and older individuals are at increased risk of the condition. Other factors that may increase your risk include frequent use of aspirin and nonsteroidal anti-inflammatory drugs (NSAIDs) such as ibuprofen (Advil, Motrin IB, others) and naproxen sodium (Aleve), as well as tobacco use and anxiety or depression.

As with ulcers, the pain is often but not always, relieved with food or antacids. It's often possible to control functional dyspepsia with diet and lifestyle changes, but medications are sometimes helpful for managing symptoms.

Plenty of theories, little proof

It's not clear what causes functional dyspepsia. Several theories have been suggested.

Stomach disorder For unknown reasons, your stomach may not be functioning or emptying normally. Functional dyspepsia has been associated with motility disorders, such as delays in gastric emptying or rapid gastric emptying. This sometimes happens after certain viral infections.

Overreaction to normal stimuli Nerve signals between your stomach and brain may be faulty, resulting in an exaggerated response to the normal changes taking place during digestion, such as how your stomach stretches and expands as it fills with food. This overreaction is known as visceral hypersensitivity.

Food sensitivity Your stomach or intestines may be overly sensitive to certain kinds of food or food ingredients. Often, but not always, these include certain spices, citrus fruits or vegetables that contain moderate to high levels of acid. Some people find that drinking coffee seems to make the symptoms worse.

Acid sensitivity Tissues that line your stomach and duodenum may be overly sensitive to normal acid levels and become easily irritated. Or, it's possible that acid-secreting cells in your stomach may produce higher than normal amounts of digestive acid. This oversupply may irritate digestive tissues.

Presence of H. pylori bacteria Even though an ulcer isn't present, your symptoms may represent irritation of stomach tissues by the *Helicobacter pylori (H. pylori)* bacteria.

Altered gut microbiome Changes to the makeup of bacteria that reside in your gut may lead to functional dyspepsia. An event such as the stomach flu (gastroenteritis) can alter the balance of bacteria in your intestines, encouraging the overgrowth of "unhealthy" bacteria while suppressing the growth of healthy bacteria. See Chapter 2 for more information.

Reaction to drugs and supplements Pain relievers such as aspirin and ibuprofen (Advil, Motrin IB, others) are known to cause ulcers and gastritis. It's possible these medications can irritate your digestive system without damaging your stomach or intestines. This may be true for other medications and supplements, including antibiotics, steroids, minerals and herbs.

Stress and anxiety Stomach pain and discomfort may be your body's way of responding to periods of stress, anxiety or depression.

Diagnosing functional dyspepsia

A doctor may diagnose a person with functional dyspepsia if diagnostic tests come back negative — indicating no disease — but the person experiences one or more of the following symptoms on a regular basis for at least three months:

- Unusual fullness and discomfort after meals
- Feeling full quickly when eating (early satiety)
- Pain in the upper abdomen
- Burning in the upper abdomen

LIFESTYLE CHANGES THE FIRST STEP

Functional dyspepsia is generally treated by examining and changing your daily routines. This may include avoiding foods that seem to worsen symptoms, controlling stress, and changing or limiting medications or supplements. Some people find that having smaller, more-frequent meals and eating low-fat foods improves their symptoms.

There's some evidence that products that contain peppermint oil or caraway oil may improve symptoms in some individuals. Further study is needed to determine the safety and potential role of these products.

Medications

If these practices don't help you, your doctor may recommend medication. Many medications used to treat ulcers are recommended for functional dyspepsia, including:

- Gas relief medications such as Mylanta and Gas-X
- Acid blockers such as cimetidine (Tagamet HB), famotidine (Pepcid AC), nizatidine (Axid AR) and ranitidine (Zantac 75)
- Proton pump inhibitors such as lansoprazole (Prevacid 24HR), omeprazole (Prilosec OTC) and esomeprazole (Nexium 24HR)
- Drugs that make the stomach empty faster
- Low-dose antidepressants to control intestinal pain
- Antibiotics to destroy *H. pylori*, if tests indicate the presence of the bacteria

Behavior therapy

Working with a counselor or therapist may relieve signs and symptoms that aren't helped by medications. A counselor or therapist can teach you relaxation techniques to lessen your symptoms, reduce stress and anxiety, and help prevent functional dyspepsia from recurring.

STOMACH CANCER

Stomach cancer generally begins in the mucus-producing cells that line the stomach. This type of cancer is called adenocarcinoma.

• • • • •

STOMACH CANCER

Key signs and symptoms:

- Severe, persistent heartburn or indigestion
- Weight loss
- Stomach pain
- Feeling full after eating only a moderate amount
- Feeling bloated after eating
- Fatigue
- Blood in vomit or stool
- Nausea and vomiting

• • • • •

For the past several decades, rates of cancer in the main part of the stomach (stomach body) have been falling. One reason is, there's a strong correlation between a diet high in smoked and salted foods and cancer of the stomach body. As use of refrigeration for preserving foods has increased worldwide, rates of this form of stomach cancer have declined. Increased use of antibiotics to treat *Helicobacter pylori* (*H. pylori*) infection may be another reason. *H. pylori* infection is associated with stomach cancer.

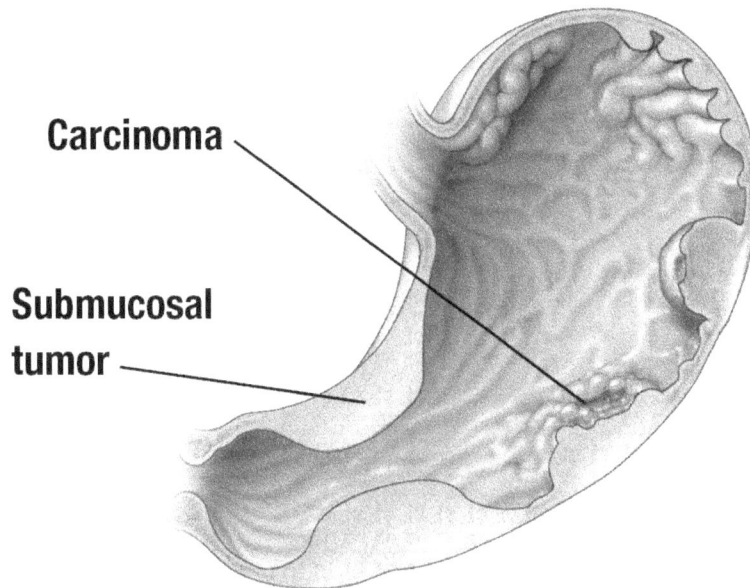

The illustration above shows cancer (carcinomas) in soft tissue lining the stomach. Swelling from cancer in deep layers of the stomach wall (submucosal tumor) can narrow the stomach body.

However, cancer of the gastroesophageal junction, where the top part of the stomach meets the lower end of the esophagus, has become more common. Gastroesophageal junction cancer is associated with gastrointestinal reflux disease (GERD), obesity and, less strongly, with smoking. GERD is a common digestive disorder caused by frequent backflow of stomach acid into the esophagus (see Chapter 10).

DIAGNOSIS AND TREATMENT

Upper endoscopy and imaging tests are most often used to diagnose stomach cancer. You can read more about these procedures in Chapter 5.

If cancer is present, additional tests may be performed to determine the extent (stage) of the cancer. This is important in devising a treatment plan. Treatment options generally depend on the stage of the cancer, your overall health and your personal preferences.

Surgery

Gastroesophageal junction cancer that hasn't spread often requires surgery to remove the part of the esophagus or stomach where the tumor is located. The goal of surgery is to remove all of the cancer and a margin of healthy tissue, if possible. Nearby lymph nodes are typically removed as well.

The goal of surgery for stomach body cancer also is to remove all of the cancer and a margin of healthy tissue. Options include:

- *Removing early-stage tumors.* Very small cancers limited to the inside lining of the stomach may be removed in a procedure called endoscopic mucosal resection. A thin, lighted tube with a camera is passed down your throat into your stomach. A doctor uses special tools to remove the cancer and a margin of healthy tissue from the stomach lining.
- *Removing a portion of the stomach (subtotal gastrectomy).* During subtotal gastrectomy, a surgeon removes only the portion of the stomach affected by cancer.
- *Removing the entire stomach (total gastrectomy).* The entire stomach and some surrounding tissue are removed. The esophagus is then connected directly to the small intestine to allow food to move through your digestive system.
- *Surgery to relieve signs and symptoms (palliative surgery).* Among individuals with advanced stomach cancer, removing part of the stomach may relieve signs and symptoms of a growing tumor. Surgery can't cure advanced stomach cancer, but it can make you more comfortable.

If all or part of your stomach is removed as part of your treatment, you may experience digestive problems, such as abdominal pain, diarrhea and malnutrition.

Radiation therapy

In gastroesophageal junction cancer, as well as cancer of the stomach body, radiation therapy may be used before surgery (neoadjuvant radiation) to shrink a tumor so that it's more easily removed. Radiation therapy may also be used after surgery (adjuvant radiation) to kill any cancer cells that might remain in the area.

Oftentimes, radiation and chemotherapy are administered at the same time (chemoradiotherapy), typically before surgery.

Depending on where the radiation is administered, radiation therapy can cause diarrhea, indigestion, nausea and vomiting, and pain and difficulty swallowing. To avoid swallowing difficulty, you may have a feeding tube placed in your stomach through a small incision in your abdomen while your esophagus heals.

Chemotherapy

Similar to radiation therapy, chemotherapy may be given before surgery (neoadjuvant chemotherapy) to help shrink a tumor so that it can be more easily removed. It's also used after surgery (adjuvant chemotherapy) to kill any cancer cells that might remain in the body. Chemotherapy side effects depend on which drugs are used.

Targeted drugs

Targeted therapy drugs attack abnormalities within cancer cells or they direct your immune system to kill cancer cells (immunotherapy). Targeted drugs used to treat stomach body cancer include the medications trastuzumab (Herceptin), ramucirumab (Cyramza), imatinib (Gleevec), sunitinib (Sutent) and regorafenib (Stivarga).

Several targeted drugs are under study for the treatment of gastroesophageal junction cancer, but only two — ramucirumab and trastuzumab — have been approved for this use.

Targeted drugs are often used in combination with standard chemotherapy medications. Tests of your cancer cells can indicate if these treatments are likely to work for you.

CHAPTER 12

Crohn's disease and ulcerative colitis

Inflammatory bowel disease (IBD) is an umbrella term for a group of chronic conditions in which the body's immune system is overactive, causing injury to parts of the digestive system. The two most common forms of IBD are Crohn's disease and ulcerative colitis.

People with Crohn's disease or ulcerative colitis may have abdominal pain, diarrhea, rectal bleeding, sores around the anus, weight loss and decreased energy. They may also experience symptoms involving organs other than the digestive tract, including the skin, eyes, joints, liver, urinary bladder and vagina. Symptoms can be mild or severe and can worsen and improve without medical intervention.

But there is good news if you have IBD. Although the disease can't be cured, it can often be managed very well. Several therapies can control your symptoms, and possibly even produce a long-term remission — a period of time when the disease isn't active.

SIMILAR BUT DIFFERENT

Crohn's disease and ulcerative colitis share many of the same signs and symptoms. In fact, they can behave so similarly that one condition is sometimes mistaken for the other.

Both conditions inflame the inner lining of the digestive tract. Both can take an unpredictable course, such as severe flare-ups that may be long term, followed by extended periods of remission. And both may require a complex drug therapy regimen, often using nearly identical medications.

Despite these similarities, the two conditions exhibit several key differences:

- *Crohn's disease.* Crohn's disease can occur anywhere in your digestive tract, from your mouth to your anus, although its most common location is the small intestine. It can develop in different locations simultaneously, typically in patches. Inflammation may settle into the deepest layers of tissue in affected areas.
- *Ulcerative colitis.* Ulcerative colitis is limited to the colon and rectum. The inflammation often begins in the rectum and then spreads in long, continuous stretches into the colon. The disease differs from Crohn's in that only the thin lining of the inner surface is inflamed and typically deeper tissues aren't affected.

Although Crohn's disease and ulcerative colitis can occur at any age, the diseases are most frequently diagnosed between ages 15 and 35. They also tend to develop after age 50. Men and women are equally susceptible. Men are more likely than women to be diagnosed with ulcerative colitis at a later age.

● ● ● ● ●

INFLAMMATORY BOWEL DISEASE (IBD)

Key signs and symptoms:

- Diarrhea
- Abdominal pain and cramping
- Blood in stool
- Fatigue
- Reduced appetite
- Weight loss
- Fever
- Pain or drainage near or around the anus

● ● ● ● ●

IBD can affect people of any racial or ethnic group. Research involving people of various ethnicities who have immigrated to the United States suggests that environmental influences may be a bigger factor in risk of the disease than are race and ethnicity. The disease tends to be more common in urban areas and more prevalent in northern climates.

Together, Crohn's disease and ulcerative colitis affect approximately 1.6 million people in the United States, including up to 80,000 children. As many as 70,000 new cases of IBD are diagnosed each year.

● ● ● ● ●

The endoscopic image at left is a healthy interior of the small intestine with even coloration and well-spaced, circular folds. The image at right shows the small intestine with a pattern of inflammation characteristic of Crohn's disease. The mucous membrane forms bumpy nodules along the margins.

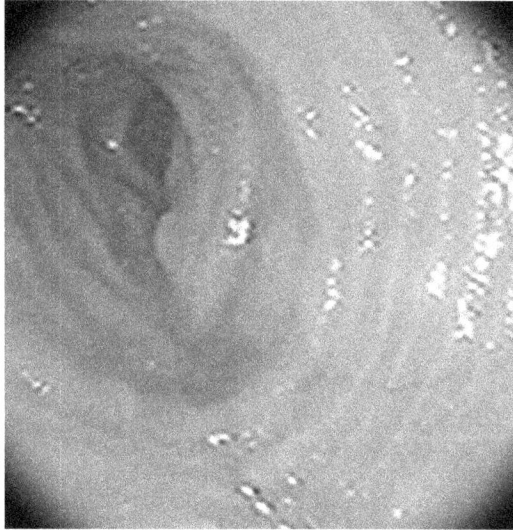

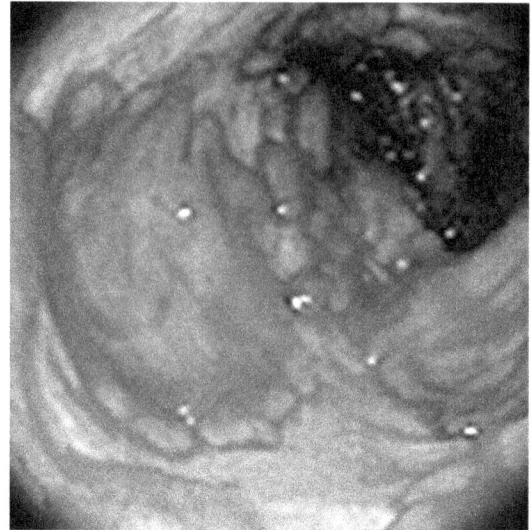

The endoscopic image at left shows typical folding and tissue coloration in the transverse colon. The image at right reveals ulcerative colitis extending in long, continuous stretches into the colon. The inflammation develops only in the thin lining of the inner surface.

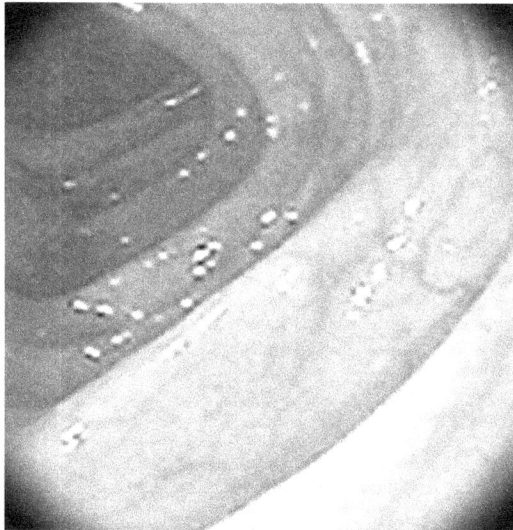

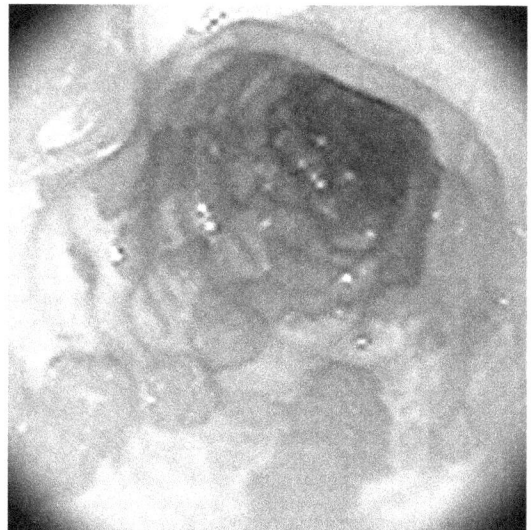

• • • • •

IN SEARCH OF A CAUSE

The exact cause of IBD remains unknown; however, researchers believe that four factors play a major role in its development. Among most individuals who develop IBD, a combination of factors is likely involved.

Genetic component

Studies show that 5 to 20 percent of people with Crohn's disease or ulcerative colitis have an immediate family member — parent, brother, sister or child — with IBD. Children of parents with IBD are at greater risk than the general population, especially if both parents have the disease.

More than 200 genes and genetic mutations connected to IBD have been identified. Mutations in one particular gene — known as the NOD2 (CARD15) gene — occur frequently in people with Crohn's disease. Up to 20 percent of people with IBD may have a mutation to this gene. Having the mutation, however, doesn't guarantee you'll develop the disease. For disease to occur, other factors must come into play.

Environmental trigger

Both Crohn's disease and ulcerative colitis are more prevalent in developed countries and in cities than in rural areas. This has led some experts to speculate that environmental factors, such as diet, may play a role. However, researchers haven't yet identified any particular foods that may increase disease risk. Smoking is a known risk factor for Crohn's disease, but not ulcerative colitis. Active smokers are more than twice as likely as nonsmokers to develop Crohn's disease.

Another theory is that people living in cleaner environments may in essence be victims of good hygiene and public health measures. As a result, they become more vulnerable to infections later in life. There's also some speculation that certain medications, such as antibiotics, aspirin, ibuprofen (Advil, Motrin IB, others) and naproxen sodium (Aleve), may play a role.

Contrary to past belief, researchers no longer believe that stress and other mental health issues are the culprits — although they may aggravate symptoms.

Immune system response

One theory holds that Crohn's disease and ulcerative colitis are linked to infection from an unknown virus or bacterium. Typically, inflammation is a result of your body's immune system trying to fight off invaders. The fact that medications used to suppress the immune system are proving to be remarkably effective at controlling the signs and symptoms of IBD is bolstering this theory.

Another possibility is that the immune system is mistaking beneficial bacteria that normally live in the intestinal tract as a threat and attacking them.

Intestinal bacteria

The human gut harbors a complex and abundant array of microorganisms, collectively called the gut microbiome. These organisms, including several types of bacteria, play a role in a variety of functions, including digestion and the body's immune system response (see Chapter 2).

In recent years, thanks to advances in technology, researchers have found that some individuals with IBD have different types of (altered) bacteria in their intestinal tracts not normally present in healthy individuals. This has led to speculation that the altered bacteria may play a role in the development of IBD.

● ● ● ● ●

IS YOUR CROHN'S DISEASE MILD, MODERATE OR SEVERE?

Mild Crohn's disease

- Four or fewer diarrheal bowel movements daily
- Minimal abdominal pain or no pain at all
- Healthy weight
- Normal temperature, pulse and red blood cell count
- Few, if any, complications

Moderate Crohn's disease

- Four to six diarrheal bowel movements daily
- Moderate abdominal pain
- Additional complications

Severe Crohn's disease

- Six or more diarrheal bowel movements daily
- Severe abdominal pain
- Underweight
- Fever, rapid pulse, low red blood cell count, high white

blood cell count

- Additional complications

• • • • •

SIGNS AND SYMPTOMS

Both Crohn's disease and ulcerative colitis produce a variety of signs and symptoms, which may appear suddenly or develop gradually.

Crohn's disease

With Crohn's disease, one or more of the following complications may occur in mild to severe forms.

Diarrhea The intestines respond to inflammation in the same way they respond to infection. Intestinal cells may secrete extra amounts of salt and water, overwhelming the capacity of the intestinal tract to absorb fluid. At the same time, muscles in the intestinal walls may contract more frequently. The result is diarrhea.

Cramping Persistent inflammation in the intestinal tract can cause scar tissue to form, which contributes to the swelling and thickening of intestinal walls. Intestinal channels may narrow, blocking the passage of food waste. This can lead to cramping. In rare cases, vomiting may occur.

Bleeding As food waste passes through the intestinal tract, it may touch or rub against inflamed tissue and the tissue may bleed. Inflamed tissue may also bleed without food waste. The blood expelled with your stool may appear bright red in the toilet bowl or dark in color and mixed in with stool.

Weight loss and fatigue Inflammation in the small intestine makes it difficult to absorb sufficient nutrients to maintain a healthy weight and normal energy level. That is why people with more severe disease often experience weight loss. Excessive blood loss also can produce fatigue. Malabsorption of nutrients may be the reason why children with Crohn's disease tend to have stunted growth.

Ulcers Chronic inflammation can produce open sores (ulcers) in the intestinal tract. Some people develop a string of disconnected ulcers throughout the tract, even in the mouth, esophagus or anus. Typically, Crohn's-related ulcers develop in the lower small intestine (terminal ileum), colon and rectum.

Fistulas Ulcers may burrow completely through the intestinal wall and create a fistula — an abnormal, tubular connection between organs or to the surface of the skin. Often, fistulas connect one loop of the small intestine to another. When a fistula develops between the small intestine and colon, food particles take a shortcut through the opening and arrive in the colon before their nutrients have been fully absorbed.

Sometimes, a fistula can develop into a pocket of infection called an abscess. Treatment of an abscess may involve medication or surgery.

Other complications Not all complications are confined to the gastrointestinal tract. Crohn's disease can cause additional problems, including:

- Inflammation, swelling, stiffness and pain in your joints

- Skin rashes or sores
- Anal skin tags that mimic hemorrhoids
- Inflammation of your eyes
- Kidney stones
- Gallstones

It's uncertain what causes these complications. Some researchers believe they're all linked to an immune system response in parts of the body other than the digestive tract. When the disease is treated, some of these signs and symptoms will disappear.

Colorectal cancer Crohn's disease that affects the colon and longstanding ulcerative colitis involving more than the rectum increase the risk of colorectal cancer.

During the first eight to 10 years after diagnosis, the risk of colorectal cancer isn't any higher than in people who don't have IBD. But after this period of time, cancer risk increases among individuals with extensive ulcerative colitis and Crohn's disease.

For people with distal ulcerative colitis — involvement of the rectum, sigmoid colon and perhaps the descending colon, but not higher — the risk of cancer increases after 15 years of disease.

An analysis of published studies found that up to 18 percent of people with IBD may develop colorectal cancer by the time they've had the disease for 30 years. Other factors that may increase risk of colorectal cancer include the extent of colon involvement, the severity of disease and the earlier in life a person is diagnosed.

Ulcerative colitis

Similar to Crohn's disease, ulcerative colitis can cause diarrhea, bleeding, cramping and abdominal pain, as well as complications such as skin rash, arthritis and eye inflammation. However, ulcerative colitis is more often associated with liver disease than with kidney stones, gallstones or anal skin tags. With ulcerative colitis, your stool often is mixed with blood, in addition to mucus or pus.

Toxic megacolon is a serious complication of ulcerative colitis that can occur in some individuals. The inflamed colon becomes immobilized and distended, unable to expel stool and gas. Signs and symptoms include abdominal pain and swelling, fever, and weakness. You may also become groggy or disoriented. Left untreated, the colon may rupture and bacteria from the colon infects the abdominal cavity, a condition called peritonitis that can be fatal. A ruptured colon requires emergency surgery.

As mentioned earlier, long-term ulcerative colitis that involves more than just the rectum increases the risk of colorectal cancer. Regular colonoscopy screenings are recommended after eight to 10 years of the disease.

DIAGNOSING IBD

There's no single test your doctor can rely on to definitively diagnose Crohn's disease or ulcerative colitis. Like many other digestive conditions, signs and symptoms may be associated with any number of other diseases. Inflammatory bowel disease is most often diagnosed following a series of tests that are able to rule out other probable causes.

Diagnostic tests that may help confirm Crohn's disease or ulcerative colitis include the following. You can read more about many of these tests in Chapter 5.

Blood tests

Blood tests identify certain proteins (biomarkers) that can be useful for detecting inflammation. Blood biomarker tests include C-reactive protein (CRP) and erythrocyte sedimentation rate (ESR). Both of these tests can indicate the presence of inflammation somewhere in your body, although neither can pinpoint its exact location.

Stool studies

Sometimes a stool sample is requested to check for infectious organisms that may be associated with chronic diarrhea. Recent travel outside the United States is often an indication for a stool study. A fecal calprotectin test is useful in assessing the degree of inflammatory activity.

Colonoscopy

This endoscopic exam is highly sensitive for diagnosing ulcerative colitis and Crohn's disease of the colon and the final section of the small intestine (terminal ileum). Areas of inflammation interspersed with areas of normal tissue suggests Crohn's disease. A continuous area of inflammation suggests ulcerative colitis. For more on this procedure, see here.

During the test, a doctor may also retrieve tissue samples (biopsies) to be examined under a microscope. Granulomas in the samples may be found in Crohn's disease, but often they're not present. Granulomas are small groupings of inflammatory cells that attempt to surround and destroy bacteria and other foreign bodies. Granulomas are not a feature of ulcerative colitis.

Capsule endoscopy

This test is sometimes used to help diagnose Crohn's disease involving the small intestine. You swallow a capsule that has a camera and battery within it. The images from the camera are transmitted to a receiver worn on a belt. The capsule passes out of the body in your stool.

Computerized tomography (CT)

The test looks at the entire bowel, as well as tissues outside the intestines. CT enterography (CTE) is a special CT scan that provides better images of the small intestine. During this exam, an oral agent and an intravenous (IV) contrast agent is administered to better outline the intestines. CTE has replaced barium X-rays in most medical centers.

Magnetic resonance imaging (MRI)

A magnetic resonance image is particularly useful for evaluating a fistula around the anal area or viewing the small intestine. MR enterography is a specialized test, similar to CT enterography, that can provide a more detailed picture of the small and large intestine.

In about 10 percent of people with chronic colitis, it can be difficult to determine if they have Crohn's disease of the colon or ulcerative colitis. In these cases, a person may be given a diagnosis of indeterminate colitis.

● ● ● ● ●

IS YOUR ULCERATIVE COLITIS MILD, MODERATE OR SEVERE?

Mild ulcerative colitis

- Four or fewer diarrheal bowel movements daily
- Occasional blood in stool
- Normal temperature, pulse and red blood cell count
- Few, if any, complications

Moderate ulcerative colitis

- Four to six diarrheal bowel movements daily
- Blood in stool fairly regularly
- Additional complications

Severe ulcerative colitis

- Six or more diarrheal bowel movements daily
- Frequent blood in stool
- Tender abdomen
- Fever, rapid pulse, low red blood cell count, high white blood cell count

- Additional complications

• • • • •

MEDICATIONS

Medications can't cure IBD, but they can effectively reduce signs and symptoms in most people and improve quality of life. The primary goal of medication therapy is reducing inflammation in the intestinal tract, because that's what triggers most of the problems.

Doctors rely on several categories of medications that help control inflammation in different ways. Some of these drugs may work well for some people but not for others. So, it may take time to discover what works best for you.

Medications for Crohn's disease

There are two general approaches to drug treatment for Crohn's disease: step-up therapy and top-down therapy. With step-up therapy, medications that are less potent and associated with fewer side effects, such as corticosteroids and aminosalicylates, are used first. If these drugs are ineffective, stronger medications are prescribed. Top-down therapy, which is the preferable approach, starts with more potent medications, such as biological therapy or immunomodulators, early in the course of the disease.

Step-up therapy is most often used in individuals with mild Crohn's disease and top-down therapy in people with moderate to severe disease.

The most commonly prescribed drugs for Crohn's disease fall into five basic categories. See this chart.

•   •   •   •   •

CROHN'S DISEASE MEDICATIONS

Drug class	Generic name (brand name)	Indications	Route of delivery
Corticosteroids	• Budesonide (Entocort EC) • Prednisolone • Prednisone	For mild to moderate Crohn's and to control disease flares. Budesonide is a newer nonsystemic steroid. The medications shouldn't be used long term.	Oral, rectal or IV infusion
Aminosalicylates (5-ASA)	• Balsalazide (Colazal, Giazo) • Mesalamine (Delzicol, Rowasa, others) • Olsalazine (Dipentum)	Not FDA approved for Crohn's disease, but sometimes prescribed for mild to moderate disease of the colon.	Oral or rectal
Biological therapies	• Adalimumab (Humira) • Certolizumab pegol (Cimzia) • Infliximab (Remicade) • Ustekinumab (Stelara) • Vedolizumab (Entyvio)	For moderate to severe Crohn's disease. Also effective for maintaining remission and for tapering off cortico-steroids. The medications are sometimes combined with an immunomodulator.	IV infusion or injection
Immunomodulators	• Azathioprine (Azasan, Imuran) • Mercaptopurine (Purinethol,	For moderate to severe disease and individuals whose symptoms worsen when discontinuing corticosteroids. Prior	Oral or injection

	Purixan) • Methotrexate (Rasuvo, Trexall, others)	testing may be required before taking these drugs.	
Antibiotics	• Ciprofloxacin (Cipro) • Metronidazole (Flagyl)	To treat infections of Crohn's disease, such as abscesses.	Oral or IV infusion

Sources: Crohn's & Colitis Foundation and MayoClinic.org

● ● ● ● ●

Medications for ulcerative colitis

Similar to Crohn's disease, some medications used to treat ulcerative colitis have been around for many years. Others, such as biological therapies, are newer. The most commonly prescribed drugs for ulcerative colitis fall into five basic categories. See thischart.

● ● ● ● ●

ULCERATIVE COLITIS MEDICATIONS

Drug class	Generic name (brand name)	Indications	Route of delivery
Aminosalicylates (5-ASA)	• Balsalazide (Colazal, Giazo) • Mesalamine (Delzicol, Rowasa, others) • Olsalazine (Dipentum)	For mild to moderate ulcerative colitis. Also used to maintain disease remission.	Oral or rectal

	• Sulfasalazine (Azulfidine)		
Corticosteroids	• Budesonide (Uceris) • Prednisolone • Prednisone	For mild to severe ulcerative colitis and to control disease flares. The medications shouldn't be used long term.	Oral, rectal or IV infusion
Biological therapies	• Adalimumab (Humira) • Golimumab (Simponi) • Infliximab (Remicade) • Vedolizumab (Entyvio)	To treat moderate to severe ulcerative colitis. Also effective for maintaining remission when tapering off corticosteroids. May be combined with an immunomodulator.	IV infusion or injection
Synthetic small molecule	• Tofacitinib (Xeljanz)	For moderate to severe disease. Not used in combination with biologicals or immunomodulators.	Oral
Immunomodulators	• Azathioprine (Azasan, Imuran) • Cyclosporine (Neoral, Sandimmune, Gengraf) • Mercaptopurine (Purinethol, Purixan)	For disease that doesn't respond adequately to aminosalicylates and corticosteroids and to reduce dependency on corticosteroids. Cyclosporine shouldn't be used long term.	Oral or injection

Sources: Crohn's & Colitis Foundation and MayoClinic.org

• • • • •

Other medications

In addition to medications to control inflammation from Crohn's disease and ulcerative colitis, a doctor may prescribe medications to help relieve other troublesome signs and symptoms. Depending on how severe these signs and symptoms are, your doctor may recommend one or more of the following drugs:

Pain relievers For mild pain, a doctor may recommend acetaminophen (Tylenol, others). Avoid aspirin, ibuprofen (Advil, Motrin IB, others) or naproxen sodium (Aleve). They may aggravate rather than reduce the signs and symptoms of IBD. For moderate to severe pain, a prescription drug may be more effective. Opioid medications should be avoided.

Iron supplements Blood loss from intestinal bleeding can cause iron deficiency anemia. Iron supplements help restore adequate blood levels of iron and cure this type of anemia. In addition to oral supplements, iron formulations also may be administered intravenously (IV).

Vitamin B-12 injections Vitamin B-12 is absorbed in the terminal ileum, a section of the small intestine commonly affected by Crohn's disease. If Crohn's is preventing the absorption of this vitamin, you may need B-12 shots. Vitamin B-12 helps prevent anemia, promotes normal growth and development, and is essential for proper nerve function.

Calcium and vitamin D supplements Crohn's disease and steroid medications used to treat it can increase your risk of osteoporosis. To help maintain bone mass, you may need to take a calcium supplement with added vitamin D.

●　●　●　●　●

WHAT ABOUT PROBIOTICS?

Probiotics are live bacteria that are similar to the beneficial ("good") bacteria that reside in your intestines. Beneficial bacteria may help keep the growth of harmful ("bad") bacteria in check. If the balance of good and bad bacteria is thrown off, harmful bacteria can overgrow and cause symptoms such as diarrhea and cramping.

It's believed that probiotics can help restore the balance of good bacteria in your gut. They're available as dietary supplements and they're naturally present in foods such as yogurt, miso and tempeh.

Currently, there's no strong evidence that probiotics heal or can treat symptoms of IBD. However, some people think they help. More research is needed to determine what role, if any, probiotics may play in managing IBD symptoms.

● ● ● ● ●

LIVING WITH IBD

Your experience with inflammatory bowel disease may include extended periods of remission, when the condition isn't as troublesome. Typically, however, the signs and symptoms return, and you again face the discomfort and concern of living with the disease. In addition to the medication your doctor prescribes, the following steps can help you manage your signs and symptoms and lengthen the time between flare-ups.

• • • • •

IBD AND OBESITY

People with inflammatory bowel disease (IBD) are often thought of as being underweight and malnourished. For many, that's not true. In fact, a recent study found that 15 to 40 percent of individuals with Crohn's disease or ulcerative colitis are overweight or obese.

If you have IBD and are overweight, it's important to try to lose some weight. Among other reasons, obese individuals with IBD are at greater risk of cardiovascular disease. In addition, being overweight may add to the complexity of your disease, including increased infections and hospitalizations and a reduced response to medication.

Trying to lose weight while also managing the symptoms of your disease may be challenging. The best approach is to consult with your doctor and meet with a registered dietitian to develop an eating and exercise plan to keep you healthy while you shed some pounds.

• • • • •

Manage your diet

There's no firm evidence that the types of food you eat contribute to inflammatory bowel disease. However, certain foods and beverages appear to aggravate signs and symptoms, especially during a disease flare.

It's also important to understand that what applies to someone else may not apply to you. Some people with IBD may need to restrict their diets all of the time, others only some of the time, and still others almost never.

If you suspect that a certain kind of food may make your condition worse, experiment with different foods and beverages to see if eliminating one or adding another helps you feel better. Do your experimenting carefully, and keep a food diary to help you identify troublesome foods. Here are some steps you can try:

Limit dairy products Some people with Crohn's disease and ulcerative colitis are able to reduce diarrhea, pain and gas when they limit their consumption of dairy products. These people may be lactose intolerant (see here). They aren't able to digest the lactose in dairy products because their bodies don't produce enough of the enzyme that breaks the substance down for absorption. If you find that dairy products seem to worsen your signs and symptoms, talk with a registered dietitian about designing a healthy, low-lactose diet.

Take care with fiber High-fiber foods, such as fruits, vegetables and grains, are the foundation of a healthy diet. But for some people with IBD, fiber can have a laxative effect, worsening diarrhea. Fiber may also increase gas and cramping. For these reasons, some people with Crohn's disease are advised to limit fiber in their diets.

Experiment with high-fiber foods to see if you're able to tolerate some better than others. In general, you may have more problems with foods in the cabbage family, such as broccoli and cauliflower, as well as foods such as nuts, seeds and popcorn. Raw fruits and vegetables also may be more bothersome than cooked versions.

If fiber remains a problem, you may need to restrict certain vegetables, fruits and grains in your diet. A dietitian can help you replace the nutrients that these foods provide.

Reduce fat People with severe Crohn's disease sometimes need to reduce the fat in their diets because their small intestines are no longer able to absorb fat. Instead, the fat passes through the digestive tract, causing or worsening diarrhea. Reducing fat generally isn't a problem, but if you're unable to maintain a healthy weight, talk with your doctor about increasing calories without increasing fat.

Drink plenty of fluids Beverages offset fluid loss from diarrhea. Drink at least eight 8-ounce glasses of fluid daily. Avoid beverages that contain alcohol, which can promote urination and fluid loss.

Other dietary suggestions These steps also may help improve your symptoms:

- Eat smaller meals at more frequent intervals.
- Eat more bland, soft foods, which may be easier to tolerate than spicy foods.
- Reduce the amount of greasy, fried foods in your diet, which can cause diarrhea and gas.
- Avoid carbonated beverages if excessive gas is a problem.
- Restrict caffeine if you experience severe diarrhea; caffeine can act as a laxative.

Consider multivitamins

Because IBD can interfere with the normal absorption of nutrients and because people with IBD may have a limited diet, your doctor may recommend that you take a multivitamin containing essential vitamins and minerals. Don't take any supplements without your doctor's supervision because ingredients in the supplement may interfere with your medication or your body's ability to absorb nutrients.

Consider curcumin for ulcerative colitis

Curcumin is a component of the Indian spice turmeric. You can purchase curcumin as tablets without a prescription. Studies found that tablets containing 95 percent curcumin taken at a dose of 3 grams daily may be beneficial when added to standard medication, such as aminosalicylates (5-ASA). Ask your doctor if you should consider taking curcumin.

Reduce stress

Stress doesn't cause inflammatory bowel disease, but it may worsen the signs and symptoms and trigger flare-ups. Many people with IBD report an increase in digestive problems when they're under moderate to severe stress.

Stress alters normal digestion. The stomach empties more slowly and acid-secreting cells release more digestive juices. Stress also speeds or slows the passage of food through the intestines, although much is still unknown about why this happens.

Some forms of stress can't be avoided. But stress can be managed with exercise, adequate rest and relaxation therapies, such as deep breathing, listening to music or practicing meditation.

Quit smoking

Smoking worsens symptoms of Crohn's disease. People with Crohn's disease who smoke are more likely to have relapses and need medications and repeat surgeries.

Seek support

Beyond the physical manifestations, Crohn's disease and ulcerative colitis can cause deep emotional scars. Chronic diarrhea may lead to embarrassing accidents. Some people become so humiliated socially that they isolate themselves, rarely leaving home. And when they do go out, they're often anxious and fearful. When IBS is left untreated, these factors — isolation, humiliation, anxiety — can severely affect quality of life and lead to depression.

Many people with IBD find emotional support simply by learning more about their disease. If you haven't done so already, schedule a time with a doctor to discuss your fears and frustrations and find answers to your questions about your condition. You might also consider joining a support group. Organizations such as the Crohn's & Colitis Foundation have chapters across the country. A doctor or another medical professional can help you locate a chapter near you.

Some people find it helpful to consult a psychologist or psychiatrist regarding their anxieties. Try to locate a professional who's familiar with inflammatory bowel disease and who understands some of the emotional difficulties it produces.

SURGERY

For most people with IBD, medication and lifestyle changes provide a significant improvement in their signs and symptoms. But some people eventually require surgery to treat IBD. A surgeon can provide information about the benefits and the risks so that you are fully aware of potential consequences of the procedure.

Crohn's disease

With Crohn's disease, removal of the damaged portion of the small intestine or colon can often provide years of relief, but surgery cannot cure the condition. The disease typically recurs, often requiring additional surgeries to remove more sections of diseased intestine.

During surgery for Crohn's disease, damaged portions of intestine are removed and healthy sections are reconnected. The surgeon may also place thin rubbery cords (setons) in fistulas, drain abscesses and open scar tissue (strictureplasty) that's blocking the intestinal passage.

Ulcerative colitis

Ulcerative colitis is different — surgery can cure the disease. However, the procedure requires complete removal of the colon and rectum. Surgery to remove the colon and rectum is call proctocolectomy.

Two options With the traditional approach to this surgery, an opening (stoma) about the size of a quarter is made in the lower right corner of the abdomen, near the waistline. After removal of the colon and rectum, the last portion of the small intestine (ileum) is attached to the abdominal wall to create a stoma. A plastic or latex bag (ileostomy bag) to collect waste is attached to the skin around the stoma with adhesive. You need to empty this bag several times a day and change it once or twice weekly.

The traditional approach is often the procedure of choice among individuals who don't have good control of the anal sphincter muscle and individuals who want to undergo only one operation.

Another surgical option is ileoanal anastomosis, which eliminates the need to wear an ileostomy bag. This surgery requires two or three operations.

First, a surgeon removes the colon and the innermost lining of the rectum. A J-shaped pouch is constructed from the end of the small intestine (ileum) and is attached directly to the anus and supported by remaining layers of rectal tissue (see this illustration). Waste is stored in the pouch and expelled normally, though bowel movements are more frequent and looser with an average of six formed or loose bowel movements a day.

During the first stage of surgery, the colon is removed, a J pouch is constructed, and a temporary ostomy is made using a loop of small intestine that's attached to an opening in the abdominal wall. An ileostomy bag is used to collect feces. This diverts the feces away from the ileal pouch until the new area of intestine has had time to heal. The ileostomy is closed during a second operation, which usually takes place about three months after the first.

In some individuals with IBD, including people who are undernourished or taking biological therapy drugs, three operations may be needed to complete an ileoanal anastomosis. In the first operation, a surgeon removes the colon and creates a temporary end ileostomy. Three months later, a second operation is performed to create the J pouch and place a temporary ileostomy. During a third operation approximately three months later, the temporary ileostomy is closed.

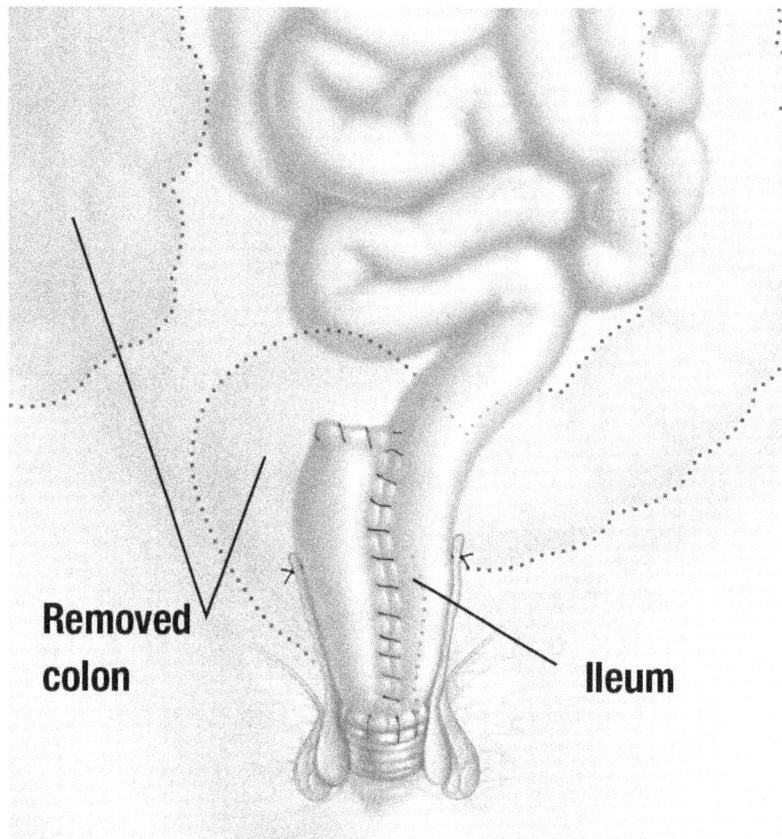

Removed colon

Ileum

In a procedure called ileoanal anastomosis, a surgeon removes the colon and innermost lining of the rectum, creates a J-shaped pouch out of the last section of the small intestine (ileum), then reattaches the pouch near the anal sphincter. Leaving the anal sphincter and rectal muscles intact allows near-normal passage of stool.

PREVENTING COMPLICATIONS

If you have IBD, it's important that you see a doctor regularly to monitor the effects of your medication and to watch for potential complications.

Laboratory monitoring

You may undergo periodic blood tests, including blood counts, to monitor for complications of disease or side effects from your medications. Because many individuals with IBD are iron deficient, blood iron levels are checked. Blood tests can also check for deficiencies in other nutrients such as vitamin B-12 and folate. In some cases, stool tests are performed to monitor disease activity.

Vaccinations

Individuals with IBD who take cortico-steroids, immunosuppressant medications or biological therapies are at increased risk of infections. Therefore, it's important that you are up to date on your vaccinations. This includes vaccinations for flu (influenza), pneumonia and shingles.

● ● ● ● ●

WHAT IS SHORT BOWEL SYNDROME?

Short bowel syndrome is a disorder that affects people who've had large portions of their small intestines surgically removed as a result of illness, such as Crohn's disease. The condition also can affect babies who are born with a short intestine or children and adults with a damaged small intestine that needs to be removed.

The small intestine is approximately 9 to 12 feet in length in a full-grown adult. Nearly all digestion of food and absorption of water and nutrients takes place in the small intestine. As a result, losing significant portions of the small intestine can have negative health effects.

When the small intestine has been shortened and the body is unable to absorb adequate water and nutrients to stay healthy, the condition is called short bowel syndrome. Effects of this condition can range from mild to life-threatening, depending on the location and how much of the small intestine is missing.

The most common symptom of short bowel syndrome is chronic diarrhea, which can cause malnutrition, dehydration and weight loss. Other symptoms may include abdominal pain, bloating, intestinal gas, heartburn, fatigue, weakness and food sensitivities.

For some people, short bowel syndrome is a temporary problem. Eventually, the small intestine adjusts to its shortened length. Others require treatment — often special diets and oral or intravenous nutritional supplements — to achieve adequate nutrition, manage signs and symptoms of the disorder, and prevent complications.

● ● ● ● ●

Cancer screening

Individuals with IBD are at increased risk of certain cancers, including colorectal cancer. Depending on the extent and duration of your disease, more-frequent cancer screenings may be recommended.

Osteoporosis screening

Many people with Crohn's disease or ulcerative colitis are at increased risk of bone loss. Periodic screenings for osteoporosis may be recommended, depending on age, health and use of corticosteroid medication.

Mental health screening

Because many individuals with IBD experience anxiety and depression, your doctor may inquire about your mental health.

• • • • •

IBD AND COLORECTAL CANCER SCREENING

Both Crohn's disease and ulcerative colitis can increase the risk of colorectal cancer. If you've experienced extensive inflammatory bowel disease of the colon for eight or more years, your doctor may recommend a colonoscopy exam every one to two years.

Fortunately, despite the increased risks, only a small percentage of people with IBD develop colorectal cancer.

●　●　●　●　●

CHAPTER 13

Diverticular disease

Many people develop small, bulging pouches in their digestive tracts as they get older. The pouches form when the inner layer of tissue in the intestinal walls pushes through weak spots in the outer, muscular layer.

Each pouch is called a diverticulum, from Latin words meaning "a small diversion from the normal path." The name for more than one diverticulum is diverticula. Diverticula, which can vary in size, often resemble a series of small balloons bulging outward (see this illustration).

Diverticula can form anywhere in your digestive tract, including the throat, esophagus, stomach and small intestine. But the most common location is your large intestine (colon), particularly on the left side in sections known as the descending colon and sigmoid colon.

The general term for this condition is diverticular disease, or diverticulosis. Diverticula by themselves generally don't cause problems, but sometimes the pouches become inflamed or infected, causing severe abdominal pain. When inflammation or infection develops in a diverticulum, the condition becomes known as diverticulitis.

DIVERTICULOSIS

Diverticulosis is relatively common and becomes more prevalent with age. More than half of people older than age 60 have diverticula somewhere along their digestive tracts, most often in their colons. The pouches — which are often about the size of a marble — ordinarily don't cause any problems, and many people don't even know they have them.

A minority of people with diverticulosis experience mild abdominal cramps, bloating, gas, diarrhea or constipation. However, these signs and symptoms are more likely related to other conditions, such as irritable bowel syndrome, and not to diverticulosis. Bleeding isn't typically a sign of diverticulosis, but it can occur in some people (see here).

● ● ● ● ●

DIVERTICULAR DISEASE

Key signs and symptoms:

- Pain in the lower left abdomen
- Abdominal tenderness
- Fever
- Nausea and vomiting
- Constipation or diarrhea

● ● ● ● ●

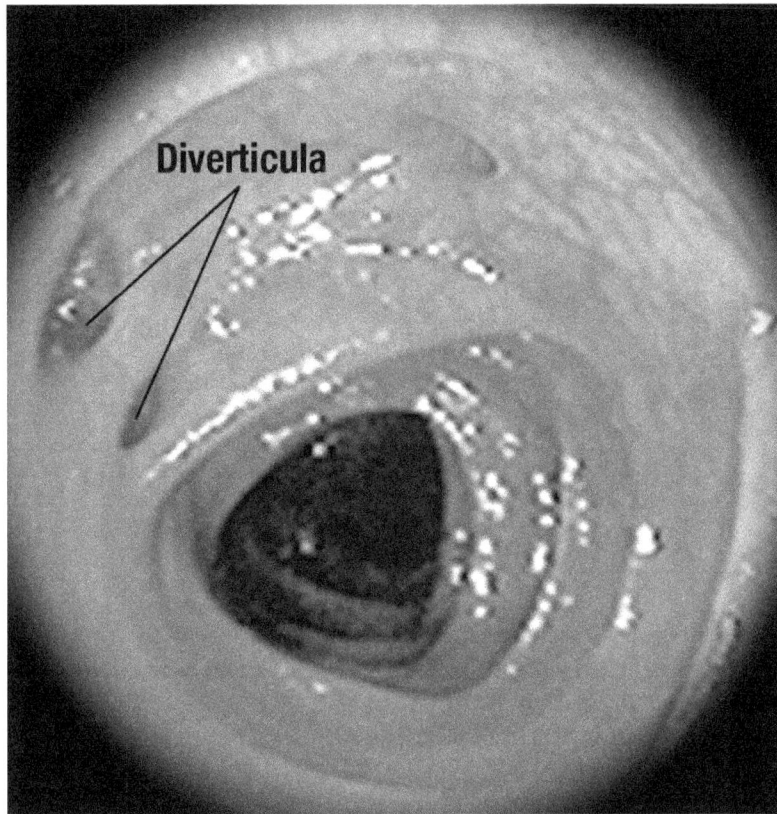

Diverticula

Pressure problems

The reason some people develop diverticula in their digestive tract while others don't isn't well-understood. The trigger appears to be strong pressure that's exerted within the digestive tract. This pressure forces inner layers of tissue to bulge outward through weak spots in the outer layers.

The colon is ringed by layers of muscle that regularly relax and contract. This action, called peristalsis, helps propel food waste through the digestive tract to the rectum. Blood vessels penetrate natural defects in the outer layers of the colon walls to deliver essential nutrients to the inner layers. These locations are structurally weaker than the rest of the colon wall and may be susceptible to outpouching.

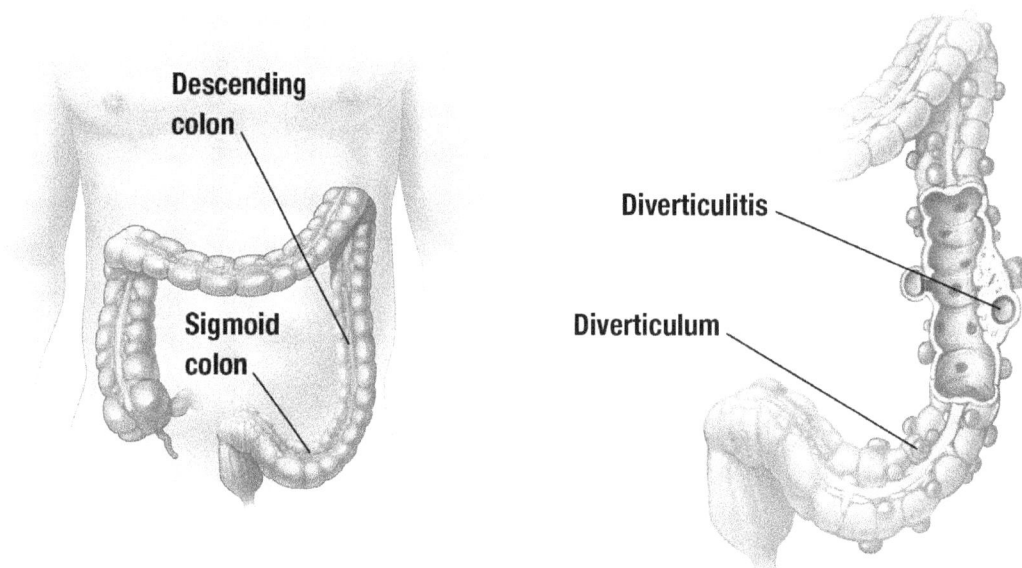

The most common locations for a small pouch (diverticulum) to form is in the descending and sigmoid sections of the colon. When a pouch becomes inflamed or infected, the condition is called diverticulitis. In this endoscopic image of the colon, diverticula are evident in the intestinal walls.

For example, when you strain to pass stool, you increase the pressure within your colon. This pressure can cause inner tissue to bulge through weakened spots, forming diverticula.

Several factors seem to play roles in the formation of diverticula:

Age Research suggests that as you age, your colon's outer muscular wall begins to thicken, causing the inner passageway of the colon to narrow. The narrowing increases the level of pressure in your colon, raising the risk of pouch formation.

Thickening of the outer wall also makes the colon less flexible, so it can't move food waste through as quickly. Waste stays in the colon longer, where it exerts pressure on the inner layers of tissue.

Diet Diverticular disease is most common in industrialized nations where the average diet is high in refined carbohydrates and low in fiber. In countries where people eat a high-fiber diet — often in places that are not as industrialized — the disease is rare.

Too little fiber in your diet contributes to small, hard stools or soft, mushy stools that are more difficult to pass through your intestinal tract. This increases the pressure in your colon. The highest pressures occur in the sigmoid colon, where most diverticula are found.

A diet high in fat or red meat also is associated with an increased risk of diverticular disease.

Physical inactivity Studies show that vigorous physical activity reduces the risk of diverticular disease. The less exercise you get, the greater your risk.

Obesity At least one large study found that obesity is associated with an increased risk of diverticular disease, as well as diverticular bleeding.

Tobacco use Smokers have a greater risk than do individuals who don't smoke.

Medications Some medications appear to increase the risk of diverticular disease, including nonsteroidal anti-inflammatory drugs (NSAIDs), steroids and opiates.

● ● ● ● ●

WHEN A POUCH BLEEDS

A few people with diverticulosis will experience painless rectal bleeding. The blood may be dark and mixed with stool, but more often it's bright red and plainly visible in the toilet bowl. The bleeding, which can appear suddenly, generally results from a weakened blood vessel that bursts.

Most often, the bleeding is short-lived and stops by itself, but sometimes it can be severe, requiring immediate medical attention. If there's noticeable blood with your bowel movements, seek immediate medical care.

For severe or persistent bleeding, you may need tests to identify the location of the bleeding. Occasionally, the only way to stop the bleeding is surgery to remove a segment of the colon where the bleeding pouch is located.

● ● ● ● ●

Treatment begins with self-care

The key to managing diverticular disease is reducing the pressure inside your colon. Often, this can be accomplished with routine steps you take at home. It's important to establish daily habits that keep your digestive tract healthy and functioning smoothly. Following are self-care steps for managing diverticular disease:

Eat more fiber High-fiber foods, such as fresh fruits and vegetables and foods made from whole grains, soften stool and help it pass more quickly through the colon. This reduces pressure inside your digestive tract and helps prevent episodes of diverticulitis.

For more information on how much fiber you should eat each day, <u>see here</u>.

People with mild signs and symptoms often find that after a week or two of consuming more fiber their condition begins to improve. However, avoid a large, sudden increase in dietary fiber, which can lead to gas, cramping, bloating and diarrhea. Gradually increase your fiber intake over several weeks.

If you find it difficult to consume the recommended amount of daily fiber, talk to your doctor about use of a natural fiber supplement. These include over-the-counter products such as psyllium (Metamucil) and methylcellulose (Citrucel). These products also help prevent constipation.

Drink plenty of fluids Fiber acts as a sponge in your colon, absorbing water into stool. As you increase the amount of fiber you eat, make sure you also drink plenty of liquid to replace lost fluid and prevent constipation. Each day, drink at least eight 8-ounce glasses of water or other nonalcoholic beverages.

Respond to bowel urges Anytime you need to pass stool, don't delay a trip to the bathroom. Delaying a bowel movement leads to harder stools, requiring more force to expel them and increasing pressure within your colon.

Exercise regularly Exercise promotes normal bowel function and reduces pressure inside your colon. Try to exercise 30 to 60 minutes on most days of the week.

DIVERTICULITIS

When inflammation or infection develops in a diverticulum, the condition becomes known as diverticulitis. Most people experience only minor inflammation, called simple (uncomplicated) diverticulitis. Others, meanwhile, can develop complications, including an abscess or a fistula, that may require surgery.

A cause of diverticulitis may be a small portion of stool becoming trapped in one of the pouches. The stool blocks the blood supply to the pouch and makes it susceptible to the invasion of bacteria. A small tear (perforation) also can develop in a diverticulum, leading to infection and, sometimes, a collection of pus.

Generally, inflammation or infection is limited to the area directly around the diverticulum. In rare cases, the pouch ruptures through a large perforation, spilling intestinal waste into your abdominal cavity. This can lead to an inflammation of the thin membrane that lines the abdominal cavity (peritonitis). This condition is usually very painful and often accompanied by fever and chills. Peritonitis is a medical emergency that demands immediate attention to fight the infection and treat the underlying condition.

Diverticulitis typically causes pain, fever, chills and nausea. The pain often is abrupt and severe, but some people experience mild pain that gradually worsens over several days.

Symptoms of diverticulitis are similar to those of appendicitis, except that the pain is usually in the lower left side of your abdomen, instead of the lower right. Less common signs and symptoms include vomiting, bloating, rectal bleeding, frequent urination, and difficulty or pain while urinating.

●　●　●　●　●

DON'T WORRY ABOUT SEEDS AND NUTS

You may have heard that eating nuts, popcorn or foods containing seeds, such as raspberries, strawberries or kiwis, is dangerous because the food particles and tiny seeds can become lodged in a diverticulum and cause inflammation or infection.

Recent research has found these foods aren't associated with an increased risk of diverticulitis. In addition, you don't want to forgo eating healthy fruits and vegetables that contain seeds for fear of infection. The nutrients and fiber these foods provide outweigh any increased risk of diverticulitis.

● ● ● ● ●

MAKING A DIAGNOSIS

Because the presence of diverticula alone generally doesn't cause signs and symptoms, most people learn they have diverticulosis during testing for other intestinal conditions or routine screening exams for colorectal cancer. Imaging tests such as colonoscopy, sigmoidoscopy, computerized tomography (CT) or colon X-ray may reveal one or more of the pouches. For more on these imaging procedures, see Chapter 5.

Diverticulitis, on the other hand, is typically diagnosed during an acute episode when signs and symptoms such as abdominal pain, fever and nausea compel you to see a doctor. The doctor likely will check your abdomen for areas of tenderness.

You may receive blood tests to check for signs of infection. An elevated number of white blood cells and tenderness in the lower left abdomen may signal diverticulitis. Other tests, such as a liver enzyme test, also may be performed to rule out other causes of abdominal pain.

Imaging tests such as a CT scan may help detect the inflammation or infection and confirm the diagnosis. During acute episodes of diverticulitis, tests such as colonoscopy, sigmoidoscopy, barium enema and CT colonography should not be performed.

TREATING DIVERTICULITIS

Acute episodes of diverticulitis signal the development of inflammation or infection in one of the diverticula. Seek medical care if you have a temperature above 100 F, experience worsening or severe abdominal cramps, or can't tolerate food or fluids.

Treating an attack of diverticulitis will depend on how severe your signs and symptoms are and whether this is your first attack. If signs and symptoms are mild, you may be able to manage the attack at home with changes to your diet and possibly a course of antibiotics to fight the infection. In case of more-severe symptoms, you may need to be hospitalized.

Hospitalization is more likely in people experiencing vomiting, high fever, high white blood cell count, or a possible bowel obstruction or in individuals at risk of peritonitis. You're also more likely to be hospitalized if you are older, are taking steroids, or have another disease or a weakened immune system.

Nonsurgical treatments include:

- ***Rest and restricted diet.*** A few days of rest allows time for the infection to heal. A liquid or low-fiber diet reduces contractions in your colon, which aids healing. In case of severe nausea and vomiting, you may have to avoid all food and take fluids intravenously. Once your signs and symptoms improve — often in two to three days — you can begin eating food.
- ***Antibiotics.*** Antibiotics kill bacteria causing the infection. Antibiotics may be administered intravenously (IV) in a hospital or taken in pill form at home.
- ***Painkillers.*** For moderate to severe pain, your doctor may recommend an over-the-counter or prescription analgesic for a few days until the pain improves.

Nonsurgical practices often are an effective treatment for a first attack of diverticulitis. Unfortunately, recurrent episodes are less likely to respond to simple measures.

Recurrent diverticulitis

Approximately 20 to 50 percent of individuals experience recurrent bouts of diverticulitis. You may be at an even greater risk if your first attack of diverticulitis occurred at a younger age. You can help prevent a second attack by eating more fiber, drinking plenty of liquids and getting plenty of exercise.

Among individuals who experience repeat episodes, antibiotics may be used to treat the condition, or your doctor may recommend surgery to remove the affected portion of the colon. Surgery generally prevents additional episodes of diverticulitis.

Your doctor will weigh your individual circumstances in determining the best approach to prevent recurrent disease.

Surgery

Surgery may be needed to treat your condition if one of the following complications occurs during an attack:

- An infection resulting from a ruptured pouch (peritonitis) that spills its contents into your abdominal cavity
- Blockage in your colon or small intestine caused by scar tissue
- Collection of pus in a pouch (abscess)
- Formation of a fistula, an abnormal passageway between two organs

Peritonitis requires emergency surgery and it may require the use of a temporary colostomy bag worn on the outside of the body to collect stool. Other problems, such as narrowing of the colon or formation of a fistula, may require surgery after the inflammation has subsided, usually about six to eight weeks after the attack.

An abscess can be drained, often without surgery, using a CT-guided needle to collect the pus. This procedure often takes place at the time of the attack. Surgery may still be needed later to prevent a recurrence.

Surgery also may be necessary if you've experienced previous episodes of diverticulitis. To prevent future infections, your doctor may recommend that the diseased portion of the colon be removed. Two forms of surgery may be performed.

Primary bowel resection This procedure is common in individuals who don't require emergency surgery. A surgeon removes the diseased part of the colon and then reconnects the remaining, healthy segments (anastomosis). This keeps the colon passage open and allows normal bowel movements.

The extent of the inflammation in the colon and other complicating factors, such as obesity, help determine who is a candidate for traditional surgery or minimally invasive (laparoscopic) surgery.

With traditional surgery, the surgeon makes one long incision in the abdomen. With laparoscopic surgery, three or four small incisions are made. Laparoscopic surgery requires less recovery time, but it generally isn't possible in people who are obese or have extensive inflammation or infection.

Bowel resection with colostomy This approach may be necessary when there's so much inflammation that it's not possible to rejoin the colon and rectum. A colostomy is necessary to eliminate stool.

A surgeon removes the diseased section of colon, closes off the upper part of the rectum and makes an opening in the abdominal wall. The colon is connected to this opening to create the colostomy. Stool passes through the opening and into a bag attached to the abdominal wall.

A colostomy may be temporary or permanent. Several months later — after the inflammation has healed — your doctor may consider a second operation to reconnect the colon and rectum. It's important that you discuss with your doctor the benefits and risks of such an operation.

● ● ● ● ●

AM I AT RISK OF CANCER?

There's no evidence that diverticulosis or diverticulitis increases your risk of colon or rectal cancer, or the formation of precancerous growths (polyps) in the lining of the colon or rectum. However, diverticular disease can make cancer more difficult to diagnose.

After an episode of diverticulitis, your doctor may suggest a colonoscopy or another screening test to make sure that you don't have cancer or some other inflammatory disease of the colon or rectum. The screening test is done several weeks after the episode, allowing time for healing.

● ● ● ● ●

CHAPTER 14

Gallbladder disease

It's bedtime, but you can't sleep. You have persistent pain in your upper abdomen and nothing relieves it — not antacids and not pain relievers. Changing your position doesn't help. You stand up, bend over, lie down, but the pain stays. Then, you start feeling nauseated.

When the pain spreads to your lower chest and back, you visit the emergency room, worried about a heart attack. At the hospital, you learn that the problem isn't your heart but your gallbladder. You're having a gallstone attack.

GALLSTONES

Gallstones are hardened deposits of digestive fluid that can form in your gallbladder. The gallbladder is a small, pear-shaped organ on the right side of your abdomen, just beneath your liver. It holds a digestive fluid called bile that's released into your small intestine. Sometimes these hard deposits ("stones") can lodge in the neck of the gallbladder, the narrow portion of the organ that connects to the cystic duct. This obstruction blocks the flow of bile, creating pressure and inflammation in the gallbladder and causing pain and often nausea.

Gallstones are common. More than 1 million Americans are diagnosed with gallstones each year. For most people, the stones cause no symptoms and require no treatment. Among some people, however, gallstones lead to painful attacks. Gallbladder attacks account for one of the most common operations in the United States. Surgery to remove the gallbladder is called cholecystectomy.

How gallstones form

Your gallbladder is a pear-shaped sac tucked under the liver, on the right side of your upper abdomen. The gallbladder is part of the biliary system that includes the liver and an intricate network of ducts for transporting bile.

● ● ● ● ●

GALLSTONES

Key signs and symptoms:

- Upper abdominal pain
- Pain in back, chest or right shoulder blade
- Nausea and vomiting

● ● ● ● ●

Bile is a digestive fluid produced in your liver. The gallbladder serves as a reservoir for bile until the fluid is ready for use in the small intestine. The composition of bile includes bilirubin, a greenish-yellow waste product from the liver that gives the fluid its color. That's why, if bile backs up into your blood, it can cause your skin and eyes to turn yellow (jaundice). Bile also contains cholesterol, bile salts and the chemical lecithin. Together, the bile salts and lecithin keep cholesterol dissolved in solution, allowing it to be excreted out of your body.

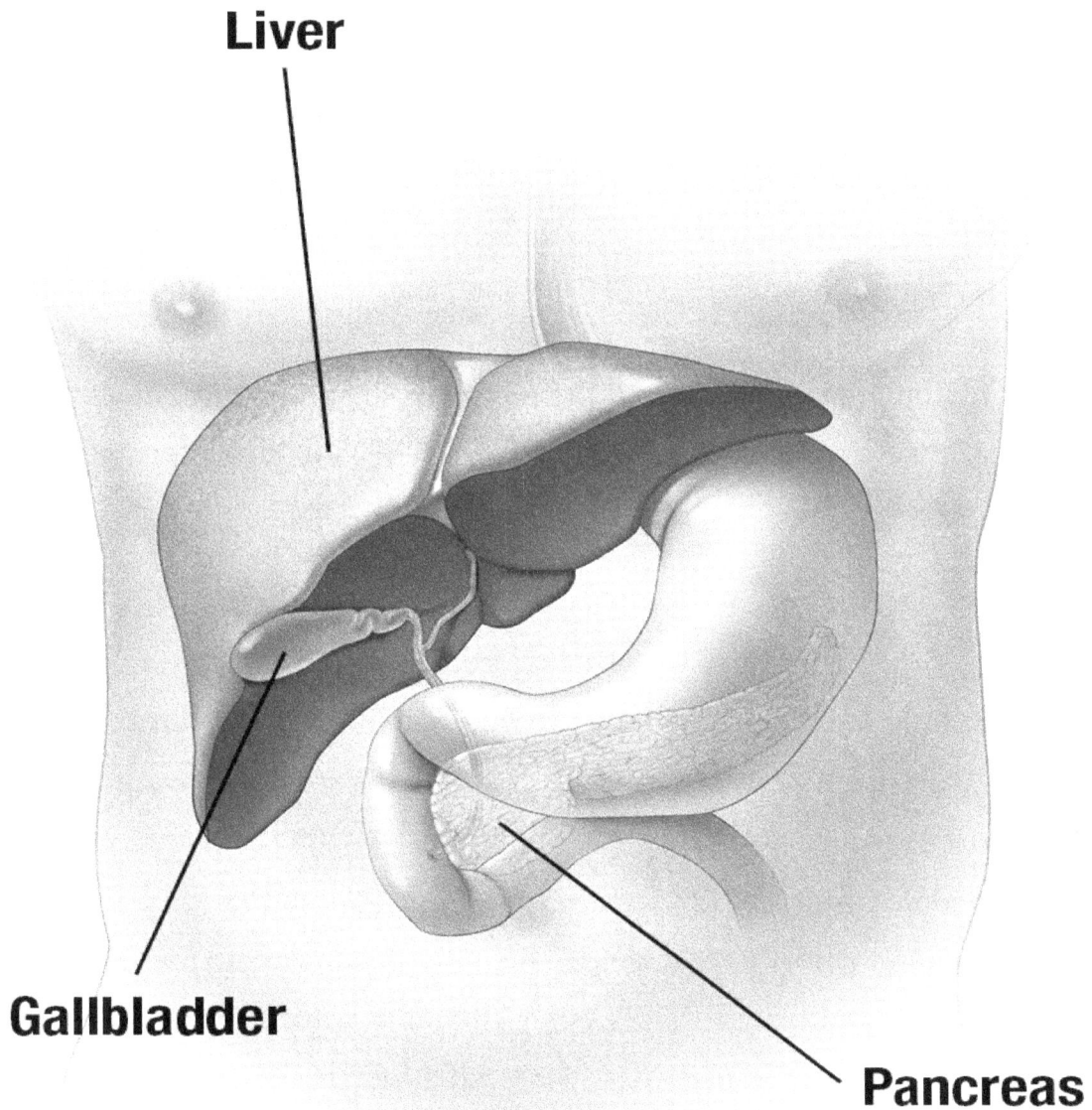

Liver

Gallbladder

Pancreas

The primary function of bile is helping break down fat molecules in the food you eat. When you eat a meal containing fat or protein, your gallbladder takes action. The organ contracts and empties the bile it holds in reserve through small tubes called bile ducts that lead to your upper small intestine (duodenum). Once in the duodenum, bile helps your small intestine digest and absorb fat and the fat-soluble vitamins A, D, E and K. Without the action of bile, these nutrients would be flushed out of your system as waste.

When bile becomes chemically imbalanced, it forms into hardened particles, which can form into stones as small as a grain of sand or bigger than a golf ball. Some people have just one stone, while others have multiple stones that may number in the hundreds or even thousands, sometimes referred to as gravel, sand or sludge.

Multiple factors may contribute to the formation of gallstones, many of which aren't well-understood. Factors that may lead to stone formation include:

- *Excess cholesterol.* Normally, your bile contains enough chemicals to dissolve the cholesterol excreted by your liver. But if your bile contains more cholesterol than can be dissolved, the extra cholesterol may eventually form into stones. Obesity, genetics and rapid weight loss may contribute to this process.
- *Gallbladder doesn't empty correctly.* Your gallbladder may fail to contract and empty as it should. This may occur during pregnancy or from prolonged fasting. The longer bile stays in your gallbladder, the more concentrated it becomes. Bile that's too concentrated can become sludgy and form stones.
- *Excess bilirubin.* Certain conditions, such as liver cirrhosis, may cause too much of the chemical bilirubin to exist in bile, potentially contributing to the formation of gallstones.

Types of stones

Not all gallstones have the same composition. Gallstones are composed of a mixture of cholesterol, calcium salts of bilirubinate or palmitate, proteins, and mucin, a constituent of mucus. Gallstones are broadly classified into the following varieties:

- *Cholesterol stones.* Cholesterol stones account for about 80 percent of all gallstones. They're composed primarily of cholesterol produced in your liver that bile is unable to keep dissolved. They often contain other components and usually appear yellow in color.
- *Pigment stones.* Pigment stones form when bile contains too much bilirubin. Pigment stones are generally small and dark brown or black in color. Some are associated with excess production of bilirubin due to excessive red blood cell destruction, and others from severe scarring of the liver (cirrhosis).

Stones that escape from the gallbladder and lodge in the bile ducts are known as secondary or retained duct stones. Primary bile duct stones actually form in the bile ducts. The stones are usually soft and brown, made of decomposed bile, and occur when a bile duct is narrowed because of infection, trauma, surgery or disease.

GALLSTONE ATTACK

Gallstones usually settle at the bottom of the gallbladder and don't cause any problems. Some people associate gallstones with heartburn, indigestion or bloating. However, there's no evidence that gallbladder disease causes these signs and symptoms.

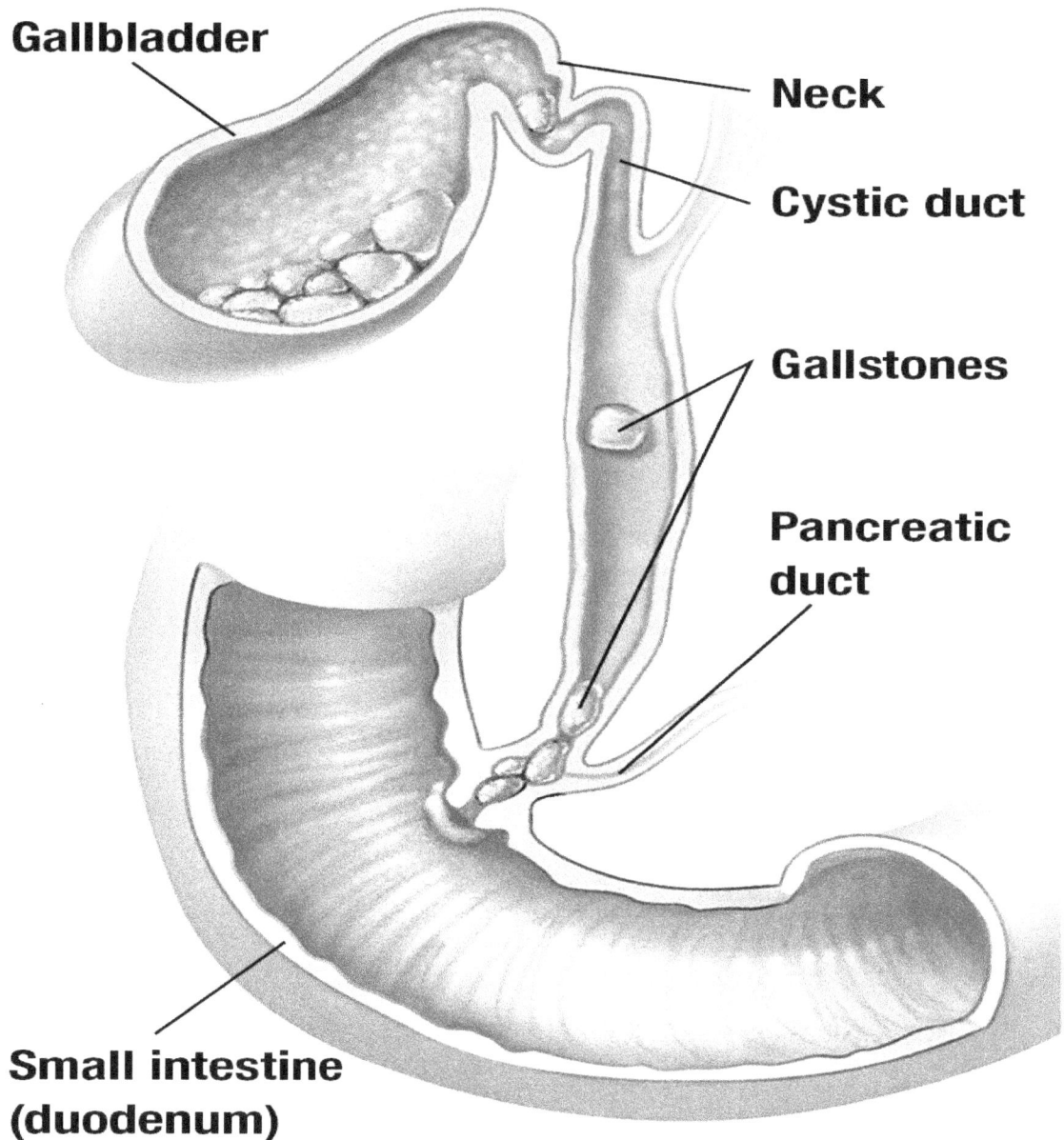

Gallbladder

Neck

Cystic duct

Gallstones

Pancreatic duct

Small intestine (duodenum)

A gallstone attack can occur when stones lodge in a bile duct or the gallbladder neck.

It's when the stones migrate up to the neck (outlet) of the gallbladder that problems may develop. When your gallbladder expels bile into the biliary system, some of the stones may be carried along with the fluid.

The smallest stones usually pass through the bile ducts, enter the small intestine and leave your body without incident. But larger gallstones can get stuck at the entrance to the cystic duct, within a bile duct or at the entrance to the small intestine.

When a gallstone blocks the flow of bile from the gallbladder, it can cause nausea and steady pain. This is what's known as a gallbladder attack. The attack may last from several minutes to several hours.

Usually, a stone lodged at the entrance to the cystic duct will drop back down to the bottom of your gallbladder. That reopens the passage and generally signals the end of the attack. If the stone doesn't work its way free, inflammation and infection may occur within the gallbladder (cholecystitis). Once you've had a gallbladder attack, your risk of another attack is increased.

Other signs and symptoms of a gallbladder attack may include fever, chills, nausea, vomiting, belching, bloating and feeling especially full after meals (early satiety).

Complications can occur when:

- Gallstones collect at the entrance to the small intestine and block the pancreatic duct, causing inflammation of the pancreas (pancreatitis).
- The cystic duct remains blocked, and infection causes the gallbladder to rupture, although rupture is rare.
- A stone lodged in a bile duct blocks bile flow from the liver, which may cause jaundice, as well as fever, chills, blood infection (bacteremia), inflammation of the bile duct system (cholangitis) or pancreas (pancreatitis) and a potentially life- threatening immune system response to a bacterial infection (sepsis).

Individuals with a history of gallstones are at increased risk of gallbladder cancer. But cancer of the gallbladder is rare, so even with an elevated risk the chance of developing it is still very small.

ARE YOU AT RISK?

The reasons why gallstones develop in some people and not in others is unclear. Factors that may put you at increased risk include:

Age and being female

The risk of gallstones increases with age. One reason may be that your liver tends to secrete more cholesterol into bile as you age.

Women are more likely than men to have gallstones. However, with age, the difference between the two decreases. In one study, the prevalence of gallstones was two to three times greater in women age 50 or younger compared with men the same age, but after age 50, the difference was less than twice as great.

Women may be at greater risk because of the hormone estrogen, which exists in much higher amounts in women than in men. Estrogen causes the liver to excrete more cholesterol into bile, increasing the likelihood of stone formation.

Family history

Gallstones often run in families, pointing to a possible genetic link. One study involving twins suggests that approximately 25 percent of gallstone disease risk is determined by an underlying genetic predisposition.

Pregnancy

Pregnancy is a risk factor for the development of cholesterol stones. Increased levels of reproductive hormones during pregnancy can produce a change in bile composition and cause delayed gallbladder emptying. Both actions promote stone formation.

Obesity

Studies indicate obese people have a greater risk of developing gallstones than people at a healthy weight. Excess cholesterol tends to accumulate in the bile of people who are overweight. Excess weight also decreases bile salt formation, as well as the ability of your gallbladder to contract and empty.

Rapid weight loss

Fasting and rapid-weight-loss diets also increase your risk of gallstone formation. The reason why isn't completely understood. One possibility might be that rapid weight loss alters the levels of bile salts and cholesterol and throws your bile chemistry out of balance.

Diabetes

Diabetes is associated with an increased risk of cholesterol stones, but how it exaggerates risk isn't well-understood. The mechanism of insulin resistance that keeps blood sugar (glucose) from entering the body's cells is believed to play a key role.

Medications

Some medications may increase a person's risk of gallstones. These include fibrate medications used to lower blood triglyceride levels, the antibiotic ceftriaxone taken to fight infection, somatostatin analogues used to control hormone production, and hormone replacement therapy to control estrogen levels. Women taking oral contraceptives may be at a slightly increased risk during the first few years of use.

MAKING A DIAGNOSIS

If your doctor suspects that your abdominal pain may be caused by gallstones, you'll probably undergo one or more tests to locate the stones. They generally include an ultrasound examination and blood tests. (For more details, see Chapter 5).

Gallbladder images

Your doctor may recommend an abdominal ultrasound or a computerized tomography (CT) scan to create pictures of your gallbladder. These images can be analyzed to look for signs of gallstones. An ultrasound examination can detect stones in your gallbladder with high accuracy. A computerized tomography (CT) scan of your abdomen can sometimes reveal gallstones that contain high levels of calcium.

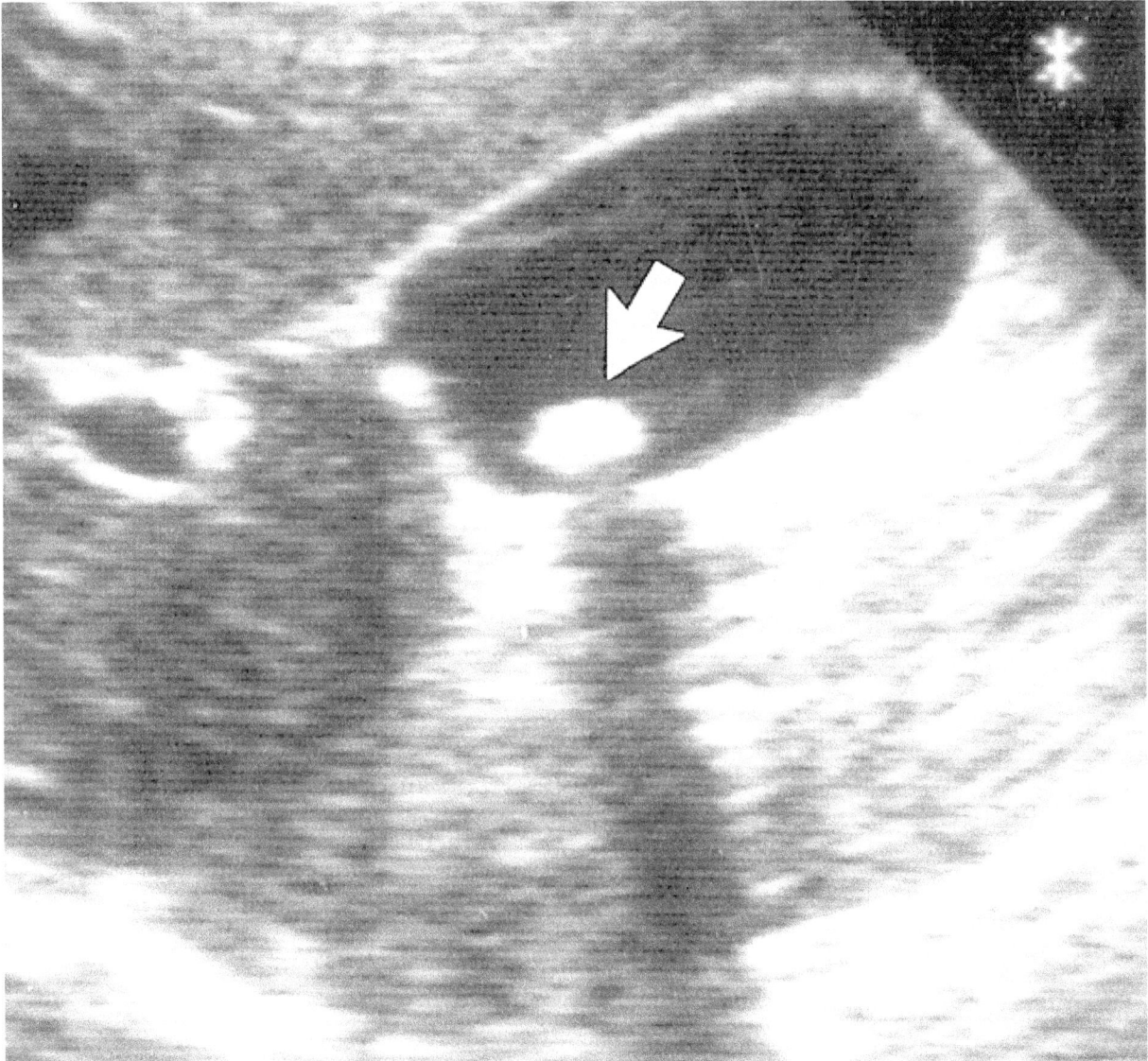

Ultrasound image of a large gallstone (arrow) inside the gallbladder

Bile duct exams

Tests that use a special dye to highlight your bile ducts on images may help your doctor determine whether a gallstone is causing a blockage. Tests may include a hepatobiliary iminodiacetic acid (HIDA) scan, magnetic resonance cholangiopancreatography (MRCP) or endoscopic retrograde cholangiopancreatography (ERCP). The test your doctor recommends will be based on a number of factors, including the probability of finding a stone in the bile duct.

A HIDA scan, which is less reliable, uses a radioactive tracer to track the flow of bile from your liver to your small intestine. A small amount of tracer is injected intravenously and absorbed by the liver. The scan will show when bile infused with the tracer reaches your gallbladder.

MRCP is an imaging technique that uses magnetic resonance imaging (MRI) to visualize the biliary and pancreatic ducts in a noninvasive manner. The procedure can help determine if gallstones are lodged in any of the ducts surrounding the gallbladder.

ERCP allows your doctor to examine your bile ducts for blockage. While you're sedated, a flexible tube with an attached camera (endoscope) is threaded through your digestive tract to the opening of the common bile duct in your upper intestine (duodenum). Dye injected from a catheter inside the scope enters the duct to outline the biliary system on X-ray images. Gallstones discovered using ERCP often can be removed during the procedure.

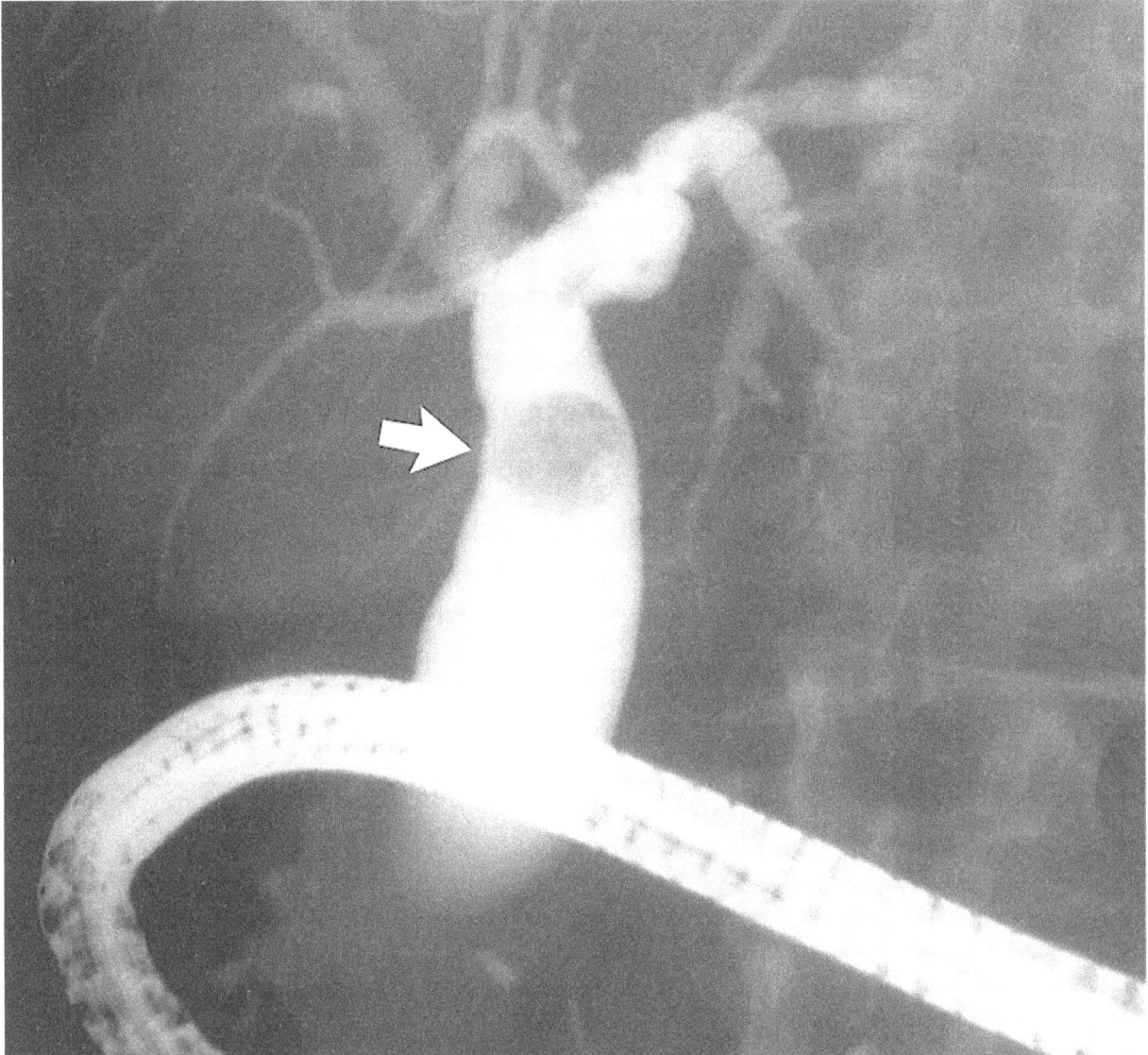

This ERCP image reveals a large gallstone (arrow) wedged in a dilated bile duct. The flexible endoscope used for the imaging test appears in the foreground.

Blood tests

Blood tests may reveal an infection, jaundice, pancreatitis or other complications caused by gallstones.

TREATMENT OPTIONS

Often, the best treatment for stones that aren't causing problems ("silent stones") is to do nothing more than watch and wait. Silent stones usually are discovered by accident, during diagnostic testing for other conditions.

In case of an acute attack, the first step is often medication to relieve the pain. Pain relievers such as nonsteroidal anti-inflammatory drugs (NSAIDs) often can control gallbladder pain. For severe pain, prescription medications may be administered intravenously in the hospital, followed by oral medications taken at home. Your doctor also may recommend surgery to remove the gallbladder to prevent future attacks.

Gallbladder removal may be advised when there's evidence of inflammation or infection in the organ or indications of possible precancerous growths (polyps) or cancer. Fortunately, the liver can directly supply bile to the small intestine when the gallbladder is removed. When surgery isn't possible, other options may be used.

● ● ● ● ●

CAN YOU PREVENT GALLSTONES?

Some home remedies recommend drinking olive oil, apple juice or lemon juice to stimulate your gallbladder to empty out small stones. However, these practices have demonstrated no beneficial effect. To date, no diet has been shown to prevent gallstones. However, there are some indications that taking vitamin C supplements, eating nuts rich in monounsaturated and polyunsaturated fats, and consuming coffee may reduce gallstone formation.

Other steps you can take to lower your risk of gallstones include:

- *Maintain a healthy weight.* If you're overweight, take steps to gradually lose weight. It's one of the most important things you can do to prevent gallstones. A good approach is to eat three well-balanced meals that are high in fiber, calcium and other essential nutrients and low in saturated fats. Eating meals at the same time each day helps promote gallbladder emptying.
- *Exercise.* Exercise helps you to maintain a healthy body weight. Researchers speculate that physical activity also may help stabilize the delicate chemical balance of bile, helping to keep cholesterol dissolved in solution and inhibiting the formation of stones.
- *Avoid extreme diets.* Stay away from diets that involve a low intake of calories and rapid weight loss. When you don't eat for a long time or lose weight rapidly, the body metabolizes fat, causing the liver to secrete extra cholesterol into bile, putting you at risk of gallstones.

● ● ● ● ●

Surgery

Surgery to remove the gallbladder is called a cholecystectomy. It's generally safe and effective, and one of the most common surgical procedures performed in the United States. Complete removal of the gallbladder is the preferred option because removing just the gallstones is often a temporary fix — new stones can form and attacks recur.

Cholecystectomy is performed in one of two ways:

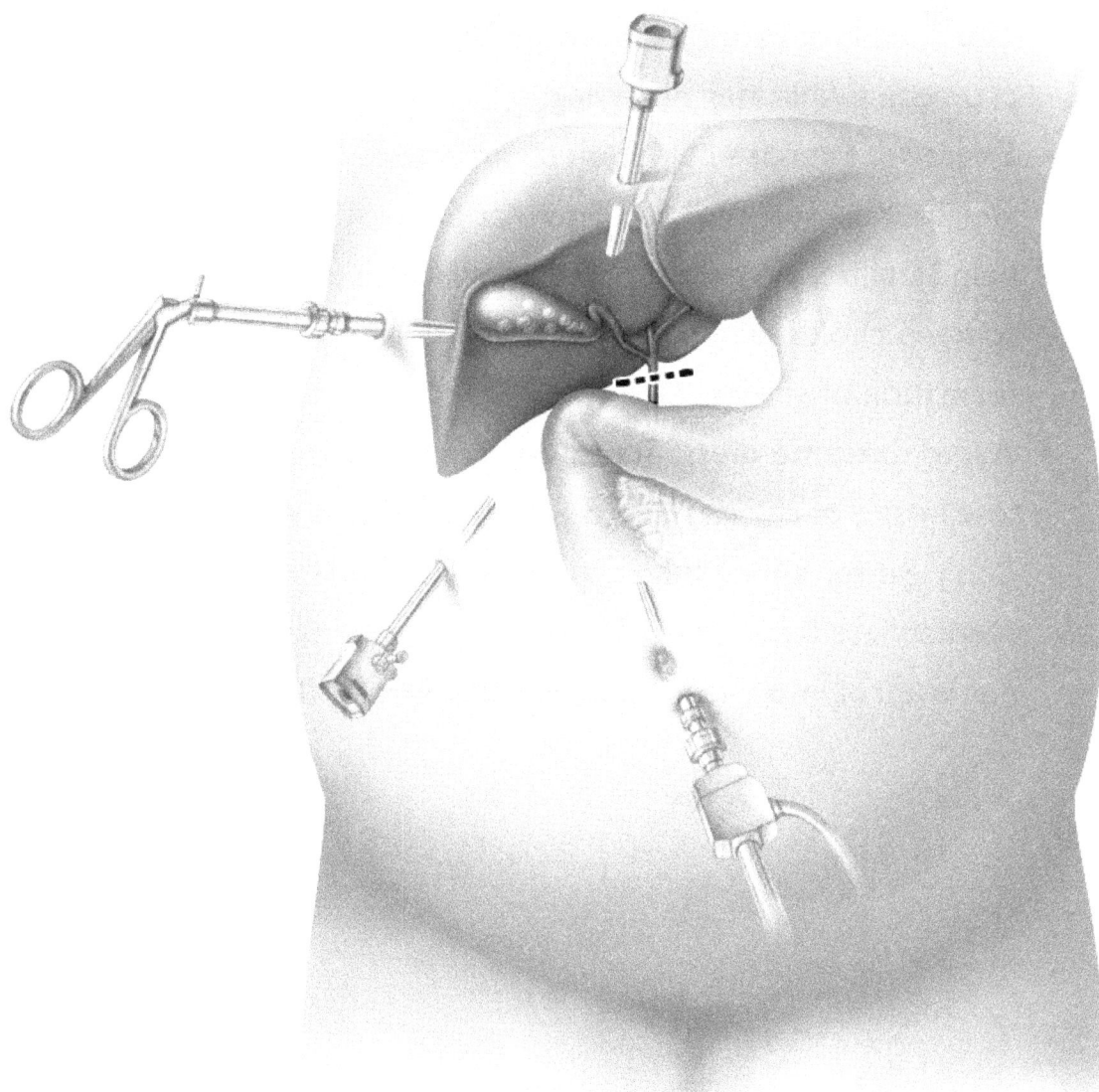

Special surgical tools are inserted through four small incisions in your abdomen during laparoscopic cholecystectomy.

Laparoscopic surgery The majority of gallbladder surgeries are done laparoscopically. With laparoscopic surgery, several small incisions are made in your abdomen instead of one large one (see the illustration below).Instruments inserted through the incisions include an endoscope equipped with a camera for viewing the gallbladder and another equipped with a cutting device to remove the gallbladder.

Recovery time is shorter than with open surgery because the incisions are small and the surgeon doesn't have to cut through abdominal muscles, which take longer to heal. Other advantages include less pain and less scarring.

Open surgery With open surgery, the gallbladder is removed through a large abdominal incision. A surgeon may recommend this approach if your gallbladder walls are thick and hard, or there's scar tissue from earlier abdominal operations. Recovery typically is longer.

Other options

Your doctor may recommend other approaches if you have complications or concerns that make surgery inadvisable.

Bile acid dissolution therapy This option involves taking bile acid tablets that dissolve cholesterol stones over several months or years. It may be effective for individuals with small stones. The tablets don't work on pigmented stones or stones that are heavily surrounded by calcium. Unfortunately, gallstones often form again once the treatment is stopped. To keep the stones from coming back, you may need to take the medication indefinitely.

Percutaneous removal This procedure, performed in highly specialized medical centers, involves inserting a small flexible tube (catheter) into the gallbladder to drain and relieve the obstruction caused by the stones. The hole through which the catheter is placed is gradually enlarged over a period of weeks and the stones are removed through the hole. However, gallstones commonly recur over a period of a few years.

Shock wave therapy In very rare instances, a procedure that uses shock waves to break up the gallstones into very small fragments may be performed. The fragments are then dissolved with medication. The procedure can be uncomfortable and it doesn't always work.

LIFE WITHOUT A GALLBLADDER

Most people who have surgery to remove their gallbladders get along well without them. Your liver continues to produce enough bile to digest the fat consumed in your diet. But instead of being stored in your gallbladder, bile flows out of the liver and empties directly into your small intestine.

You don't need to change your eating habits after surgery. However, with bile flowing more frequently into your small intestine, you may experience more bowel movements and your stools may be softer. Often, these changes are temporary. Over time your intestines adjust and bowel movements become more normal.

In some people, additional bile in the small intestine leads to a condition called bile-salt associated diarrhea. If the amount of bile in the small intestine is excessive, medication may be prescribed to treat the problem.

GALLBLADDER AND BILE DUCT CANCERS

Gallbladder cancer is rare. It's most common in people who've had gallstones, but even in this group, the cancer is very uncommon. Other factors that increase your risk of gallbladder cancer are being female — the cancer is more common in women — advancing age and other gallbladder conditions, such as chronic infection or gallbladder polyps.

● ● ● ● ●

GALLBLADDER CANCER

Key signs and symptoms:

- Abdominal pain and bloating
- Fever
- Weight loss
- Nausea
- Yellowing of skin and eyes (jaundice)

● ● ● ● ●

Most gallbladder cancers are adenocarcinomas. These are cancers that start in the glandular cells that line the inner surface of the gallbladder. When a tumor is discovered early, your chance of finding a cure is good. But because the disease causes few signs and symptoms, it's rarely diagnosed in the early stages. When signs and symptoms do develop, they're generally a result of the cancer invading adjacent structures, such as the bile ducts, and causing jaundice.

Cancer of the bile ducts (cholangiocarcinoma) may involve the network of tiny bile channels within the liver or occur in ducts located outside the liver. Primary sclerosing cholangitis, an inflammatory condition associated with ulcerative colitis, is a known risk factor.

Diagnosis and treatment

Early-stage cancer is often found incidentally during surgery to remove gallstones. Ultrasound imaging may identify gallbladder cancer, but often when the disease is in a late stage. Other imaging techniques, such as computerized tomography (CT) or magnetic resonance imaging (MRI) provide little help in detecting early-stage gallbladder cancer but may be useful in determining how advanced the cancer is. An imaging procedure called cholangiography that looks into the bile ducts can show if a person has a tumor that's blocking a bile duct.

Surgery to remove the gallbladder may cure early-stage cancer but is ineffective for the later stages. Gallbladder cancer that extends beyond the gallbladder and into the liver is sometimes treated with surgery to remove the gallbladder, as well as portions of the liver and bile ducts that surround the gallbladder. For advanced cancer, the focus of treatment is on relieving pain and improving quality of life through medications or radiation therapy.

Cancer of the bile ducts usually grows slowly, spreads gradually and is often not diagnosed until advanced stages. It's generally treated with chemotherapy and surgery to remove the tumor. Treatment may also include radiation therapy. If surgery isn't possible, your doctor may place a tiny tube (stent) to keep the cancerous duct open, preventing blockage and relieving jaundice.

The prognosis for gallbladder cancer and cancer of the bile ducts depends on how advanced the cancer is and the extent to which it has spread.

CHAPTER 15

Pancreatic disease

It's a stomachache like you've never felt before. Severe pain that bores right through your upper abdomen, from the chest to the back. Lying flat on your back causes your stomach to hurt more, but leaning forward and doubling over offers some relief. Your breathing becomes shallow because taking deep breaths causes even more pain. These symptoms are typical of pancreatitis, an inflammation of the pancreas.

The pancreas is a very important part of your digestive system. The organ is a long, flat gland tucked behind your stomach. The pancreatic duct connects the pancreas to the common bile duct leaving your gallbladder. The combined duct empties into the upper section of the small intestine (duodenum).

The pancreas has two main functions:

- It produces digestive juices and enzymes that help break down fats, carbohydrates and proteins in your small intestine.
- It secretes the hormones insulin and glucagon into your bloodstream, along with somatostatin, a hormone that helps control their function. The primary role of these hormones is to regulate how your body metabolizes sugar (glucose).

When the pancreas becomes inflamed, digestive functions are disrupted. There are two forms of pancreatitis — acute and chronic. The pain of acute pancreatitis is often sudden, severe and steady, and lasts for days. In contrast, chronic pancreatitis occurs in intermittent episodes and the pain often builds gradually. Chronic pancreatitis can occur over many years.

Most cases of pancreatitis are mild, but some people experience moderate to severe pancreatitis that doesn't permanently damage the pancreas or other organs.

• • • • •

PANCREATITIS

Key signs and symptoms:

- Upper abdominal pain and tenderness
- Abdominal pain that radiates to the back
- Abdominal pain that feels worse after eating
- Fever
- Nausea and vomiting
- Rapid pulse

• • • • •

ACUTE PANCREATITIS

Each year, acute pancreatitis results in about 275,000 hospitalizations in the United States. For unknown reasons, it appears the condition is becoming more common. The main symptom is steady pain in the upper abdomen that springs up suddenly. The pain often radiates to the back and chest and usually persists for hours or days without relief.

Acute pancreatitis is thought to be caused by digestive enzymes that your body activates too soon. Normally, the enzymes produced in the pancreas are manufactured in an inactive form. Only after they're transported through the pancreas and into the upper small intestine do they become active. If these enzymes are activated while still in the pancreas, they irritate and inflame the gland, sometimes destroying delicate pancreatic tissues.

Eating or drinking alcohol typically makes the symptoms worse. Many people with acute pancreatitis sit up and bend forward or curl up in a fetal position because these positions seem to relieve the pain.

People with pancreatitis often feel and look extremely sick. They frequently experience nausea and vomiting. Other signs and symptoms may include a high fever, difficulty breathing and abdominal swelling (distention). The pain may become so severe that hospitalization is necessary.

Causes of acute pancreatitis

Acute pancreatitis can occur for various reasons but, in some cases, its cause remains unknown. The two most common causes are gallstones and excessive alcohol use.

Gallstones Many people with acute pancreatitis have gallstones. Sometimes, the stones migrate out of the gallbladder and move through the common bile duct. They may become lodged at the junction with the pancreatic duct, near the entrance to the upper small intestine (duodenum), blocking the flow of pancreatic juices into the digestive tract and triggering an attack of pancreatitis that may be mild to severe. Usually, blockage of the duct is temporary, and the stones spontaneously pass into the duodenum. However, the pancreas remains inflamed despite passage or removal of the stones.

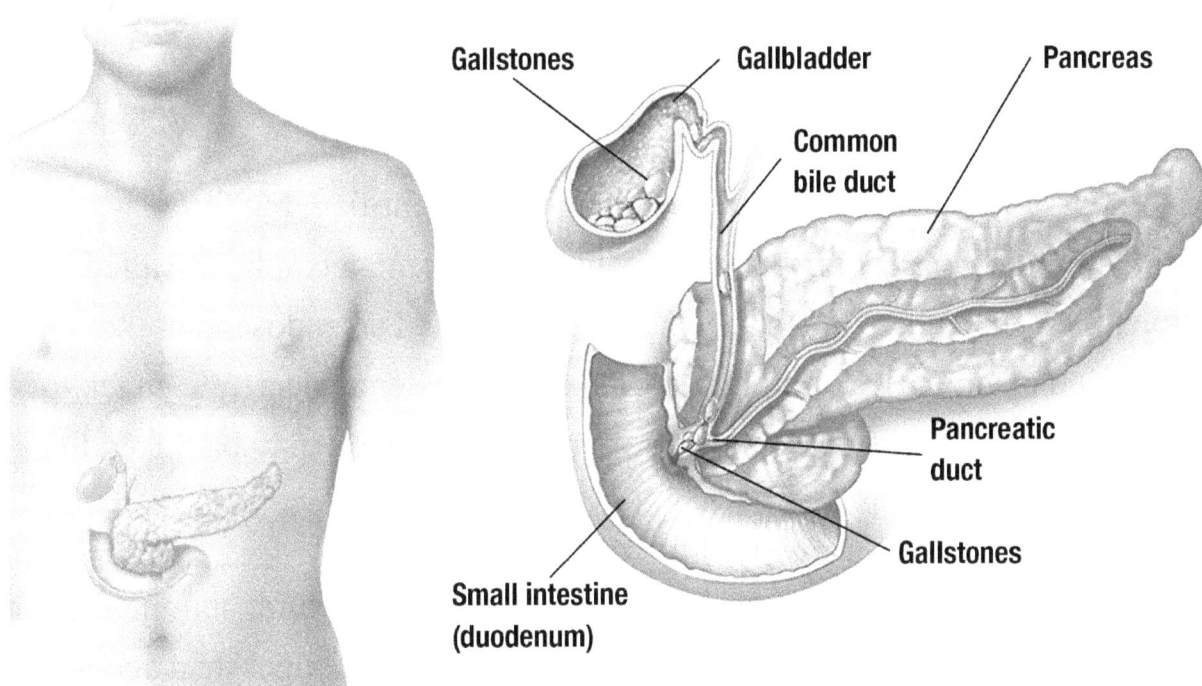

Gallstones that leave the gallbladder and block the pancreatic duct are a common cause of acute pancreatitis. Digestive juices produced by the pancreas become trapped, inflaming delicate tissues.

Alcohol Heavy alcohol use over several years is another leading cause of acute pancreatitis. Alcohol is responsible for approximately 25 to 35 percent of cases of acute pancreatitis in the United States. It's unclear how alcohol damages the pancreas. A common theory is that it directly injures pancreatic tissues. Genetic and environmental factors also may influence the development of pancreatitis. Many individuals who consume large amounts of alcohol also smoke.

Less common causes Other factors that may lead to acute pancreatitis include:

- Certain medications, including certain diuretic blood pressure,

autoimmune, antibiotic and cancer drugs
- Hereditary conditions such as high blood triglyceride levels
- Injury to the abdomen
- Major abdominal surgery or certain invasive diagnostic tests
- Family history of acute pancreatitis

Many possible causes for pancreatitis have been identified, but for a surprising number of individuals, no cause is apparent, a condition called idiopathic pancreatitis. Your doctor may recommend an endoscopic ultrasound examination approximately six weeks after a pancreatic attack to see if a cause is more apparent. It's possible some attacks may be linked to gallstones that, initially, are too small to identify.

Idiopathic pancreatitis may also be associated with a structural abnormality or a genetic mutation. It's recommended that individuals younger than age 35 who experience an attack of idiopathic pancreatitis undergo genetic testing.

●　●　●　●　●

AUTOIMMUNE PANCREATITIS

Autoimmune pancreatitis (AIP) is a newly recognized, chronic inflammation thought to be caused by the body's immune system attacking the pancreas. There are two subtypes of AIP:

Type I. This type is also called IgG4-related pancreatitis and is part of a disease called IgG4-related disease (IgG4-RD) that often affects multiple organs including the pancreas, bile ducts in the liver, salivary glands, kidneys and lymph nodes. In the United States, about 80 percent of people with autoimmune pancreatitis have type 1. These individuals are often male and older than age 60.

Type 2. This type is also known as idiopathic duct-centric pancreatitis. It seems to affect only the pancreas, although about one-third of people with type 2 AIP have associated inflammatory bowel disease, such as ulcerative colitis. Type 2 is most common in people age 40 or older and occurs in men and women equally.

Autoimmune pancreatitis is rare and it can be mistakenly diagnosed as pancreatic cancer. The two conditions have similar signs and symptoms, but very different treatments, so it's important to distinguish one from the other.

The most common sign of AIP is painless jaundice, caused by blocked bile ducts. AIP can also cause weight loss. Many people with autoimmune pancreatitis have masses in the pancreas and other organs or general enlargement of the pancreas. Because its signs and symptoms are very similar to those of pancreatic cancer, it can be difficult to diagnose. To make an accurate diagnosis and determine which type of AIP you have, your doctor likely will order blood and imaging tests.

The disease is typically treated with steroid therapy. Among people who don't respond to steroids, medications that alter the body's immune response (immunomodulatory medications) may be prescribed. Surgery generally isn't necessary for autoimmune pancreatitis.

● ● ● ● ●

Complications of acute pancreatitis

Acute pancreatitis can lead to a variety of complications, such as destruction of part of the pancreas, inflammation and fluid buildup in and around the gland, and the failure of other organs, including the heart, lungs and kidneys. Serious complications include:

Necrotizing pancreatitis Severe inflammation of the pancreas can cause tissue within the pancreas to die (necrotize). Fluid that contains dead tissue may collect within the pancreas. As the fluid accumulates, it may obstruct neighboring organs.

Infected pancreatic necrosis Necrotizing pancreatitis can lead to an infection that produces a high fever and worsening illness. Treatment generally involves procedures to drain the infected fluid and remove the dead tissue.

Organ failure Severe pancreatitis may be associated with the failure of other organs — notably the kidneys, lungs and heart — and the body's blood coagulation system. These complications, which can be accompanied by infection, are the most life-threatening. Fortunately, multiple organ failure is rare.

Kidney failure If the kidney failure is severe and persistent, it can be treated with dialysis.

Breathing problems Chemical changes in the body that affect lung function can cause the level of oxygen in blood to fall to dangerously low levels.

DIAGNOSING ACUTE PANCREATITIS

If your doctor suspects acute pancreatitis, he or she will check your abdomen for pain and tenderness and perform diagnostic tests. Tests and procedures used to diagnose acute pancreatitis include:

- Blood tests to look for elevated levels of pancreatic enzymes
- Computerized tomography (CT) to look for masses and determine the extent of the inflammation
- Abdominal ultrasound to look for gallstones, stones in the common bile duct and inflammation
- Endoscopic ultrasound to look for inflammation, masses and blockages in the pancreatic duct or bile duct
- Magnetic resonance imaging (MRI) to look for abnormalities in the gallbladder, pancreas and ducts

Your doctor may recommend other tests, depending on your particular situation. If you have two of three main signs and symptoms of pancreatitis — characteristic pain, significantly elevated pancreatic enzymes and imaging that shows inflammation or damage to pancreatic tissue — a diagnosis of pancreatitis is likely.

TREATING ACUTE PANCREATITIS

Treatment of acute pancreatitis usually requires a hospital stay. If you have complications, you may be admitted to the intensive care unit. Treatment generally focuses on hydration with intravenous fluids, controlling the pain, and identifying and treating the complications.

Initially, until a diagnosis is made, you may be asked to avoid eating. After it's been determined that you have pancreatitis, you may be allowed to eat, as tolerated. If eating is difficult, a feeding tube may be inserted for a short period. As your symptoms improve, your doctor will likely recommend that you start eating orally again. Early re-initiation of food is often associated with improved outcomes.

If your attack is caused by gallstones blocking the common bile duct, your doctor may recommend a procedure called endoscopic retrograde cholangiopancreatography (ERCP) to remove the stones. A long tube containing a camera is passed down your throat and into your upper intestine to examine your pancreas and bile ducts. The camera sends pictures of your digestive tract to a monitor. In addition to diagnosing problems in the bile and pancreatic ducts, ERCP may be used to make repairs or remove smaller stones.

If you have gallstones, it's likely you'll also need surgery to remove your gallbladder. In addition, endoscopic procedures or surgery are sometimes necessary to drain fluid from your pancreas or remove diseased tissue.

If alcohol is the cause, treatment may include therapy to stop drinking. Abstaining from drinking alcohol helps reduce the chances of future attacks. However, it doesn't guarantee a cure. If you smoke, it's also important that you quit smoking.

Mild cases of acute pancreatitis generally improve in a few days. Moderate to severe cases may take longer to resolve. Once the inflammation is under control, you may begin drinking clear liquids and eating bland foods again. With time, you can go back to your normal diet.

CHRONIC PANCREATITIS

Chronic pancreatitis differs from acute pancreatitis in that the inflammation occurs over many years. Chronic pancreatitis can be more difficult to diagnose because the damage occurs slowly and it may take a while before the signs and symptoms appear. In the early stages of chronic pancreatitis, you may experience mild to severe episodes similar to acute pancreatitis.

On occasion, a complication of acute pancreatitis, such as damage to the pancreatic duct, can lead to chronic pancreatitis. Sometimes, young adults with cystic fibrosis and associated gene abnormalities have episodes of acute pancreatitis that eventually develop into chronic pancreatitis. In addition, some people are born with a hereditary form of pancreatitis that can cause acute attacks during childhood or adolescence but eventually develops into chronic pancreatitis.

While some people with chronic pancreatitis experience no pain, many have intermittent periods of mild to moderate abdominal pain. The pain may be sharp and last for a few hours, or it may be a continuously dull ache that lasts for weeks. In addition to pain, other symptoms of chronic pancreatitis include nausea and vomiting, fever, bloating, and gas. Eating or drinking alcohol may worsen symptoms.

While acute pancreatitis often resolves spontaneously without long-term complications, the chronic form often causes permanent organ damage. As the inflammation persists, it slowly destroys tissue in the pancreas. The gland becomes less able to produce enzymes and hormones necessary for digestion.

An inadequate supply of digestive enzymes and hormones leads to poor absorption of nutrients, particularly fat. Malabsorption of nutrients is what causes weight loss and the passage of fat-containing stools that are loose, foul smelling and oily in appearance. Eventually, the cells that produce insulin become impaired, resulting in diabetes. Malabsorption and diabetes often don't appear until almost all of the gland has been destroyed.

Causes of chronic pancreatitis

Some of the most common causes of chronic pancreatitis include:

- Heavy alcohol use
- Recurrent episodes of acute pancreatitis
- A family history of chronic pancreatitis
- Genetic abnormalities
- Blockage of the pancreatic duct
- Cystic fibrosis
- Very high triglyceride levels

Complications of chronic pancreatitis

Complications of acute pancreatitis, such as tissue death (necrosis), infection and organ failure, rarely occur in chronic pancreatitis. Complications of chronic disease include:

Pseudocysts Cystlike, fluid-filled blisters called pseudocysts may form on the pancreas or extend from the gland after an attack of acute pancreatitis. If the cyst is small, no special treatment is necessary. If it is large and becomes infected or causes bleeding, intervention is necessary. Your doctor may drain the cyst through an endoscopic- or radiologic-guided catheter, or you may need surgery to remove the cyst.

Diabetes Damage to insulin-producing cells in your pancreas from chronic pancreatitis can lead to diabetes, a disease that affects the way your body uses blood sugar.

Malnutrition Both acute and chronic pancreatitis can cause your pancreas to produce fewer of the enzymes that are needed to break down and process nutrients from the food you eat. This can lead to malnutrition, diarrhea and weight loss, even though you may be eating the same foods or the same amount of food.

Pancreatic cancer Long-standing inflammation in your pancreas caused by chronic pancreatitis is a risk factor for developing pancreatic cancer.

DIAGNOSING CHRONIC PANCREATITIS

To confirm a diagnosis of chronic pancreatitis, your doctor will likely take samples of blood and stool. Blood tests can help determine the cause of pancreatitis as well as identify inflammation. The stool test measures fat content in your feces. When fat isn't absorbed in the small intestine, it is passed in stool.

Your doctor may have you undergo X-ray, computerized tomography (CT), magnetic resonance imaging (MRI) or endoscopic procedures to look for evidence of a blockage in the pancreatic duct or common bile duct or scarring in the pancreas. You may also need additional tests if your doctor is concerned about the possibility of other diseases, such as pancreatic cancer.

Having chronic pancreatitis puts you at a slightly higher risk of pancreatic cancer.

TREATING CHRONIC PANCREATITIS

The main goals of treatment for chronic pancreatitis are to control pain and treat malabsorption problems. Unlike acute pancreatitis, in which pain often disappears within a few days to weeks, with chronic pancreatitis, pain lingers. In fact, persistent pain may be the greatest challenge of managing the condition.

Your doctor may prescribe supplements containing pancreatic enzymes, in addition to conventional pain relievers. This therapy is thought to increase the levels of digestive enzymes that are active in your upper intestine (duodenum). This decreases the demand for the secretion of enzymes from the pancreas, reducing accompanying pain and pressure within the organ.

For severe pain that can't be controlled, treatment options include surgery to remove damaged tissue or procedures to block pain signals or deaden nerves transmitting the pain.

Malabsorption therapy

Enzyme supplements containing pancreatic lipase and other digestive enzymes (Creon, Pancreaze, others) can help treat malabsorption caused by pancreatitis. The tablets replace enzymes no longer produced by the pancreas, helping to restore normal digestion of fat, protein and carbohydrates.

Depending on the amount of enzymes in the supplements, you may take up to three to five tablets with your meals — one to two tablets after a few bites of food, one tablet at the end and the rest spread throughout the meal. Supplements should also be taken with snacks.

Diabetes

Chronic pancreatitis may cause diabetes. Treatment is similar to that of type 2 diabetes and usually involves maintaining a healthy diet and getting regular exercise. Some people also need insulin injections. Your doctor can explain how to manage the condition and prevent complications.

LIVING WITH CHRONIC PANCREATITIS

Unlike acute pancreatitis, in which people recover completely, chronic pancreatitis often causes problems that come and go. Even if you don't have lingering signs and symptoms, it's important to keep your pancreas healthy.

- *Alcohol.* If you can't voluntarily stop drinking alcohol, seek treatment. Abstaining from alcohol may not reduce the pain, but it will reduce your risk of dying of your disease.
- *Smoking.* In people with pancreatitis, smoking reduces pancreatic function, hastens the development of stones that block the pancreatic duct and increases the risk of pancreatic cancer. If you smoke, stop.
- *Meals.* The more food you eat during a meal, the greater the amount of digestive juices your pancreas must produce. Instead of large meals, eat smaller, more frequent meals.
- *Pain.* Talk with your doctor about your options for controlling pain.

Prescription and over-the-counter pain relievers are effective, but they carry risks of side effects, including dependency and stomach problems.

PANCREATIC CANCER

The American Cancer Society estimates that in 2019 about 56,770 people will be diagnosed with pancreatic cancer and about 45,750 will die of pancreatic cancer. While pancreatic cancer accounts for only about 3 percent of all cancers in the United States, it's responsible for about 7 percent of all cancer deaths.

● ● ● ● ●

PANCREATIC CANCER

Key signs and symptoms:

- Pain in the upper abdomen
- Weight loss
- New-onset diabetes
- Fatigue
- Yellowing of skin and eyes (jaundice)
- Depression

● ● ● ● ●

Pancreatic cancer often spreads rapidly to nearby organs. The cancer doesn't cause symptoms right away, and when they do develop, they're often vague.

Risk factors

It's unclear what causes most pancreatic cancers. Risk factors include:

- Chronic inflammation of the pancreas (pancreatitis)
- Diabetes
- Family history of certain genetic syndromes, such as BRCA2, p16 and the genes responsible for Lynch syndrome
- Family history of pancreatic cancer
- Obesity
- Smoking
- Age, especially if you're over age 65

Diagnosis

If your doctor suspects pancreatic cancer, he or she may have you undergo one or more of the following tests:

- ***Imaging tests that create pictures of your internal organs.*** These tests help your doctors visualize your internal organs, including the pancreas. Techniques used to diagnose pancreatic cancer include ultrasound, computerized tomography (CT) scans, magnetic resonance imaging (MRI) and, sometimes, positron emission tomography (PET) scans.
- ***Use of a scope to create ultrasound pictures of your pancreas.*** Endoscopic ultrasound (EUS) uses an ultrasound device to make images of your pancreas from inside your abdomen. The device is passed through a thin, flexible tube (endoscope) down your esophagus and into your stomach in order to obtain the images.
- ***Removal of a tissue sample for testing (biopsy).*** During a biopsy, a

small sample of tissue is removed and examined under a microscope. Your doctor may obtain a sample of tissue from the pancreas by inserting a needle through your skin and into your pancreas (fine-needle aspiration). Or he or she may remove a sample during EUS, guiding special tools into the pancreas.

- ***Blood test.*** Your doctor may test your blood for specific proteins (tumor markers) shed by pancreatic cancer cells. One tumor marker test used in pancreatic cancer is called CA19-9. But the test isn't always reliable, and it isn't clear how best to use the CA19-9 test results. Some doctors measure your levels before, during and after treatment.

● ● ● ● ●

IDENTIFYING THE CANCER EARLIER

Researchers believe that pancreatic cancer develops in a series of steps known as pancreatic intraepithelial neoplasia (PanIN). Early in the process, changes occur in a small number of genes, and the duct cells of the pancreas look fairly normal. In later steps, changes develop in several genes and the duct cells appear more abnormal.

Researchers are using this information in hopes of developing tests to identify the cancer in its earlier stages. One of the most common DNA changes affects the KRAS oncogene, which affects regulation of cell growth. New diagnostic tests are often able to recognize this mutation in samples of pancreatic juice collected during an endoscopic retrograde cholangiopancreatography (ERCP) procedure.

For now, genetic tests to detect changes in certain genes — such as KRAS — are options for people with a strong family history of pancreatic cancer. They're not recommended for widespread testing among people at average risk without symptoms.

Research is taking place on several other fronts. Among individuals older than age 50 who develop diabetes, studies indicate that about 1 percent have pancreatic cancer. Researchers are actively investigating how to use this information to help diagnose pancreatic cancer earlier.

Researchers are also looking to see if groups of proteins found in the blood might be used to find pancreatic cancer early. Some early results with this approach have been promising, but more studies are needed to confirm its usefulness.

● ● ● ● ●

TREATING PANCREATIC CANCER

Treatment may include surgery, radiation, chemotherapy or a combination. Researchers are finding the order in which the treatments are given is important. For people who are candidates for surgery, chemotherapy and radiation (chemoradiation) administered before surgery, called neoadjuvant therapy, may be the most appropriate. For some people, chemotherapy makes surgery feasible, which otherwise wouldn't be possible.

When pancreatic cancer is advanced and these treatments aren't likely to offer any benefit, the goal of treatment is to make you as comfortable as possible.

Types of surgery used in people with pancreatic cancer include:

- ***Surgery for tumors in the pancreatic head.*** If your cancer is located in the head of the pancreas, your doctor may recommend an operation called a Whipple procedure (pancreaticoduodenectomy). The Whipple procedure is a technically difficult operation to remove the head of the pancreas, the first part of the small intestine (duodenum), the gallbladder and part of the bile duct. In some situations, part of the stomach and nearby lymph nodes may be removed as well. The surgeon reconnects the remaining parts of your pancreas, stomach and intestines to allow you to digest food.
- ***Surgery for tumors in the pancreatic body and tail.*** Surgery to remove the left side (body and tail) of the pancreas is called distal pancreatectomy. The surgeon may also remove your spleen.
- ***Surgery to remove the entire pancreas.*** In some people, the entire pancreas may need to be removed. This is called total pancreatectomy. You can live relatively normally without a pancreas but do need lifelong insulin and enzyme replacement.
- ***Surgery for tumors affecting nearby blood vessels.*** Many people with advanced pancreatic cancer aren't eligible for the Whipple procedure or other pancreatic surgeries if their tumors involve nearby blood vessels. At some medical centers in the United States, highly specialized and experienced surgeons will safely perform these operations with removal and reconstruction of parts of blood vessels in select patients.

Chemotherapy is often combined with radiation therapy. Chemoradiation is typically used to treat cancer that has spread beyond the pancreas, but only to nearby organs and not distant regions of the body. At specialized medical centers, chemoradiation may be used before surgery to help shrink the tumor. Sometimes it's used after surgery to reduce the risk that pancreatic cancer may recur.

In people with advanced pancreatic cancer, chemotherapy may be used to control cancer growth and prolong survival.

CHAPTER 16

Liver disease

The liver is your largest single internal organ and possibly the most complex. It consists of two main lobes, and its specialized cells are connected by the body's biliary system — an intricate system of bile ducts and blood vessels.

The liver is a hardworking and multitasking organ that goes about its duties without drawing much attention to itself. For that reason, it may be easy to ignore the liver until something goes wrong. Signs and symptoms that people often chalk up to stomach or intestinal problems, such as lack of appetite, weight loss and nausea, may actually stem from a liver disorder.

Due to its complexity and frequent exposure to many potentially harmful substances, the liver is vulnerable to infection, inflammation and blockage. There are more than 100 liver diseases and conditions, and at times the damage that occurs to the organ can be hard to reverse.

WHAT DOES THE LIVER DO?

The liver plays a critical role in your body's metabolic, digestive and regulatory systems. You might think of it as the body's main manufacturing center.

Production

The liver processes most of the nutrients absorbed from your intestines and converts them into forms that can be used by your body. The liver also manufactures cholesterol, blood-clotting factors, specific proteins such as albumin and bile, a fluid that's essential for the digestion of fat. In addition, it regulates the composition of your blood, in particular, the amounts of sugar (glucose), protein and fat that enter your bloodstream.

Waste

The liver filters waste from your blood. It converts some potentially harmful substances, drugs and toxins into forms that are less harmful and can be removed from your body via bile and, subsequently, stool.

Storage

The liver stores nutrients such as iron, vitamins and carbohydrates (glycogens) for later use and makes them available when needed.

Liver

Bilary system

Gallbladder

Stomach

Small intestine

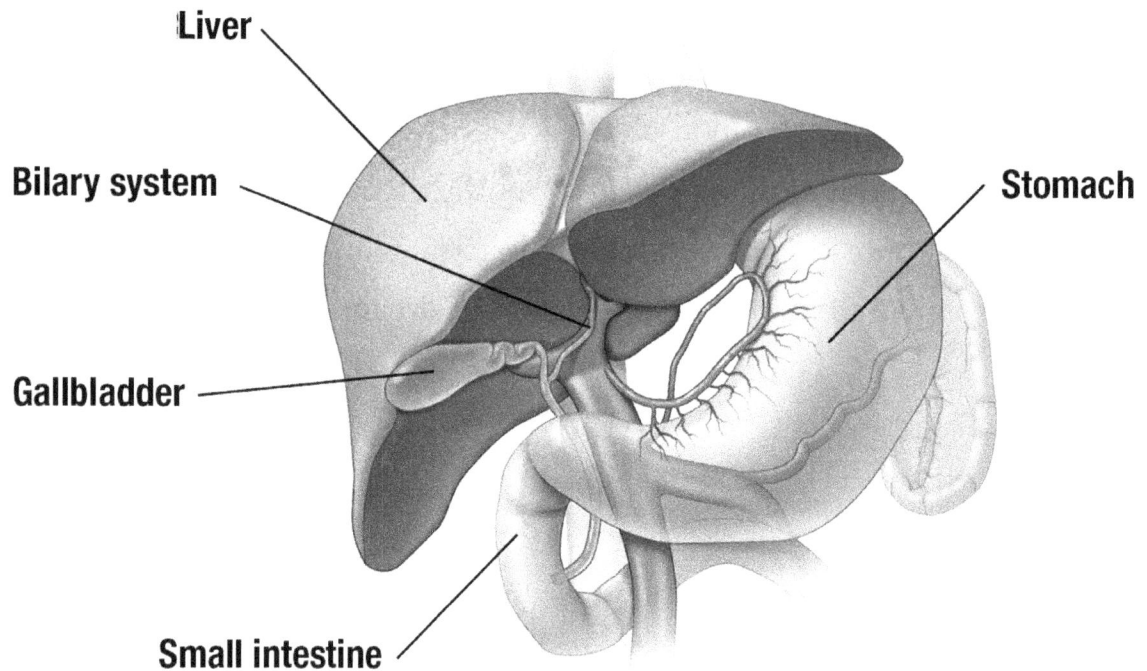

LIVER DISEASE

Liver problems include a wide range of diseases and conditions that damage liver tissue or impair its function. These conditions may be associated with a variety of factors, such as an infection, trauma or exposure to toxins. They may also stem from inflammation or scarring of the liver.

If your liver isn't functioning properly, your body may not be getting the nutrients it needs. This can lead to weight loss and fatigue. A buildup of waste and toxins in your blood can cause yellowing of your skin and eyes (jaundice), as well as loss of appetite, nausea and, sometimes, vomiting. Other indications of possible liver disease include swelling of the ankles, fluid accumulation in the abdominal cavity (ascites), bruising and confusion (hepatic encephalopathy).

Diagnosing liver disease

For some liver conditions, fatigue and jaundice are early indicators. For others, weight loss or abdominal discomfort may be the most common symptoms.

If your doctor suspects liver disease, he or she may ask you a series of questions regarding your health and lifestyle. A physical examination is typically the next step in making a diagnosis. Your doctor will likely feel (palpate) your upper abdomen for evidence of an enlarged, shrunken or hardened liver. He or she will also look for other signs and symptoms of liver disease, such as swelling of the abdomen, legs and ankles, and jaundice.

In addition, you'll likely undergo tests to measure certain enzymes or proteins in your blood. Blood tests for liver disease, called liver tests or liver function tests, can identify a variety of abnormalities:

- ***Liver cell and bile duct damage.*** If liver cells are inflamed or damaged, the enzymes normally found in those cells will leak into the bloodstream and show up in test results. Two tests that check for elevated enzyme levels are the alanine aminotransferase (ALT) and aspartate aminotransferase (AST) tests. The enzyme alkaline phosphatase is produced primarily by cells located in small bile ducts in your liver. Its levels may increase with conditions that affect the ducts or liver.
- ***Reduced liver function.*** When your liver is impaired, usually because of severe injury, it's not able to produce protein (albumin) as it normally does, or provide certain blood clotting factors (prothrombin). Albumin level and prothrombin time tests measure these functions. Low albumin and elevated prothrombin indicate reduced liver function.
- ***Increased bilirubin.*** Bilirubin is a substance produced by the normal

breakdown of red blood cells. If your liver isn't removing bilirubin, this test detects elevated levels that circulate in your bloodstream. Certain blood diseases also can increase bilirubin levels in blood.

For some liver diseases, blood tests provide a clear enough indication to make a diagnosis. For others, your doctor may order additional tests that show images of the liver, and he or she may take samples of liver tissue (biopsy) for laboratory examination. The samples can help identify specific diseases. They may also indicate the severity of liver inflammation and whether there's any permanent liver damage.

INFECTIOUS HEPATITIS

The most common liver disease is hepatitis, an inflammation of the liver. If an organ becomes inflamed, it's trying to fight an infection or heal an injury. In addition to causing pain and swelling, inflammation disrupts your liver's ability to filter harmful substances from your body.

When that happens, waste products such as bilirubin build up in your bloodstream, causing your skin and eyes to turn yellow (jaundice). If the inflammation continues without treatment, your liver may become permanently damaged. There are several forms of hepatitis.

●　●　●　●　●

HEPATITIS

Key signs and symptoms:

- Fatigue
- Nausea and vomiting
- Loss of appetite
- Unexplained weight loss
- Low-grade fever
- Dark urine
- Yellowing of skin and eyes (jaundice)

● ● ● ● ●

Hepatitis A

Hepatitis A is a highly contagious liver infection caused by the hepatitis A virus. The virus is one of several types of hepatitis viruses that cause inflammation and affect your liver's ability to function.

Signs and symptoms such as fatigue and nausea typically don't appear until you've had the virus for a few weeks. But not everyone with hepatitis A develops them.

Transmission Common routes of transmission of hepatitis A include:

Contaminated food and water Hepatitis A most commonly spreads when you eat or drink something contaminated with fecal matter, even tiny amounts. This can happen when you consume food handled by someone who doesn't thoroughly wash his or her hands after using the toilet.

Other routes of transmission include drinking contaminated water, eating raw shellfish harvested from contaminated water, or eating unpeeled fruit or vegetables rinsed in contaminated water. Outbreaks of hepatitis A have been traced to contaminated irrigation water used to grow foods such as strawberries, green onions and other produce.

Contact with an infected person Hepatitis A can spread by way of close contact with a person infected with the virus, even if that person has no signs or symptoms. The virus doesn't spread through sneezing or coughing.

Treatment No specific treatment exists for hepatitis A. Your body will clear the virus on its own. In most cases of hepatitis A, the liver heals within six months and people have a complete recovery.

Unlike other types of viral hepatitis, hepatitis A doesn't cause long-term liver damage, and it doesn't become long-lasting (chronic). In rare cases, hepatitis A can cause a sudden loss of liver function, especially in older adults or people with chronic liver diseases.

Treatment usually focuses on keeping you comfortable and controlling your signs and symptoms. You may need to:

- *Rest.* Many people feel tired and sick and have less energy.
- *Manage nausea.* Try snacking throughout the day rather than eating full meals. To get enough calories, eat more high-calorie foods. For instance, drink fruit juice or milk rather than water. Drinking plenty of fluids is important to prevent dehydration if vomiting occurs.
- *Avoid alcohol and limit medications.* Your liver may have difficulty processing medications and alcohol. Don't drink alcohol. Talk to your doctor about the medications you take, including over-the-counter drugs.

To reduce the risk of passing hepatitis A to others while you're actively infected:

- ***Wash your hands thoroughly after using the toilet and changing diapers.*** Scrub vigorously for at least 20 seconds and rinse well. Dry your hands with a disposable towel.
- ***Don't prepare food for others.*** You can easily pass the infection to others.

Immunization The hepatitis A vaccine is typically given to children between their first and second birthdays. It's also given to people at risk of hepatitis A. The vaccine is administered in two doses. The first injection is followed by a booster shot six months later.

The Centers for Disease Control and Prevention recommends a hepatitis A vaccine for the following people:

- Children who didn't receive the childhood vaccine
- Children and adults traveling to countries where the disease is common
- Laboratory workers who may come in contact with hepatitis A
- Men who have sex with men
- People who use any type of illegal drugs, not just injected ones
- People who receive treatment with clotting-factor concentrates
- People with chronic liver disease
- People who work or travel in parts of the world where hepatitis A is common
- People in contact with an international adoptee from a country where hepatitis A is common

• • • • •

PREVENTING HEPATITIS

The following precautions may help you avoid viral forms of hepatitis.

Immunization

There are effective vaccines for hepatitis A and B. Depending on the type of vaccine used, you may require two or three injections. Since hepatitis A is a risk when traveling to most parts of the world, consult your doctor regarding a hepatitis A vaccine before traveling.

Almost anyone can receive the vaccine for hepatitis B, including infants, older adults and those with compromised immune systems. Children born to mothers infected with hepatitis B can be vaccinated soon after birth.

Food preparation

Since hepatitis A and E can spread through contaminated food and drink, follow these safe-food-handling habits:

- Thoroughly wash all fruits and vegetables.
- Cook foods thoroughly — freezing doesn't kill a virus.
- When visiting developing countries, use only bottled water for drinking, cooking and brushing your teeth, or tap water that's been boiled for at least 10 minutes.

Workplace precautions

In health care settings, follow all infection control procedures, including washing hands and wearing gloves. In child-care settings, which are high-risk areas for hepatitis A infections, wash your hands thoroughly after changing or handling diapers.

Other precautions

These good health habits also can reduce your risk of hepatitis:

- Wash your hands often and thoroughly.
- If you have sexual relations with multiple partners — a risk factor for hepatitis B and C — use a latex condom with each sexual contact.
- Don't share drug syringes.
- If you undergo acupuncture, make sure the needles are sterilized.
- Avoid body piercing and tattooing unless you can be sure the instruments and dyes are safe (dedicated to one person only).
- Don't share toothbrushes, razors, nail clippers or other items that may come into contact with blood.

● ● ● ● ●

Hepatitis B

This hepatitis virus, also highly contagious, is found in blood and semen, and is commonly transmitted through unprotected sexual contact or by sharing contaminated syringes and needles during intravenous drug use. At greatest risk are people with multiple sexual partners, users of illicit drugs and hospital workers exposed to blood.

At birth, a newborn can be infected with hepatitis B if the mother is already infected. However, some people are infected without any known risk factor. Hepatitis B is not spread through hugging, sneezing, coughing, consuming food or water, or sharing eating and drinking utensils.

Most adults with hepatitis B recover fully, even if their signs and symptoms are severe. For some people, hepatitis B infection becomes chronic, meaning it lasts more than six months. Having chronic hepatitis B increases your risk of developing liver failure, liver cancer or cirrhosis — a condition that permanently scars the liver. Infants and children are more likely to develop a chronic (long-lasting) hepatitis B infection.

Treatment If you know you've been exposed to the hepatitis B virus and aren't sure if you've been vaccinated, call your doctor immediately. An injection of an antibody (immunoglobulin) given within 12 hours of exposure to the virus may help protect you from getting sick with hepatitis B. Because this treatment only provides short-term protection, you should also get the hepatitis B vaccine at the same time, if you never received it.

Acute hepatitis B infection If your doctor determines your hepatitis B infection is acute — meaning it's short-lived and will go away on its own — you may not need treatment. Instead, your doctor might recommend rest, proper nutrition and plenty of fluids while your body fights the infection. In severe cases, antiviral drugs or a hospital stay is needed to prevent complications.

Chronic hepatitis B infection Most people diagnosed with chronic hepatitis B infection need lifelong treatment to reduce the risk of liver disease and prevent them from passing the infection to others. Treatment for chronic hepatitis B may include:

- **Antiviral medications.** Several antiviral medications — including entecavir (Baraclude), tenofovir (Viread), lamivudine (Epivir) and adefovir (Hepsera) — can help fight the virus and slow its ability to damage your liver. These drugs are taken by mouth. Other drugs to treat hepatitis B also are being developed.
- **Interferon injections.** Interferon alfa-2b (Intron A) is a man-made version of a substance produced by the body to fight infection. It's used mainly for young people with hepatitis B who wish to avoid long-term treatment or women who want to get pregnant within a few years, after completing a course of therapy. Interferon shouldn't be used during pregnancy.
- **Liver transplant.** If your liver has been severely damaged, a liver transplant may be an option. During a liver transplant, a surgeon removes your damaged liver and replaces it with a healthy liver. Most transplanted livers come from deceased donors, though a small number come from living donors who donate a portion of their livers.

● ● ● ● ●

HEPATITIS B VACCINE

A vaccine is available that can prevent hepatitis B infection. The hepatitis B vaccine is administered at birth and given as three or four injections over a six-month period. The vaccine is recommended for:

- Newborns
- Children and adolescents not vaccinated at birth
- Sexual partners of someone who has hepatitis B
- Anyone who has a sexually transmitted disease
- Men who have sexual contact with other men
- People who have multiple sexual partners
- People who live with someone who has hepatitis B
- Health care workers, emergency workers and other people who come into contact with blood or body fluids
- Staff and residents of facilities for developmentally disabled persons
- People in correctional facilities
- People who share needles, syringes or other drug-injection equipment
- People with chronic liver disease, kidney disease, HIV infection or diabetes
- Travelers to regions with a high hepatitis B infection rate
- Anyone who wants to be protected from hepatitis B

See here for information on other ways to prevent hepatitis B infection.

• • • • •

Hepatitis C

Hepatitis C is the most common cause of viral hepatitis. An estimated 3.5 million people in the United States are living with hepatitis C, and about half don't know they're infected because they don't have symptoms.

The rate of hepatitis C infection has fluctuated over time, but remains high. Hepatitis C infection rates have increased among young adults in the United States, likely reflecting the epidemic of opioid and injection drug use. Hepatitis C also remains a concern among people born between 1945 and 1964, many of whom don't know they're infected.

Unlike hepatitis A and B, there is no vaccine for hepatitis C.

Transmission Hepatitis C is spread primarily through blood and blood products and contaminated needles. Users of illicit drugs who share needles or syringes account for many of the new infections.

Individuals most at risk of hepatitis C infection are current or former injection drug users, including individuals who injected only once many years ago. The virus is most commonly spread by:

- Sharing needles, syringes, or other equipment to prepare or inject drugs
- Needlestick injuries in health care settings
- Being born to a mother with hepatitis C

Less commonly, a person can get hepatitis C virus by way of:

- Sharing personal care items that come in contact with another person's blood, such as razors or toothbrushes
- Having sexual contact with a person with hepatitis C
- Getting a tattoo or body piercing in an unregulated setting

Other individuals at increased risk are those who received a blood transfusion or organ transplant before 1992, received clotting factor concentrates before

1987 or received hemodialysis treatments for a lengthy period.

The hepatitis C virus isn't spread by sharing eating utensils, breast-feeding, hugging, kissing, holding hands, coughing or sneezing. It's also not spread through food or water.

Acute vs. chronic Hepatitis C infection starts with an acute phase. Acute hepatitis C usually goes undiagnosed because it rarely causes symptoms. When signs and symptoms are present, they may include jaundice, along with fatigue, nausea, fever and muscle aches. Acute symptoms typically appear one to three months after exposure to the virus and last two weeks to three months.

Acute hepatitis C infection doesn't always turn chronic. Some people clear the virus from their bodies after the acute phase, an outcome known as spontaneous viral clearance. For others, the infection becomes long-lasting. Chronic hepatitis C often remains a "silent" infection for many years until it damages the liver enough to cause signs and symptoms such as:

- Easy bruising and bleeding
- Fatigue
- Poor appetite
- Yellow discoloration of the skin and eyes (jaundice)
- Dark-colored urine
- Itchy skin
- Fluid buildup in your abdomen (ascites)
- Swelling in the legs
- Weight loss
- Confusion, drowsiness and slurred speech (hepatic encephalopathy)
- Spider-like blood vessels on your skin (spider angiomas)

Hepatitis C infection that continues for many years can cause significant complications such as scarring of the liver (cirrhosis) and liver failure. A small number of people may develop liver cancer.

●　●　●　●　●

SCREENING FOR HEPATITIS C

A simple screening test can pinpoint hepatitis C antibodies or the virus in blood, often identifying the disease before signs and symptoms develop and serious liver damage occurs. Health officials recommend that you have a screening test if you:

- Were born from 1945 to 1965
- Currently inject drugs
- Ever injected drugs, even just once many years ago
- Received clotting factor concentrates produced before 1987
- Were ever on long-term hemodialysis
- Have persistently abnormal alanine aminotransferase (ALT) levels
- Have HIV infection
- Received blood from a donor who later tested positive for the hepatitis C virus
- Received a transfusion of blood, blood components or an organ transplant before July 1992
- Are a health care or public service worker who's been exposed to hepatitis C-positive blood
- Were born to a hepatitis C-positive mother

- Have had sexual relations with anyone diagnosed with hepatitis C infection
- Spent time in prison
- Have had an abnormal liver function test with no identifiable cause

● ● ● ● ●

Treatment Once a diagnosis of hepatitis C is made, it's important to identify the variant of the virus you have. There are several forms of the virus — called genotypes — each of which must be treated differently. In the United States, genotype 1 is the most common.

In contrast to just a few years ago, today hepatitis C is often curable with the right medications, taken daily for several months. People who haven't been treated for hepatitis C before are cured more than 90 percent of the time. People in which earlier treatment was unsuccessful or who have cirrhosis have a slightly lower cure rate. But cure rates are improving with newer treatments.

Medications Hepatitis C infection is treated with a variety of antiviral medications intended to clear the virus from your body. The goal of treatment is to have none of the virus detected in your body at least 12 weeks after completing drug therapy.

Researchers have made significant advances in treatment for hepatitis C using new, "direct-acting" antiviral medications. Treatment often includes two or three medications combined into one pill. As a result, people experience better outcomes, fewer side effects and shorter treatment times — some as short as eight weeks. Examples of combination drugs include sofosbuvir and ledipasvir (Harvoni), sofosbuvir and velpatasvir (Epclusa), sofosbuvir, velpatasvir and voxilaprevir (Vosevi), and glecaprevir and pibrentasvir (Mavyret).

The choice of medications you receive and the length of treatment depend on a variety of factors including the virus genotype, existing liver damage and other medical conditions you may have.

Liver transplantation If you've developed serious complications from chronic hepatitis C infection, liver transplantation may be an option (see here).

In most cases, a liver transplant alone doesn't cure hepatitis C. The infection is likely to return, requiring treatment with antiviral medication to prevent damage to the transplanted liver. Several studies have demonstrated that new, direct-acting antiviral medication regimens are effective at curing post-transplant hepatitis C. Treatment with direct-acting antivirals can also be effective in appropriately selected patients before liver transplantation.

Hepatitis D and E

These forms of hepatitis are rare. To get hepatitis D, a bloodborne virus, you must already have hepatitis B. Hepatitis D survives by attaching itself to the hepatitis B virus. Hepatitis E is a foodborne virus. Most cases reported in the United States involve travelers to parts of the world where the disease is prevalent, such as the Middle East, Asia, Mexico and South America.

• • • • •

LIVING WITH HEPATITIS

Once you have hepatitis, your risk of getting another form of the virus increases. Therefore, it's important to stay healthy and avoid exposure to additional risks. Self-care strategies vary, but the following generally applies to everyone:

- **Rest.** For acute hepatitis, get adequate rest, drink plenty of fluids and eat a healthy, high-calorie diet. This strengthens your immune system to fight off the virus.
- **Avoid alcohol.** Alcohol can aggravate inflammation and speed the progression of liver disease to cirrhosis and organ failure.
- **Use medications carefully.** Many medications impair liver function, especially if taken regularly. If your liver isn't working properly, it has trouble removing toxins produced by the drugs. Inform your doctor of any medication you take, including over-the-counter drugs.
- **Maintain a healthy lifestyle.** A healthy lifestyle includes eating a balanced, nutritious diet and getting adequate exercise. In addition to improving your physical health, good nutrition and exercise can help overcome depression, a common problem for people with hepatitis.
- **Get vaccinated.** Get vaccinated against hepatitis A and B if you're not immune to these infections. Keep up to date on all of your vaccinations, including pneumonia vaccinations

and yearly flu shots.

● ● ● ● ●

ALCOHOL- OR DRUG-INDUCED HEPATITIS

Alcohol- or drug-induced hepatitis, also known as toxic hepatitis, is an inflammation of your liver in reaction to certain substances to which you're exposed. In addition to alcohol and drugs, toxic hepatitis may be caused by nutritional supplements or industrial chemicals. Exposure can occur through ingesting a chemical, breathing it in or through contact with the skin.

The most common form of toxic hepatitis occurs in people who drink excessive amounts of alcohol or who take certain medications. Inflammation stems from the toxic chemicals that your body produces as it breaks down the alcohol or drugs. Over time, these chemicals damage liver cells and interfere with your liver's ability to do its job.

In some cases, toxic hepatitis develops within hours or days of exposure to a toxin. In other cases, it may take months or years of regular use before signs and symptoms appear. The symptoms of toxic hepatitis often go away when exposure to the toxin stops. But toxic hepatitis can permanently damage your liver, leading to irreversible scarring of liver tissue (cirrhosis) and in some cases to liver failure, which can be life-threatening.

Medications that most commonly lead to drug-induced hepatitis are nonprescription pain relievers, especially if the drugs are taken frequently or combined with alcohol. They include acetaminophen (Tylenol, others), aspirin, ibuprofen (Advil, Motrin IB, others) and naproxen sodium (Aleve).

In most people, prescription medications don't cause liver problems, but in certain situations or in people with liver disease, some may be damaging. Medications linked to serious liver injury include the statin drugs used to treat high cholesterol, the combination drug amoxicillin-clavulanate (Augmentin), phenytoin (Dilantin, Phenytek), azathioprine (Azasan, Imuran), niacin (Niaspan), ketoconazole, certain antivirals and anabolic steroids. There are others.

Treatment

Doctors will work to determine what's causing your liver damage. Sometimes the cause is clear; other times it takes more detective work. In most cases, stopping exposure to the toxin causing liver inflammation will reduce signs and symptoms.

If your liver damage was caused by an overdose of acetaminophen, you'll likely receive a chemical called acetylcysteine right away. The sooner this medication is administered, the greater the chance of limiting liver damage. It's most effective if administered within 16 hours of an acetaminophen overdose.

While your liver is healing, it's important to avoid any alcohol. And don't take any medications or supplements without first checking with your doctor.

In cases when liver function is severely impaired, for some individuals a liver transplant is a potential option (see here).

NONALCOHOLIC FATTY LIVER DISEASE

Nonalcoholic fatty liver disease has become increasingly common cause of liver disease, especially in Western nations. As the number of individuals who are overweight or obese has increased worldwide, so has the prevalence of nonalcoholic fatty liver disease. In the United States, it is the most common form of chronic liver disease.

● ● ● ● ●

NONALCOHOLIC FATTY LIVER DISEASE

Key signs and symptoms:

- Enlarged liver
- Fatigue
- Upper right abdominal pain

● ● ● ● ●

With this condition, excess fat accumulates in the liver — similar to what happens in alcohol-induced hepatitis — but it occurs among individuals who drink little or no alcohol.

Most people develop a form called simple fatty liver that causes no signs or symptoms. A small number experience a more severe form of the disease called nonalcoholic steatohepatitis (NASH).

In the case of simple fatty liver, you have fat in your liver but little or no inflammation or liver cell damage. Simple fatty liver typically doesn't progress to cause liver damage or complications. With NASH, in addition to fat in your liver, you develop inflammation of the liver and liver cell damage, which can lead to scarring of the liver (cirrhosis).

Normal liver

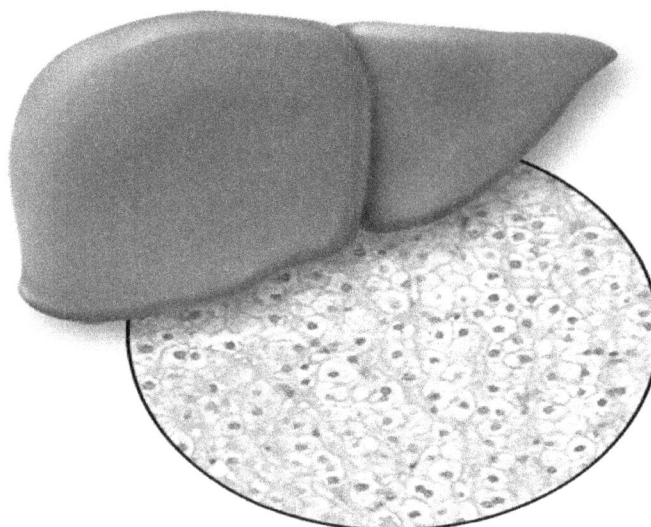

Fatty liver

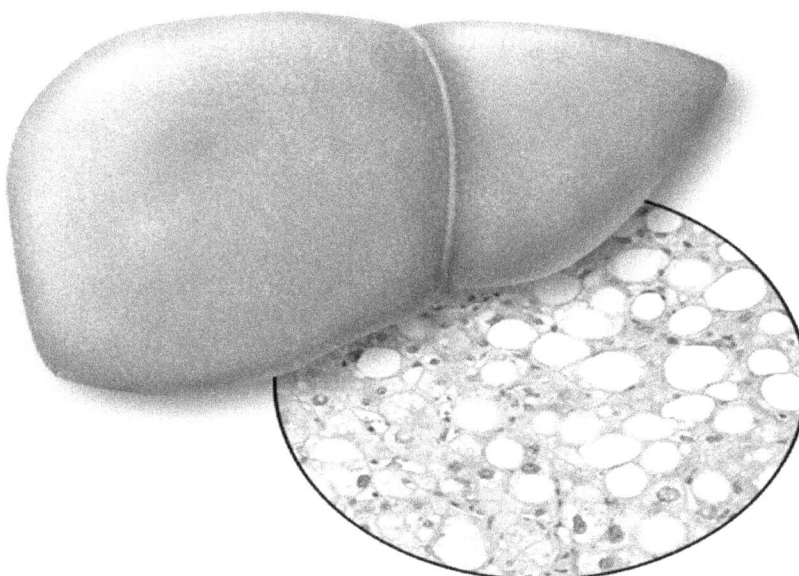

Nonalcoholic fatty liver disease can affect people of any age, even children, but it tends to occur most often in people in their 40s and 50s. It's most common in people who are obese or who have type 2 diabetes or high triglyceride levels. The condition is also closely linked to metabolic syndrome, which is a cluster of abnormalities, including increased abdominal fat, poor ability to use the hormone insulin, high blood pressure and high triglyceride levels.

Experts aren't certain why some people accumulate fat in their livers and others don't. Similarly, there's limited understanding of why some fatty livers lead to inflammation that eventually progresses to cirrhosis.

Treatment

The first line of treatment is usually weight loss through a combination of a healthy diet and exercise. Losing weight addresses the conditions that contribute to nonalcoholic fatty liver disease and can improve the health of your liver. Weight-loss surgery may be an option for individuals who need to lose a great deal of weight.

Your doctor also may recommend that you stop drinking alcohol because alcohol, especially when consumed heavily, can worsen the disease.

If you don't have diabetes, your doctor may recommend vitamin E supplements. There's some indication that vitamin E can reduce fat accumulation and liver inflammation. However, vitamin E carries some safety concerns, so it's important that you discuss the benefits and risks with your doctor. If you have diabetes, it's important to take steps to manage the disease.

For individuals with NASH who develop cirrhosis, liver transplantation may be an option. Outcomes of liver transplantation in this population group are generally very good.

AUTOIMMUNE DISEASE

Some forms of liver disease are the result of an autoimmune disorder, a condition in which your body's immune system attacks and damages its own tissues — in this case tissues within the liver.

Autoimmune hepatitis

Autoimmune hepatitis is a form of liver inflammation resulting from your immune system attacking your liver. The exact cause of autoimmune hepatitis is unclear, but researchers think it may stem from an interaction between specific genes that control functioning of your immune system and environmental factors, including exposure to particular viruses or drugs.

Signs and symptoms of autoimmune hepatitis vary from person to person and may come on suddenly. Some people have few, if any, recognized problems in the early stages of the disease, whereas others may experience fatigue, abdominal discomfort, yellowing of the skin and eyes (jaundice), itching, skin rashes, and joint pain. Left untreated, autoimmune hepatitis may lead to scarring of the liver (cirrhosis) and liver failure.

Factors that may increase your risk of autoimmune hepatitis include:

- *Being female.* Both men and women can develop autoimmune hepatitis, but the disease is more common in women.
- *A history of certain infections.* Autoimmune hepatitis may develop after you're infected with the measles, herpes simplex or Epstein-Barr virus. The disease is also linked to hepatitis A, B or C infection.
- *Heredity.* Evidence suggests that a predisposition to autoimmune

hepatitis may run in families.

- ***Having an autoimmune disease.*** People who already have an autoimmune disease, such as celiac disease, rheumatoid arthritis, Graves' disease or Hashimoto's thyroiditis, may be more likely to develop autoimmune hepatitis.

Types Doctors have identified two main forms of autoimmune hepatitis.

- ***Type 1.*** This is the most common type of the disease. It can occur at any age. About half the people with type 1 autoimmune hepatitis have other autoimmune disorders, such as celiac disease, rheumatoid arthritis or ulcerative colitis.
- ***Type 2.*** Although adults can develop type 2 autoimmune hepatitis, it's most common in girls and young women. Other autoimmune diseases may accompany this type of autoimmune hepatitis.

Diagnosis and treatment Autoimmune hepatitis is diagnosed with blood tests and a liver biopsy. When diagnosed and treated early, it often can be managed with medications that suppress the immune system. To keep your liver as healthy as possible, it's also important to avoid alcohol — even small amounts can worsen your disease and cause other damage. And don't take any medications or supplements without discussing them first with your doctor.

Regardless of which type of autoimmune hepatitis you have, the goal of treatment is to slow or stop the immune system attack on your liver. To meet this goal, you'll need medications that lower immune system activity. The initial treatment is usually glucocorticoid medication, such as prednisone. A second medication, azathioprine (Azasan, Imuran) or 6-mercaptopurine (Purinethol), may be recommended in addition to prednisone.

Doctors typically prescribe prednisone at a high dose for about the first month of treatment. Then, to reduce the risk of side effects, they gradually reduce the dose over the next several months until reaching the lowest possible dose that controls the disease. Prednisone, especially when taken long term, can cause a wide range of serious side effects. Adding another drug may help avoid prednisone side effects. However, azathioprine and 6-mercaptopurine can also produce side effects, including allergic reactions, a low white blood cell count, inflammation of the pancreas, nausea and abnormal liver blood test.

Most people need to continue taking the prednisone for several months, and many remain on it for life. Although you may experience remission a few years after starting treatment, the disease often returns if the drug is discontinued.

When medications don't halt progression of the disease or you develop irreversible scarring (cirrhosis) or liver failure, a liver transplant may be considered (see here).

Primary sclerosing cholangitis

Primary sclerosing cholangitis is a disease of the bile ducts, the tiny tubes that carry digestive juices from your liver to your small intestine. Chronic inflammation causes scars to form within the ducts. The scars make the ducts hard and narrow, eventually resulting in serious liver damage.

It's not clear what causes primary sclerosing cholangitis. An immune system reaction to an infection or toxin may trigger the disease in people genetically predisposed to it. A large proportion of people with primary sclerosing cholangitis also have inflammatory bowel disease.

In most people with primary sclerosing cholangitis, the disease progresses slowly and individuals continue to feel well for several years. When signs and symptoms develop, they often include fatigue and itching. The disease can eventually lead to liver failure, repeated infections, and tumors of the bile duct or liver.

Care for primary sclerosing cholangitis focuses on monitoring liver function, managing symptoms and, when necessary, performing procedures that temporarily open blocked bile ducts. Many medications have been studied in people with primary sclerosing cholangitis, but so far none have been found to slow or reverse liver damage associated with this disease.

A liver transplant is the only treatment known to cure primary sclerosing cholangitis. Transplants are generally reserved for people with severe complications of primary sclerosing cholangitis. Though uncommon, it's possible for primary sclerosing cholangitis to recur after a liver transplant.

INHERITED LIVER DISEASE

Some diseases of the liver are inherited, developing as a result of a genetic defect.

Hemochromatosis

Hemochromatosis is an inherited abnormality that causes your intestines to absorb too much iron from the food you eat, leading to iron overload. The extra iron enters your bloodstream and is stored in certain organs, primarily in the liver, heart and pancreas.

● ● ● ● ●

HEMOCHROMATOSIS

Key signs and symptoms:

- Chronic fatigue
- Joint pain
- Loss of sex drive (libido) or impotence
- Infertility
- Hypothyroidism

● ● ● ● ●

The most common cause is a mutation in the HFE gene that helps control iron absorption in the small intestine. You inherit one HFE gene from each of your parents. If both parents pass mutated HFE genes to you, you may develop hemochromatosis. You can't develop the disease with only one mutated gene.

Although you carry the genetic condition from birth, signs and symptoms generally don't appear until midlife — usually between ages 30 and 50 in men, and after age 50 in women. Some people never exhibit signs and symptoms. For others, early signs and symptoms mimic those of other common conditions, making the disease difficult to diagnose.

Diagnosis and treatment At any stage, even before signs and symptoms appear, your doctor can detect iron overload with blood tests. A serum transferrin saturation test measures the amount of iron in your blood. A serum ferritin test measures how much iron is stored in your liver. Because other conditions can cause elevated test results, both tests are needed to diagnose hemochromatosis. A genetic test can confirm that you're carrying two abnormal copies of the HFE gene.

Genetic testing is recommended for all first-degree relatives — parents, siblings and children — of anyone diagnosed with hemochromatosis. If a mutation is found in only one parent, then children do not need to be tested.

Hemochromatosis is treated by regularly removing blood from your body (phlebotomy). The goal is to reduce iron levels to normal. Once or twice a week, a pint of blood is withdrawn from a vein in your arm, in the same way as you make a blood donation.

After reaching a normal iron level, most people continue to need blood removed every two to four months to keep iron from accumulating again.

If hemochromatosis is discovered early, permanent damage can usually be prevented. Left untreated, the disease can lead to organ damage, particularly to the heart and liver, and in the reproductive system.

Alpha-1-antitrypsin deficiency

This disorder results from a genetic defect that causes your body to produce abnormal forms of the alpha-1-antitrypsin protein, an enzyme inhibitor that helps protect your lungs. A deficiency of this protein may lead to lung and liver disease, although most people with alpha-1-antitrypsin deficiency don't develop serious liver disease.

Wilson's disease

With this condition, your body accumulates excessive amounts of copper, leading to organ damage. Like hemochromatosis, Wilson's disease stems from a flawed gene. Nearly everyone with the disease has signs and symptoms by age 40, which may include liver tenderness, weight loss, fatigue, mild jaundice, and neurological or psychiatric problems. If caught early, Wilson's disease is treatable with medications that remove excess copper from your body.

Gilbert syndrome

This mild disorder is quite common and doesn't lead to liver damage, but jaundice may develop periodically, especially following prolonged fasting or infections such as colds or the flu.

CIRRHOSIS

Cirrhosis is the term used to describe scarring of the liver. The most common causes of cirrhosis include alcohol abuse, chronic hepatitis B or C infection, and nonalcoholic fatty liver disease.

• • • • •

CIRRHOSIS

Key signs and symptoms:

- Fatigue
- Loss of appetite and nausea
- Weight loss
- Easy bleeding or bruising
- Itchy skin
- Abdominal swelling
- Swelling in your legs, feet or ankles (edema)
- Yellowing of skin and eyes (jaundice)
- Gastrointestinal bleeding (varices)
- Sleepiness or confusion

• • • • •

Each time your liver is injured, it tries to repair itself. In the repair process, scar tissue forms. With mild cirrhosis, your liver makes repairs and continues its functions. But as more scar tissue builds up, liver function becomes increasingly more difficult. Advanced cirrhosis is life-threatening.

Cirrhosis most often results from chronic inflammation caused by alcohol abuse or hepatitis — including hepatitis B, hepatitis C and autoimmune hepatitis. Cirrhosis can also result from a variety of other conditions such as nonalcoholic fatty liver disease, hemochromatosis, Wilson's disease or alpha-1-antitrypsin deficiency.

Left untreated, cirrhosis can result in a variety of complications including high blood pressure in the veins that supply the liver with blood (portal hypertension), swelling in the legs and abdomen, bleeding, spleen enlargement, infections, malnutrition, jaundice, and buildup of toxins in the brain (hepatic encephalopathy).

Diagnosing cirrhosis

People with early-stage cirrhosis usually don't experience symptoms. Often, cirrhosis is first detected through a routine blood test or checkup.

If signs and symptoms suggest liver disease, your doctor will feel (palpate) your upper abdomen for evidence of an enlarged, firm liver. As cirrhosis advances, however, the liver may actually shrink. Swelling of your abdomen from fluid accumulation in your peritoneal cavity (ascites) may be another warning sign of the disease.

If your doctor suspects cirrhosis, he or she will likely order an imaging test of the abdomen, such as an ultrasound exam or magnetic resonance imaging (MRI). These tests also can detect stiffness or lack of elasticity in your liver due to cirrhosis. Your doctor might also order a liver biopsy, which involves use of a needle to obtain a liver tissue sample to be examined for signs of damage.

Treatment

There is no cure for cirrhosis, and the damage to your liver often is irreversible. Treatment for cirrhosis generally depends on the cause and extent of the damage. The goals of treatment are to slow the progression of scar tissue formation in the liver and to prevent or treat symptoms and complications.

In early-stage cirrhosis, it may be possible to minimize liver damage by treating the underlying cause, for example, alcohol dependency or hepatitis. People with cirrhosis caused by nonalcoholic fatty liver disease may improve their condition if they lose weight and control their blood sugar levels.

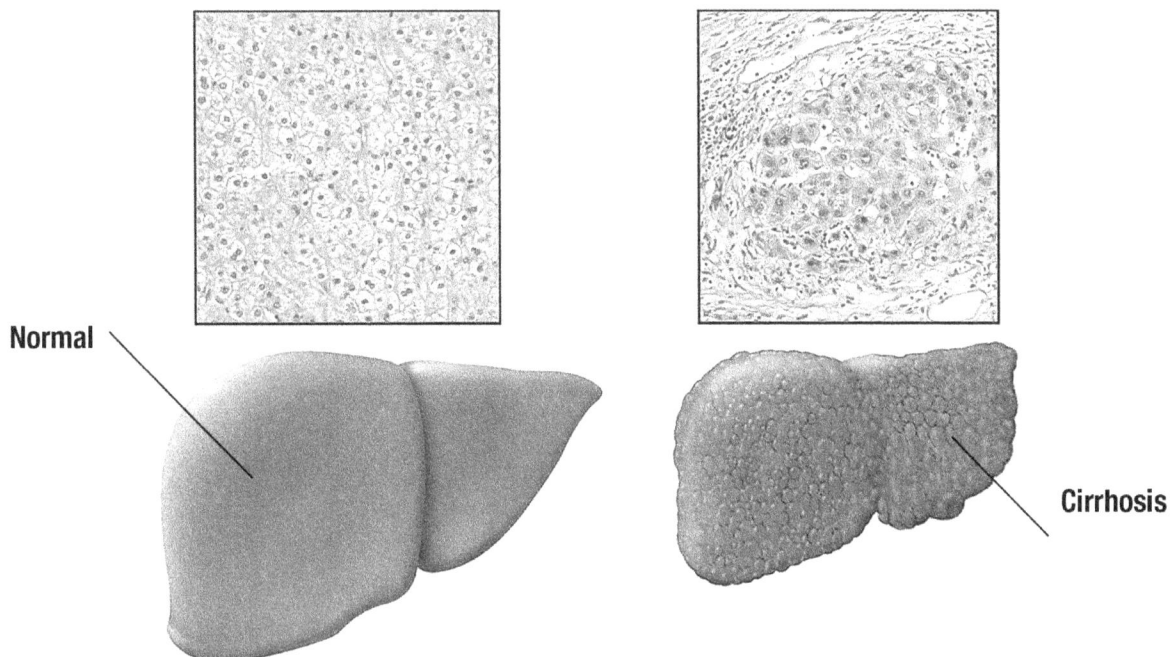

Normal

Cirrhosis

A normal liver (left), shown in cross section, shows no sign of scarring. The cirrhotic liver (right) shows extensive scarring and shrinkage.

Managing complications For more advanced cirrhosis, the focus of medical care often is on managing complications.

Preventing internal bleeding Cirrhosis can slow or block the movement of blood through your liver. This may cause the formation of small, twisted blood vessels (varices) with thin walls, most commonly in the esophagus or stomach. Because the walls are subject to high pressure, it's not uncommon for the blood vessels to start bleeding.

To stop internal bleeding, your doctor may recommend a medication to help lower the pressure within the varices. Another option is an endoscopic procedure using rubber band ligation to stop blood from flowing into the varices.

Reducing fluid retention Diuretic medications may be used to help reduce the accumulation of excess fluid in your abdomen. Your doctor may also ask you to restrict sodium intake, including cutting down on table salt, to reduce fluid retention.

Sometimes, fluid that accumulates in your abdomen can become infected, causing pain and fever. If this occurs, your doctor may insert a catheter into the abdomen to remove a fluid sample. Laboratory analysis of the sample can help identify the infecting organism and the proper antibiotic can be prescribed.

Reducing itching Antihistamines as well as cholestyramine (Prevalite) may be prescribed to reduce itching caused by toxins (bile acids) in your blood.

Advanced disease With advanced cirrhosis, you may become confused and delirious or enter a comatose state. This condition, called hepatic encephalopathy, occurs when your brain is under assault from toxins in your blood, such as ammonia, that are normally eliminated from the body by a healthy liver.

Infection and bleeding into the gastrointestinal tract can cause episodes of hepatic encephalopathy. Treatment usually requires locating the source of infection or bleeding and treating it. In addition, you may be asked to take medication to increase bowel movements and help remove ammonia and other toxins from your body. Your doctor may also recommend an antibiotic to reduce certain bacteria in your intestines that produce ammonia. This will help lower the toxic levels of ammonia.

• • • • •

HOW MUCH IS TOO MUCH?

Some people have difficulty distinguishing when "normal drinking" becomes "problem drinking." How do you know how much alcohol is too much?

Experts use many terms and definitions to define different types of alcohol-related conditions. In general, drinking is considered a problem when it starts to adversely affect your personal or professional life, you lose control over how much you consume, or it causes health concerns.

If you drink alcohol, it's recommended that you drink only a moderate amount. The National Institute on Alcohol Abuse and Alcoholism defines moderate drinking as:

- Women: No more than one drink per day
- Men: No more than two drinks per day
- People age 65 and older: No more than one drink per day

A drink is defined as:

- 12 ounces regular beer, which is usually 5% alcohol
- 5 ounces wine, which is typically about 12% alcohol
- .5 ounces distilled spirits, which is about 40% alcohol

Liver transplant In advanced cases of cirrhosis, a liver transplant may be the only treatment option. Cirrhosis is one of the most common reasons for a liver transplant.

Historically, individuals with alcoholic cirrhosis haven't been liver transplant candidates because of the risk that they will return to harmful drinking after the transplant. Recent studies, however, suggest that carefully selected candidates with severe alcoholic cirrhosis have post-transplant survival rates similar to those of liver transplant recipients with other types of liver disease.

LIVER TRANSPLANT

A liver transplant is a surgical procedure to remove a liver that no longer functions properly and replace it with a healthy liver. Liver transplantation is usually the last treatment option for people experiencing significant complications due to liver failure (end-stage chronic liver disease).

Liver failure can happen quickly or over a long period. Liver failure that occurs quickly, in a matter of weeks, is called acute liver failure. It's usually associated with medication that causes immediate liver damage.

Chronic liver failure, which is more common, occurs slowly over months and years. Chronic liver failure may be caused by a variety of conditions. The most common cause is scarring of the liver (cirrhosis), a process in which scar tissue replaces normal liver tissue and impairs liver function.

The most common causes of cirrhosis leading to the need for a liver transplant include:

- Hepatitis B and C
- Alcoholic liver disease
- Nonalcoholic fatty liver disease
- Genetic diseases affecting the liver (including hemochromatosis and Wilson's disease)
- Diseases that affect the bile ducts, such as primary biliary cirrhosis and primary sclerosing cholangitis

Types

There are two types of liver transplants — deceased donor and living donor.

Deceased donor Deceased-donor transplants are the most common. The liver to be transplanted comes from an individual who has recently died. Unfortunately, the need for donated livers far outweighs the number available. The wait for a deceased-donor liver can vary greatly.

Living donor This type is less common but is being performed more often. With a living- donor transplant, a person who is living — generally a close family member or friend — donates part of his or her liver to be transplanted into the individual who is sick.

Living-donor liver transplants were initially performed in children needing a liver transplant due to the scarcity of appropriately sized deceased-donor organs. The procedure has also become an option for adults with end-stage liver disease.

With deceased-donor liver transplants, access to a donated liver is determined primarily by the severity of your liver disease. In the case of living-donor transplantation, availability is determined by identification of a living donor who is healthy and able to safely undergo a major surgical procedure. The individual also needs to be the right size and blood type.

Surgery

How your surgery is performed will depend on the type of transplant you have.

Deceased-donor liver transplant The surgeon makes a long incision across your abdomen to access the liver. The location and size of the incision varies according to the surgeon's approach and your anatomy.

The surgeon disconnects your liver's blood supply and attached bile ducts and then removes the diseased liver. The donor liver is then placed in your body, and blood vessels and bile ducts are reattached. Surgery can take up to 12 hours, depending on your personal situation.

Living-donor liver transplant If you're receiving a liver transplant from a living donor, surgeons first operate on the donor, removing the portion of the liver to be transplanted. Next, they remove your diseased liver and place the donated liver portion into your body. Finally, they connect your blood vessels and bile ducts to the new liver.

The donor's remaining liver will grow back — regenerate itself — and return to its normal volume and capacity within a couple of months after the surgery. The transplanted liver portion placed in your body does the same. It regenerates rapidly, reaching normal volume within a couple of months.

With both types of transplants, doctors will test your liver function often and monitor you for signs of complications.

Recovery

After a liver transplant you'll need to take a number of medications to prevent organ rejection. You may need to take many of them for the rest of your life.

Medications called immunosuppressants help prevent your immune system from attacking your new liver. The medications can cause side effects including bone thinning, diabetes, diarrhea, headaches, high blood pressure and high cholesterol. Additional medications may be prescribed to help reduce the risk of other complications.

Expect six months or more recovery time before you start to feel healed. How long it takes to recover often depends upon how ill you were before your surgery.

LIVER CANCER

Liver cancer is cancer that begins in the cells of your liver. Several types of cancer can form in the liver. The most common is hepatocellular carcinoma, which begins in the main type of liver cell (hepatocyte).

Not all cancers that affect the liver are considered liver cancer. Cancer that begins in another area of the body — such as the colon, lung or breast — and then spreads to the liver is called metastatic cancer rather than liver cancer. And this type of cancer is named after the organ in which it began — such as metastatic colon cancer to describe cancer that begins in the colon and spreads to the liver. Cancer that spreads to the liver is more common than cancer that begins in the liver cells.

Most people don't show signs and symptoms in the early stages. Primary liver cancer is two to three times as common in men as in women, and it typically occurs after age 50. These factors may increase your risk:

- Chronic hepatitis B or C infection
- Cirrhosis
- Certain inherited liver diseases
- Nonalcoholic fatty liver disease
- Diabetes
- Environmental toxins, including aflatoxin, found in contaminated food
- Excessive alcohol consumption

Diagnosis

As with most other digestive cancers, primary liver cancer ordinarily produces few signs and symptoms in its early stage. By the time signs and symptoms do appear, the cancer is often advanced.

● ● ● ● ●

Key signs and symptoms:

- Upper abdominal pain
- Weight loss
- Loss of appetite
- Nausea and vomiting
- Abdominal swelling
- General weakness and fatigue
- Yellowing of skin and eyes (jaundice)

● ● ● ● ●

Blood tests to detect functional abnormalities and imaging tests — ultrasound, computerized tomography (CT) or magnetic resonance imaging (MRI) — are generally the first steps in diagnosing liver cancer. A sample of liver tissue (biopsy) may be taken and sent to a laboratory to make a definitive diagnosis.

Once liver cancer is diagnosed, your doctor will work to determine the extent (stage) of the cancer and whether it has spread.

Treatment

The goal of any treatment for cancer is to remove the cancer completely — and surgery is often the most effective recourse. The decision to have surgery will depend on the number, size and location of the tumors, and on how well your liver is functioning. If the tumors are small and have not spread beyond the liver, your doctor may be able to remove all of the cancerous tissue successfully.

For a small percentage of people with early- stage liver cancer, a liver transplant may be an option. It is also dependent on finding donated liver tissue, either from a deceased person or a live donor.

When surgery or a liver transplant isn't possible, treatment may focus on preventing further growth or spread of the tumor. The following procedures may be used:

- Blocking the main artery to the liver and injecting strong anti-cancer drugs directly to the liver (chemoembolization)
- Injecting concentrated alcohol into the tumor to destroy cancer cells (ethanol ablation)
- Freezing the tumor with an instrument containing liquid nitrogen (cryosurgery)
- Heating the tumor with energy from high-frequency radio waves (radiofrequency ablation)
- Placing beads filled with radiation into the liver. Tiny spheres that contain radiation are placed in the liver where they can deliver radiation directly to the tumor.

Traditional chemotherapy and radiation therapy also may be used to temporarily shrink liver tumors. Targeted drug therapy is another potential treatment option. Targeted drugs work by interfering with specific abnormalities within a tumor. These medications, such as the drugs sorafenib (Nexavar) and regorafenib (Stivarga), show promise but more study is needed to understand how targeted therapies may be used to control advanced liver cancer.

Researchers also are experimenting with use of a virus to kill cancer cells. With this approach, a solution containing an altered virus is injected into a tumor, where it causes cancer cells to die or to make proteins that are attacked by the body's immune system. Similar to targeted therapies, while early results have been promising, more study is needed.

CHAPTER 17
Colorectal cancer

When digestive signs and symptoms occur, often the first thing people fear is cancer. Most of the time, cancer isn't the cause — but occasionally it is. You can get cancer almost anywhere in your body, but most gastrointestinal cancers occur in the colon and rectum, where food waste moves slowly and toxins linger.

Colon cancer begins in the large intestine (colon), the final portion of your intestinal tract. Rectal cancer develops in the rectum, the last several inches of the colon. Together, they're referred to as colorectal cancer.

Colorectal cancer is the most common of all digestive cancers. In the United States, approximately 135,000 cases are diagnosed each year. Most cancers begin as small, noncancerous (benign) growths, called polyps, that develop on the inside lining of the colon. Polyps may produce few, if any, signs and symptoms, but over time some become cancerous.

SIGNS AND SYMPTOMS

Most people with colorectal cancer don't experience any signs and symptoms in the early stages of the disease. When signs and symptoms do appear, they generally vary depending on the origin of the cancer and the extent of its spread within the colon.

A cancer located in the lower portion of your colon or rectum can block the passage of stool, causing cramps. Having a bowel movement also may become more difficult. You may feel the urge to pass stool, and after having a bowel movement, you may still feel like you need to go to the bathroom. Blood mixed with stool or that appears in the toilet bowl is another warning sign of colorectal cancer.

Cancer in the upper portion of the colon can cause anemia, especially iron deficiency anemia, and fatigue due to blood loss that you may not be aware of or see. The blood may be masked because it's usually mixed in with stool and is darker in color instead of bright red.

Other signs and symptoms of cancer in the upper portion of your colon include persistent diarrhea or constipation, decreased appetite, unexplained weight loss, and abdominal pain.

Be aware that any of these signs and symptoms may be caused by other medical conditions and not necessarily by colorectal cancer. But no matter what the cause, it's important to see a doctor as early as possible for a complete evaluation.

●　●　●　●　●

COLORECTAL CANCER

Key signs and symptoms:

- Blood in stool
- Weight loss
- Weakness or fatigue
- Change in bowel habits
- Abdominal pain or discomfort

· · · · ·

ARE YOU AT RISK?

As with other digestive cancers, heredity and lifestyle factors appear to play combined roles in colorectal cancer development.

Family history

You're at greater risk of colorectal cancer if a parent, sibling or child has the disease. Inherited genetic mutations that increase the risk of colon cancer can be passed through families. However, inherited genes are linked to only a small percentage of colon cancers. Inherited genetic mutations don't make cancer inevitable, but they can increase a person's risk of cancer significantly.

The most common forms of inherited colon cancer syndromes are:

Hereditary nonpolyposis colorectal cancer (HNPCC) Also called Lynch syndrome, HNPCC increases the risk of many types of cancer, particularly colorectal cancer. The genes affected in HNPCC are responsible for correcting changes in the genetic code, but they lack the ability to make necessary repairs. An accumulation of code mistakes leads to increasing genetic damage within cells and eventually can cause the cells to become cancerous. People with HNPCC tend to develop colon cancer early in life, before age 50.

Familial adenomatous polyposis (FAP) This rare disorder is caused by a defect in the adenomatous polyposis coli gene, resulting in the development of thousands of polyps in the lining of the colon and rectum. Polyps can also occur in the upper gastrointestinal tract. Most people inherit the defective gene from a parent, but for some individuals the genetic mutation occurs spontaneously. People with untreated FAP have a greatly increased risk of developing colon cancer before age 40. Some individuals experience a milder form of the condition called attenuated familial adenomatous polyposis (AFAP). People with AFAP usually have fewer colon polyps and develop cancer later in life.

HNPCC, FAP and other inherited colon cancer syndromes can be detected through genetic testing. If you're concerned about your family's history of colon cancer, talk to your doctor about whether your family history suggests that you may be at risk of these conditions. Individuals with an inherited condition should undergo early colorectal cancer screening.

Diet

Studies of large groups of people have shown an association between a typical Western diet and an increased risk of colorectal cancer. A typical Western diet is high in fat and low in fiber.

When people move from an area where the typical diet is low in fat and high in fiber to an area where a Western diet is common, their risk of colon cancer increases significantly. It's not clear why this occurs. Researchers are studying whether a high-fat, low-fiber diet affects the microbes that live in the colon or causes underlying inflammation that may contribute to cancer risk. This is an area of ongoing investigation and research.

●　●　●　●　●

WHAT IS CANCER?

The basic characteristic of all cancers is the same — the uncontrolled growth and spread of abnormal (malignant) cells. Unlike healthy cells, cancer cells lack the controls that switch off growth or they lose their ability to undergo natural cell death (apoptosis). Cancer cells divide without restraint, crowd out neighboring cells, compete for available nutrients and interfere with normal body functions.

The result of uncontrolled cell growth often is a densely packed mass of excess tissue called a tumor. Tumors can press on nerves, block arteries, bleed, obstruct the intestinal tract or interfere with the work of nearby organs.

Cancer cells can also travel to other parts of the body via the bloodstream or lymphatic system. When cancer spreads outside its place of origin, the disease becomes much more lethal and difficult to treat.

Why cancer develops in some people and not in others isn't fully understood, but researchers are learning more about specific components that may contribute to its onset. A complex mixture of factors, including lifestyle, environment and genetics, is likely responsible for turning a healthy cell into a cancerous one.

● ● ● ● ●

Other factors

Beyond diet, several other factors may increase your risk of colorectal cancer. They include the following:

Age About 90 percent of people diagnosed with colorectal cancer are older than age 50. The disease also occurs in younger people but much less frequently.

Race Black Americans of African ancestry have a greater risk of colorectal cancer than do people of other races. They also tend to develop it at a slightly earlier age. If you're African American, your doctor may recommend you undergo colorectal cancer screening at an earlier age.

History of colorectal cancer or polyps If you've already had colon cancer or you have colon polyps, you have a greater risk of colorectal cancer in the future.

Diabetes Individuals with diabetes and insulin resistance have an increased risk of colon cancer.

Inflammatory intestinal conditions A history of ulcerative colitis or Crohn's disease involving a substantial part of the colon increases your risk of colorectal cancer, and of developing it at a younger age.

Obesity People who are obese are at increased risk of getting colorectal cancer and of dying of cancer compared with individuals at a healthy weight.

Inactivity People who are inactive tend to be at increased risk of colorectal cancer. This may be related to the fact that inactive individuals also tend to be overweight.

Smoking and alcohol Individuals who smoke or consume large amounts of alcohol are at greater risk of colorectal cancer.

Radiation therapy Radiation therapy directed at the abdomen to treat a previous cancer increases colorectal cancer risk.

● ● ● ● ●

ASPIRIN AND CANCER PREVENTION

Among people at high risk of colorectal cancer, some medications have been found to reduce the risk of precancerous polyps or colon cancer.

For instance, there's some evidence that regular use of aspirin or aspirin-like medications may be associated with a reduced risk of polyps and colon cancer. But it's not clear the length of time you would need to take aspirin and at what dose you'd need to decrease your odds of developing the disease.

Taking aspirin daily also has some risks, including gastrointestinal bleeding and ulcers. Therefore, doctors typically don't recommend this as a prevention strategy unless you have an increased risk of colon cancer or you need to take aspirin to help prevent heart disease and stroke. For people at average risk, not enough evidence exists to show that the benefits outweigh the risks.

● ● ● ● ●

SCREENING

When should you be screened for colorectal cancer? The American Cancer Society recently changed its screening guidelines. It recommends that adults at average risk of colorectal cancer start screening at age 45 instead of age 50. However, not all medical organizations have adopted these guidelines. Many still recommend that individuals at average risk begin colorectal cancer screening at age 50.

The best approach is to discuss with your doctor when you should start screening, based on your health, lifestyle and family history. Also check with your health insurance provider to see at what age your screening tests are covered.

How long should you continue to be screened? Most organizations generally recommend the following:

- Average-risk adults in good health should continue colorectal cancer screening through age 75.
- Between ages 76 and 85, screening decisions should be made in consultation with your doctor based on your prior screening history, health status and life expectancy.
- Screening generally isn't recommended beyond age 85.

Screening tests

Several screening tests can be used to find polyps or colorectal cancer. Colonoscopy is considered the gold standard for colorectal cancer detection, but other options may be used. Talk to your doctor about which test is right for you.

Stool tests Stool tests check for blood in stool, indicating possible cancer, or for DNA shed from cancer cells. If any of these tests produces a positive result, you'll need a colonoscopy exam to view the colon and rectum and look for indications of cancer.

- *Guaiac-based fecal occult blood test (gFOBT).* It uses the chemical guaiac to detect blood in the stool. For this test, performed annually, you receive a test kit from your doctor. At home, you use a stick or brush to obtain a small amount of stool after a bowel movement. You then return the test kit to the doctor or a laboratory, where stool samples are checked for the presence of blood. The test is not as reliable (sensitive) as other stool tests.
- *Fecal immunochemical test (FIT).* This test uses antibodies to detect blood in stool. It's also performed once a year in the same way as a gFOBT.
- *Stool DNA test.* This test, also known as the FIT-DNA test, combines FIT with a test that detects altered DNA in stool. Cologuard is currently the only stool DNA test approved for colorectal cancer screening in the United States. The test is intended for healthy individuals and is not approved for use in people known to have polyps or cancer. For this test, you collect an entire bowel movement in a specialized container and send it to a laboratory, where it's checked for cancer cells. If no cancer

cells are found, it's generally recommended you have the test every three years.

Flexible sigmoidoscopy For this test, a doctor inserts a short, thin, flexible, lighted tube into your rectum. He or she checks for polyps or cancer inside the rectum and lower third of the colon. The drawback of this test is that it doesn't examine the entire colon and some potentially cancerous lesions may be missed.

Flexible sigmoidoscopy is recommended every five years, or every 10 years with an annual FIT.

Colonoscopy A colonoscopy exam is similar to flexible sigmoidoscopy except it involves a longer tube, making it possible for a doctor to view the entire colon, in addition to the rectum. A tiny video camera at the tip of the tube allows the doctor to detect changes or abnormalities inside the colon, and attached cutting tools make it possible to remove polyps. Colonoscopy also is used as a follow-up test if anything unusual is found during one of the other screening exams.

If you're at average risk of colorectal cancer, it's recommended that you have a colonoscopy every 10 years. If you're at high risk, your doctor may recommend that you have the test more often.

Virtual colonoscopy Virtual colonoscopy, also known as computerized tomography (CT) colonography, uses X-rays and computers to produce images of the entire colon, which are displayed on a computer screen for a doctor to analyze. If an abnormality is detected, you'll need to follow up with a colonoscopy or sigmoidoscopy exam.

Virtual colonoscopy is recommended every five years.

CANCER STAGING

If cancer is detected during screening tests, your doctor will decide what additional tests may be necessary. Unlike some other cancers, the size of the tumor is not a major factor in determining the outcome of colo- rectal cancer. Of greater importance is how far the cancer has spread. Called staging, this testing process determines your outlook and what treatment may be appropriate for your cancer.

Additional tests may include a physical exam, tissue biopsies and a variety of imaging tests, such as computerized tomography (CT) or magnetic resonance imaging (MRI). Surgery also may be a part of the staging process.

Primary factors that a doctor takes into account during the staging process are:

- To what extent has the cancer spread through tissue layers of the colon wall, from the inner lining to the outer layer?
- Has it spread to nearby lymph nodes?
- Has the cancer spread (metastasized) to organs in other parts of the body, such as the liver or lungs?

When testing is complete, your doctor will categorize your cancer into one of five different stages. Each stage, from 0 to 4, indicates the spread of cancer on a scale of increasing severity (see this illustration).

● ● ● ● ●

Stage 0. The cancer is in its earliest stage. It hasn't grown beyond the inner layer (mucosa) of the colon or rectum.

Stage 1. The cancer has grown through the mucosa but hasn't spread outside the colon or rectal wall.

Stage 2. The cancer has grown through the wall of the colon or rectum but hasn't spread to nearby lymph nodes.

Stage 3. The cancer has spread to nearby lymph nodes but hasn't spread to other parts of the body.

Stage 4. The cancer is advanced and has spread to distant organs, such as the liver or lungs, or the lining of the abdominal cavity.

Unlike some other cancers, with colorectal cancer, the size of the cancerous tumor isn't a major factor in determining the outcome. Of greater importance is how far the cancer has spread.

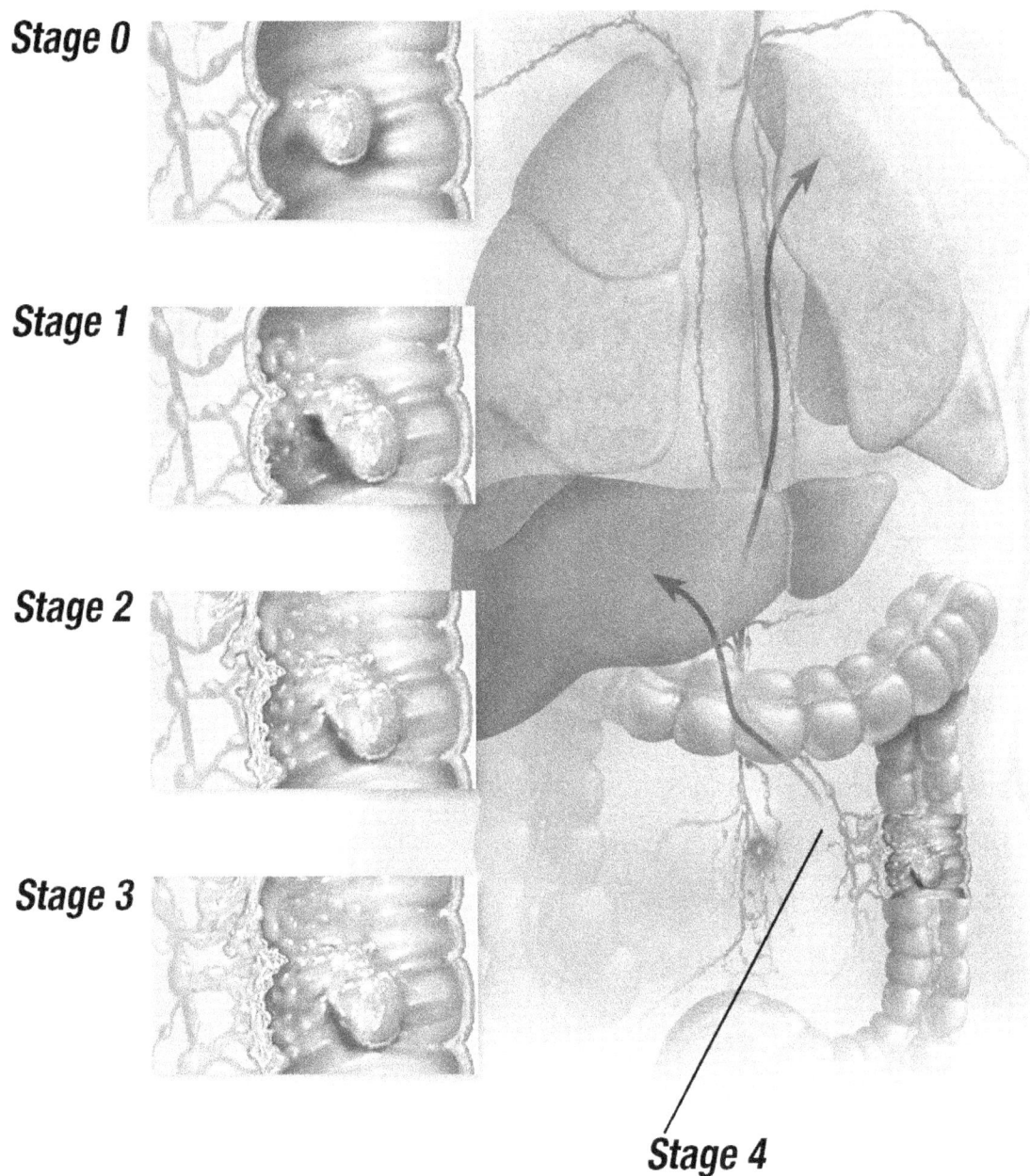

Stage 0

Stage 1

Stage 2

Stage 3

Stage 4

TREATMENT

The type of treatment your doctor recommends will depend largely on the stage of the cancer as well as your general health, other existing medical conditions, and the size and location of the tumor. Surgery, radiation therapy and chemotherapy are the primary treatments for colorectal cancer. However, other options are being studied.

Colon cancer surgery

If your colon cancer is very small, your doctor may recommend a minimally invasive approach. More-extensive cancers may require traditional open surgery.

- *Removing polyps during a colonoscopy.* If your cancer is small, localized and completely contained within a polyp and in a very early stage, your doctor may be able to remove it completely during a colonoscopy.
- *Endoscopic mucosal resection.* Removing larger polyps may require taking a small amount of the lining of the colon or rectum in a procedure called an endoscopic mucosal resection.
- *Minimally invasive surgery.* Polyps that can't be removed during a colonoscopy may be removed using laparoscopic surgery. Several small incisions are made in your abdominal wall through which a surgeon inserts instruments with attached cameras that display your colon on a video monitor. The surgeon may also take samples from lymph nodes in the area where the cancer is located.

If the cancer has grown into or through your colon, a surgeon may recommend:

- *Partial colectomy.* During this procedure, a surgeon removes the part of your colon that contains the cancer, along with a margin of normal tissue surrounding the cancer. The surgeon is often able to reconnect the healthy portions of your colon or rectum. This procedure can often be performed with a minimally invasive approach (laparoscopy).

- *Colostomy surgery.* When it's not possible to reconnect the healthy portions of your colon or rectum, you may need an ostomy. This involves creating an opening (stoma) in the wall of your abdomen and connecting the remaining bowel to the stoma for the elimination of stool. A bag fits securely over the opening to collect the waste. Sometimes an ostomy is only temporary, allowing your colon or rectum time to heal after surgery. In other cases, a colostomy may be permanent.
- *Lymph node removal.* Nearby lymph nodes are usually removed during colon cancer surgery and tested for cancer.

If your cancer is advanced or your overall health is very poor, your surgeon may recommend an operation to relieve blockage of your colon or other conditions in order to improve your symptoms, such as pain or bleeding. The purpose of this type of surgery is not to cure the cancer.

Rectal cancer surgery

Surgery for rectal cancer is different from that of colon cancer. A variety of procedures may be used to treat the cancer, depending on its size and location.

For early-, small-stage cancers that are unlikely to spread, the tumor may be removed through a local excision. This procedure does not include lymph node removal.

For rectal tumors that are located extremely close to the anal sphincter, the surgeon may need to remove both the tumor and the sphincter. After this surgery, it's no longer possible to pass stool through the anus. A colostomy connects the end of the colon to an opening (stoma) in the lower abdomen. Stool passes into a removable pouch placed over the stoma.

For tumors located above the anal sphincter, it may be possible to spare the sphincter. All or a portion of the rectum is removed. The remaining end of the colon may be shaped into a pouch that's connected to the colon. Alternatively, the end of the colon may be connected directly to the anus or remaining section of the rectum.

Radiation therapy

Radiation therapy, either alone or combined with chemotherapy, is one of the standard treatment options for the management of colorectal cancer. Radiation may be used to shrink large tumors before an operation so that they can more easily be removed; destroy cancers cells that may remain after surgery; or relieve symptoms.

Intraoperative radiation therapy (IORT) This treatment consists of a single, high dose of radiation focused directly on the original tumor site immediately after surgery before the abdomen is closed. The tight focus of the radiation beam, along with careful placement of radiation shields, protects nearby organs from radiation damage.

The main purpose of the treatment is to reduce the chance of cancer recurrence when the surgeon is unable to remove the optimal amount of healthy tissue around the tumor.

Chemotherapy

Chemotherapy for colorectal cancer is usually given after surgery if the cancer has spread to the lymph nodes. Sometimes chemotherapy may be used before surgery, with the goal of shrinking the tumor before an operation. Chemotherapy before surgery is more common in rectal cancer than in colon cancer.

Targeted drug therapy

Drugs that target specific malfunctions that allow cancer cells to grow are available to people with advanced colon cancer. They include the medications bevacizumab (Avastin), cetuximab (Erbitux), panitumumab (Vectibix), ramucirumab (Cyramza), regorafenib (Stivarga) and ziv-aflibercept (Zaltrap).

Targeted drugs may be given along with chemotherapy or alone. Some people are helped by targeted drugs, while others are not. Researchers are making progress in determining who's most likely to benefit from targeted drugs. Until more is known, doctors carefully weigh the possible benefit of targeted drugs against the risk of side effects and the cost when deciding whether to use these treatments.

Immunotherapy

Some individuals with advanced colon cancer may benefit from immunotherapy with antibodies such as pembrolizumab (Keytruda) and nivolumab (Opdivo). Immunotherapy drugs stimulate the immune system to target and attack the cancer. A specific test of the tumor tissue can help determine if there's a chance the cancer may respond to these medications.

● ● ● ● ●

COLORECTAL POLYPS

The lining inside your colon is usually smooth. But some people have growths that sprout from the lining and intrude into the channel through which food waste passes. These growths are known as polyps. Many people will have one or more polyps at any given time, but some people can have hundreds or thousands of them.

Your risk of having polyps increases with age — up to half of all Americans develop them during their lifetimes. Most polyps don't become cancerous, but some do.

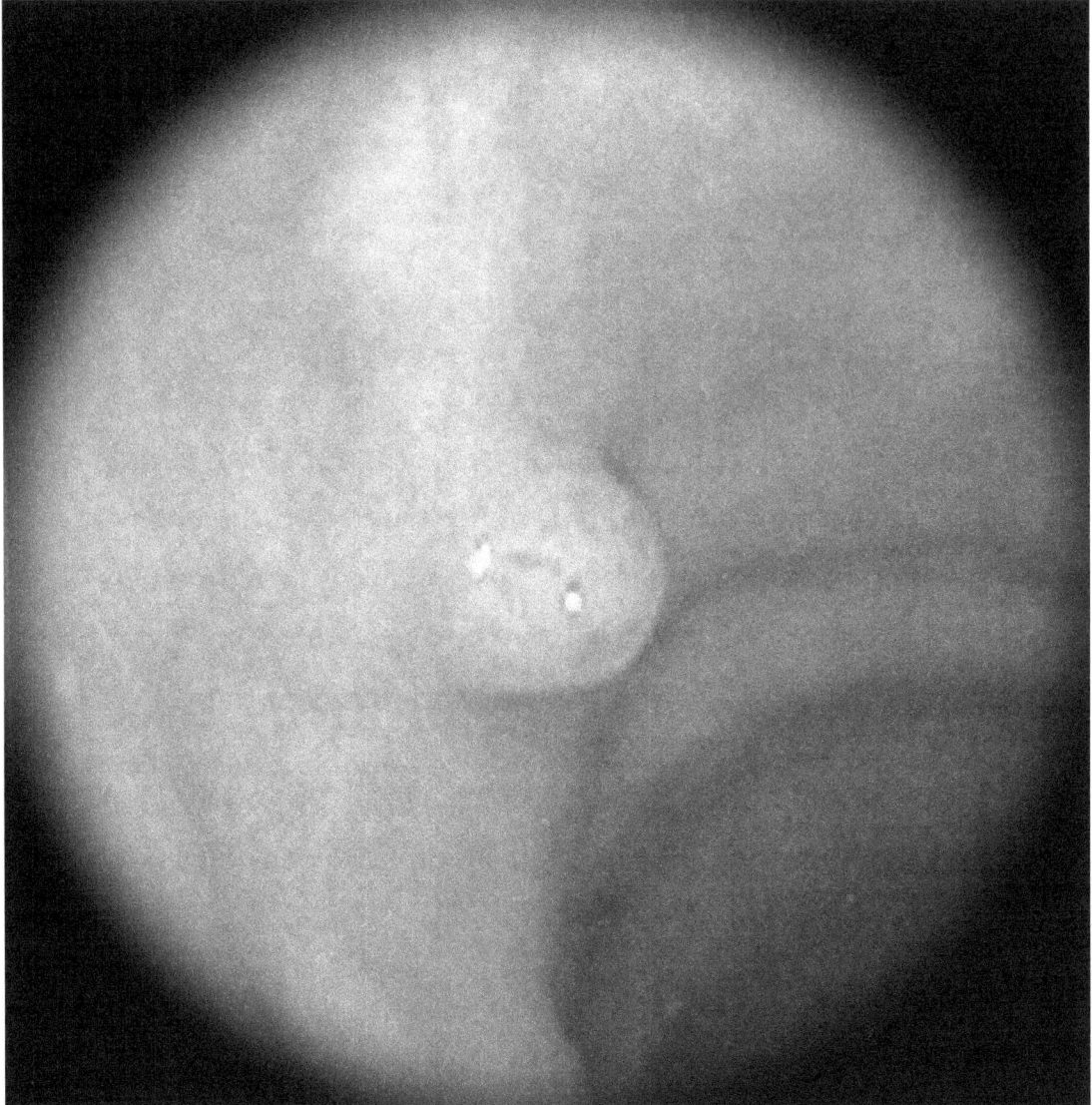

Polyps are small, noncancerous growths of various shapes and sizes that may develop in your colon and rectum.

The smaller the polyp, the less likely it is to be cancerous. The precancerous stage is a window of opportunity to detect and remove the growths, which your doctor can do relatively easily. Polyp removal is often done during screening for colon cancer using a procedure called colonoscopy.

You should have a colonoscopy examination, or an alternative form of screening test, beginning at age 45 or 50. If you have a higher than average risk of colorectal cancer, your doctor may recommend that screening begin at an earlier age.

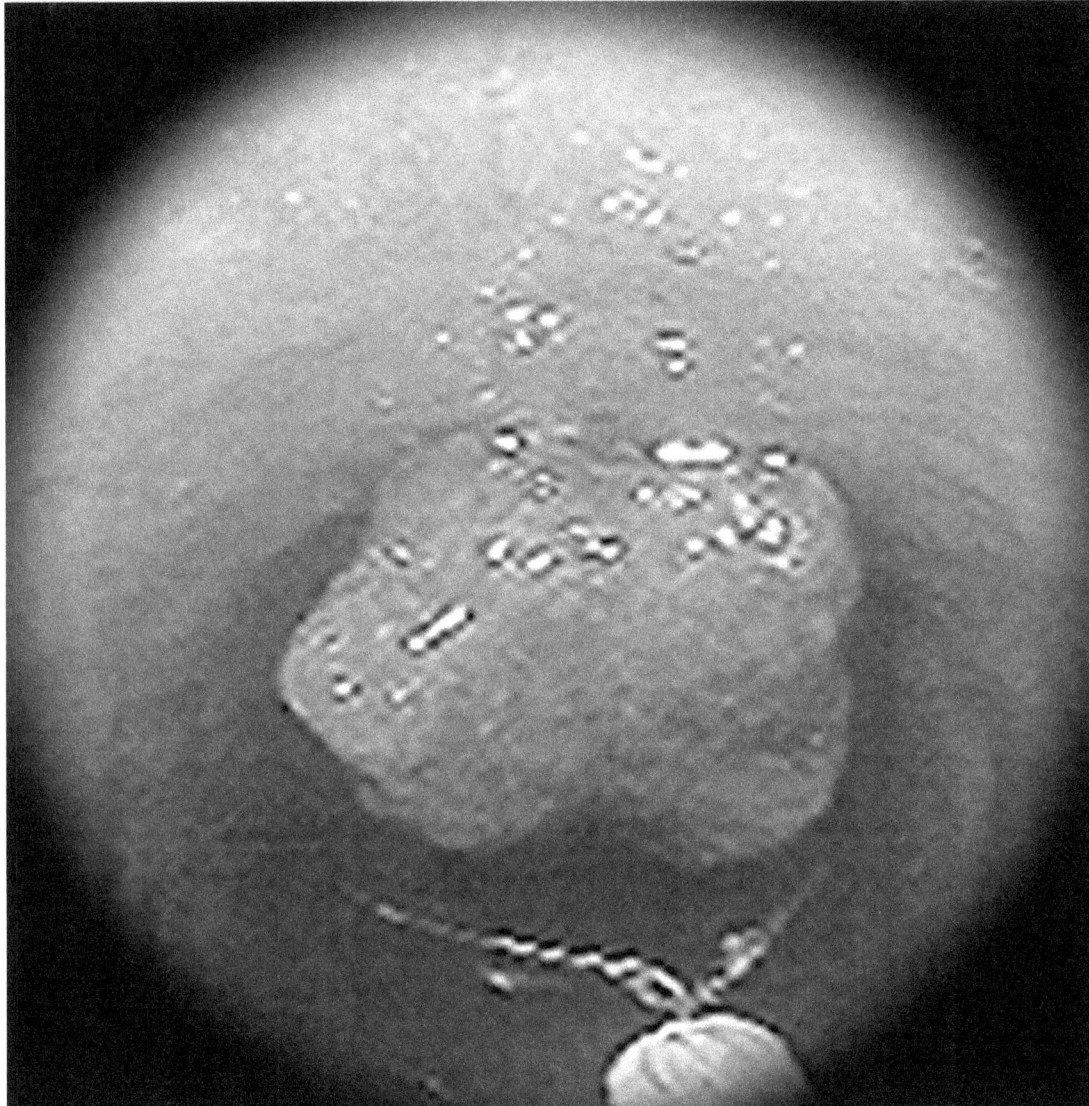

With use of an endoscope, a polyp can be removed with a thin wire.

• • • • •

FODMAP eating plan

FODMAPs are dietary sugars found in foods. They're a group of carbohydrates that often don't absorb well in the small intestine. The term "FODMAP" stands for:

- *F*ermentable
- *O*ligosaccharides — fructans and galactans, found in wheat, garlic and legumes (dried beans and peas)
- *D*isaccharides — lactose, found in dairy products (milk and others)
- *M*onosaccharides — excess fructose, found in honey and certain fruits
- *A*nd
- *P*olyols — sorbitol and mannitol and certain other low-calorie sweeteners

FODMAPs serve as a source of "food" for bacteria that live in the digestive tract. As they sit in the small intestine, FODMAPs can pull water into the intestine and bacteria can ferment the carbohydrates, causing gastrointestinal problems in people who have a sensitive gastrointestinal tract. Signs and symptoms include abdominal bloating and expansion (distention), excess gas, and abdominal pain. FODMAPs can also cause changes in bowel habits such as diarrhea and constipation.

A low-FODMAP diet is designed to relieve gastrointestinal signs and symptoms by restricting foods that are high in FODMAPs. The diet works by eliminating all foods that contain FODMAPs and then gradually adding the foods back into your diet until you determine the carbohydrates that are triggering your pain, discomfort and other symptoms.

This diet is not a diet for life. It's a tool to help you learn which foods agree with you, and which don't.

FODMAP diet

The FODMAP diet has three phases:

- Elimination
- Reintroduction
- Maintenance

Elimination During the elimination phase, you avoid all FODMAP foods for two to four weeks. See the food lists that follow. Most people begin to feel much better within a few days. But it may take weeks to feel as healthy as you can after you make this dietary change.

Reintroduction After the elimination phase, if your symptoms are under control, you may begin to eat foods that you eliminated. This is the reintroduction phase. You "reintroduce" the foods one at a time. This phase is important because you learn which foods likely caused your symptoms, and which don't cause symptoms. Many of the foods that you stopped eating during the elimination phase are good for your health. So if you can eat them again, you should.

Before you begin the reintroduction phase, it may be a good idea to return for a follow-up visit with your dietitian. He or she can give you instructions about how best to execute this next phase.

In general, there are no rules about the order you should use to reintroduce the foods. But here are some key guidelines to follow:

- Keep a food diary. Describe how you react to the food you eat. Your reaction is also called your "tolerance" for the food.
- Only reintroduce one FODMAP group at a time and one food at a time.
- Choose one food or ingredient from one food group. Then include that food or ingredient in your diet once a day for three days, starting with just half a serving the first day.
- If you eliminated a food that isn't on any of the food lists, you may try it again during this time.

Maintenance During this phase, your goal is to eat a varied diet. Include as many FODMAP foods as you wish as long as they don't produce any symptoms.

THE ELIMINATION PHASE

In this section, you'll find information on foods that you can eat during the elimination phase of the diet and foods that you want to avoid during this phase.

Sweeteners

Use allowed sweeteners in reasonable amounts. Look on the package for information about how much equals one serving. Limit your intake to just that amount. Check the ingredient lists on food and beverage labels to see which FODMAPs may be included.

Note:

- Sugar alcohols are found most often in sugar-free gum and candies. But they may also be used in other sugar-free foods and some medications.
- Other sugar substitutes don't need to be limited.

Foods allowed

- Bar sugar
- Beet sugar
- Brown sugar
- Cane sugar, cane juice, cane syrup
- Corn syrup
- Dextrose
- Evaporated cane sugars
- Glucose
- Glucose polymers
- Glucose syrup
- Glucose tablets
- Invert sugar
- Maltodextrin
- Maltose
- Maple sugar
- Maple syrup, pure
- Organic sugar
- Raw sugar
- Rice syrup

- Sucrose
- Sugar, granulated, white
- Sugar, powdered
- Sugar, raw, brown, often called turbinado

Sugar substitutes

- Aspartame (Equal, NutraSweet)
- Saccharin (Sweet N' Low)
- Sucralose (Splenda)
- Stevia (Stevia In The Raw)

Foods to avoid

- Agave syrup
- Fructose and crystalline fructose
- Fruit juice concentrate
- High-fructose corn syrup
- Honey
- Maple-flavored syrup/pancake syrup
- Molasses

Sugar alcohols

These artificial sweeteners are used in many sugar-free products, such as sugar-free gum, candy, medications, desserts, and protein drinks or bars.

- Erythritol
- Isomalt
- Maltitol
- Mannitol

- Sorbitol
- Xylitol
- Stevia made with erythritol

Miscellaneous foods

For items marked with an asterisk (*), check the product's food label to see if it contains FODMAP ingredients.

Foods allowed

- Balsamic vinegar, 1 Tbsp.
- Bouillon made from allowed ingredients
- Capers, 1 Tbsp.
- Cocoa powder, 1 Tbsp.
- Dark and milk chocolate, 1 fun size bar*
- Gelatin, regular or sugar-free
- Guar gum
- Jam or jelly*
- Miso paste
- Mustard*
- Pectin
- Soy lecithin
- Soy protein isolate
- Soy sauce, tamari
- Tabasco sauce
- Tahini paste, 1 Tbsp.
- Tapioca

- Vinegar
- Worcestershire sauce, 2 Tbsp.

Seasonings

- Cinnamon
- Ginger root and turmeric
- Green leafy herbs, either fresh or dried: parsley, oregano, cilantro, coriander, dill, marjoram, thyme, rosemary, mint
- Lemon and lime juice
- Paprika
- Pepper
- Salt
- Seed spices, such as coriander, mustard, cumin, caraway, dill seed, celery seed, sesame seed, poppy seed, nutmeg
- Vanilla extract, real or imitation

Foods to avoid

Condiments sweetened with sweeteners to avoid:

- Barbecue sauce
- Chutney
- Ketchup
- Plum sauce
- Relish
- Sweet and sour sauce
- Tomato paste
- Tomato soup

Seasonings

- Garlic powder
- Garlic salt
- Onion powder
- Onion salt

Fibers of chicory, inulin, fructo-oligosaccharide (FOS)

These ingredients are often added to foods to increase fiber. Check the ingredient lists on foods that have added fiber.

Fruit

- Eat up to three servings per day — but no more than one serving per meal — of the allowed fruits. The fruit may be fresh or frozen.
- Eat fruit with other foods. This slows your digestion of the fructose.
- Pay attention to serving size. The suggested serving for fruit is ½ cup or 1 small to medium-size piece, unless otherwise noted.

Foods allowed

- Avocado, ⅛
- Bananas, 1 medium unripe or ⅓ ripe
- Blueberries
- Cantaloupe
- Clementine
- Coconut, ¼ cup
- Cranberry
- Dragon fruit
- Grapes

- Honeydew
- Kiwi
- Lemon or lime
- Mandarin
- Orange
- Papaya
- Passion fruit
- Pineapple
- Pomegranate, ½
- Raspberries
- Rhubarb
- Strawberries
- Dried cranberries, raisins, currants, 1 Tbsp.
- Dried banana, 10 chips

Foods to avoid

- Apples
- Apricots
- Blackberries
- Boysenberries
- Canned fruit, all unsweetened and sweetened varieties
- Cherries
- Dates
- Dried fruit (other than those allowed)
- Figs
- Fruit juice, all unsweetened and sweetened varieties
- Fruit leather (fruit roll-ups and snacks)
- Grapefruit

- Mangos
- Nectarines
- Peaches
- Pears
- Persimmons
- Plums
- Prunes
- Tamarillo
- Watermelon

Vegetables

A serving size is about ½ cup cooked or 1 cup raw unless otherwise noted. Start with one serving per meal. Increase the amount you eat as long as you can tolerate it. For healthy eating, have five or more servings daily.

Foods allowed

- Alfalfa and bean sprouts
- Bamboo shoots
- Beets, 2 slices
- Bell pepper
- Bok choy
- Broccoli, 1 cup
- Brussels sprouts, ½ cup
- Cabbage: red, common or ½ cup savoy
- Carrots
- Celery, ¼ stalk

- Chili, red, green
- Chives
- Corn, ½ cob or ⅓ cup kernels
- Cucumber
- Eggplant
- Endive
- Fennel, bulb and leaves
- Ginger root
- Green beans
- Jicama
- Kale
- Lettuce: iceberg, romaine, baby lettuce, etc.
- Okra
- Olives
- Parsnip
- Potatoes, sweet, ½ cup
- Potatoes, white
- Pumpkin, ¼ cup
- Radish
- Rutabaga
- Snow peas, 5 pods
- Spinach
- Spring onion/scallion (green part only)
- Squash, butternut, ¼ cup
- Tomatoes, fresh or canned, no onion or garlic
- Turnips
- Water chestnuts
- Zucchini

- Artichoke
- Asparagus
- Cauliflower
- Chicory root or greens
- Dandelion greens
- Garlic
- Leeks
- Mushrooms
- Onions and shallots
- Sugar snap peas

Breads and grain products

Wheat, rye and barley-based foods contain the FODMAP fructans. You may substitute wheat-free and gluten-free foods that are free of other FODMAPs. Be sure to read the food labels. Eat at least four to six servings from this group per day. A serving includes ½ cup cooked grain, 1 cup dry cereal or 1 slice bread.

Note: Whole grains are good sources of fiber. Whole grains include oats, brown and wild rice, rice bran, millet, pure buckwheat, and popcorn.

Foods allowed

- Almond flour, ¼ cup
- Bread, gluten-free with allowed ingredients
- 100% buckwheat flour and cereal

- Cereals made from corn, rice, oats
- Cornmeal (polenta)
- Corn tortillas
- Grits
- Millet
- Oats, oat bran, oat flour
- Pasta made from corn, rice or quinoa
- Popcorn
- Pretzels, regular, ½ cup
- Pretzels, gluten-free
- Quinoa
- Rice: white, brown or wild
- Rice bran
- Rice flour
- Rice crackers/rice cakes
- Saltine crackers
- Soba noodles, 100% buckwheat
- Sourdough bread, wheat or white (The process of making this bread breaks down the fructans.)
- Tortilla chips

Foods to avoid

- Amaranth flour
- Barley
- Bulgur
- Coconut flour
- Couscous
- Gluten-free baked goods, breads, cereals, bars with ingredients to avoid

- Kamut
- Muesli, all varieties, including gluten- free pumpernickel
- Rye
- Wheat-based food: pasta, cereal, crackers, bread, baked goods

Meat and meat substitutes

Plain meat, poultry and fish that have no additives don't contain FODMAPs.

Foods allowed

- Chicken
- Eggs, egg substitutes
- Fish
- Game meats
- Hummus with allowed ingredients, ¼ cup
- Legumes:
- Chickpeas, ¼ cup canned
- Lentils, ½ cup canned
- Red or green lentils, ¼ cup boiled
- Edamame, 1 cup in the pod or ½ cup shelled
- Meat, lean
- Nut butters, 2 Tbsp.
- Nuts: almonds, macadamia, peanuts, pecan, pine nuts, walnuts (small handful)
- Organ meats
- Protein powders with allowed ingredients
- Seeds, unsweetened: chia, pumpkin, sesame, sunflower, 2 Tbsp.

- Shellfish
- Soy protein isolate
- Tempeh, ½ cup
- Tofu, firm only
- Turkey

Foods to avoid

- Breaded meats
- Commercially prepared meats that may contain FODMAP ingredients
- Legumes:
- Baked beans
- Dried or split peas
- Green peas
- Lima or butter beans
- Dried beans
- Pork and beans
- Refried beans
- Pinto beans
- Kidney beans
- Black beans
- Navy beans
- Nuts: pistachios and cashews
- Soy protein made from textured vegetable protein (TVP)
- Tofu, silken

Milk and milk products

For items marked with an asterisk (*), check the product's food label to see if it contains FODMAP ingredients.

Beverages and foods allowed

- Almond milk
- Coconut milk, canned only
- Flax milk
- Goat's milk yogurt
- Hard/aged cheese: cheddar, Colby, Swiss, brick, parmesan, mozzarella, others
- Hemp milk
- Kefir (99% lactose-free)*
- Lactose-free milk
- Lactose-free ice cream, lactose-free frozen yogurt*, lactose-free yogurt*
- Lactose-free cottage cheese
- Rice milk

Beverages and foods to avoid

- Goat's milk
- Coconut milk in a carton
- Cow's milk
- Foods made from cow's milk:
- Custard
- Frozen yogurt
- Ice cream
- Pudding
- Processed cheese
- Yogurt

- Soy milk

Fats

Foods allowed

- Butter
- Cooking sprays
- Cream, 1 Tbsp.
- Gravy made with allowed flours or corn starch
- Margarine
- Mayonnaise with allowed ingredients
- Oils, any type
- Sour cream, 1 Tbsp.

Foods to avoid

- Salad dressings with FODMAP ingredients

Beverages

Beverages listed with a portion size should be limited to that amount per day.

Beverages allowed

- Beer, 12 oz.
- Coffee (not chicory), 8 oz.
- Carbonated beverages, sugar-free
- Distilled spirits (also called hard alcohol): brandy, gin, vodka, whiskey,

others

- Sports drinks with allowed sweeteners
- Sugar-free powdered beverages
- Sugar-sweetened carbonated beverages made with allowed sweeteners, 8 oz.
- Tea (not chamomile, chicory, dandelion, fennel or oolong teas)
- Wine, dry: red or white, 5 oz.

Beverages to avoid

- Cider
- Coconut water
- Dessert wines: port, Marsala, Madeira, Muscat, rice, Tokay
- Fruit juices and fruit drinks
- Rum
- Tea: chamomile, chicory, dandelion, fennel and oolong

Menu ideas

With the long lists of foods that you are supposed to avoid, you may wonder what you can eat during the elimination phase of a low-FODMAP diet. Here are some meal suggestions and snack ideas to help get you started.

Breakfast

- Oat cereal such as oatmeal, oat flakes, Cheerios, others
- Corn cereal such as corn flakes, Corn Chex, others
- Rice cereal such as Rice Krispies, Rice Chex, Cream of Rice, others
- Grits

- Hash browns
- Eggs
- Ham
- Bacon
- Omelet made with aged cheese, vegetables
- Gluten-free toast with butter or margarine
- Sourdough bread, wheat or white
- Lactose-free milk, rice milk or 1 cup almond milk
- Allowed fruit, 1 serving
- Handful of nuts

Lunch

- Salad with allowed greens, cucumbers, tomatoes, aged cheese, chicken, egg, tuna
- Wine vinegar and oil salad dressing. Limit to 1 Tbsp. if balsamic vinegar is used.
- A sandwich — tuna salad, chicken salad, egg salad, grilled cheese or meat — made with gluten-free bread
- Corn tortilla with seasoned lean protein, shredded lettuce, tomatoes, shredded cheese
- Nachos with cheese
- Homemade soup with allowed ingredients
- No-bean chili with shredded cheese and corn chips
- Leftovers from another meal
- Allowed fruit, 1 serving

Dinner

- Lean meat

- Meatloaf made from lean ground meat, with egg, oatmeal and allowed seasonings
- Chicken
- Turkey
- Fish
- Shellfish
- Stir fry with allowed foods
- Steamed rice: white, brown or wild
- Potato: baked, boiled or mashed
- Quinoa
- Rice or corn pasta
- Allowed vegetables
- Allowed fruit, 1 serving

Snacks

- Aged cheese
- Lactose-free yogurt
- Corn chips, plain
- Allowed nuts (small handful)
- Potato chips, plain
- Popcorn
- Popcorn cakes
- Raw vegetables such as carrots, cherry tomatoes, cucumber and other allowed vegetables
- Rice cakes
- Peanut butter, 2 Tbsp.
- Rice crackers
- FODMAP-friendly salsa and hummus

THE REINTRODUCTION PHASE

After four to six weeks of the elimination diet, if your symptoms have improved, you may start to introduce foods that contain FODMAPs.

If your symptoms haven't improved, ask yourself if you're following the diet closely. If you don't fully understand the diet, meet with your dietitian to review the diet again. Or, you might be among the 1 in 4 people for whom this diet doesn't work. Ask yourself if other factors could be contributing to your symptoms, such as stress or anxiety.

How to begin

There are no firm rules about which foods you start with or the order in which you try the food again. However, if you want to figure out which foods caused your symptoms, there are guidelines about how you reintroduce the foods.

- Reintroduce one FODMAP group, such as fructans, at a time. Use one food from that group at a time. See the upcoming lists of FODMAP groups.
- Keep a food diary. Write down each food you reintroduce and how much you ate. Note whether you had any symptoms after you ate from that food group.
- Wait about three days (72 hours) before you move on to the next food.
- The food groups that follow list foods according to which type of FODMAP they contain. Introduce one food from whichever group you decide to start with.

- Start with a half-portion on the first day. Then try one portion on day two and again on day three.
- If you have symptoms — meaning that you don't tolerate that food — stop eating it. Wait for the symptoms to go away. Then try other foods in that FODMAP group. Later, you can retry the poorly tolerated food in a smaller amount.

Add more foods from the same FODMAP group. Continue to add foods from this group until you are ready to try another group. You don't have to try all foods in each group. Eat those you like.

Before starting a new group

Before you start a new FODMAP group, go back to the basic diet. Stop all foods from the first group. Wait about three days (72 hours) before you introduce another food group into your diet.

Continue to do this until you have introduced all the food groups. If at any time you try a food that you react to, stop eating that food. Try it again later in a smaller amount to see if you react any differently.

If a food has more than one FODMAP in it, wait to try it until after you've separately tried food from each of the FODMAP groups. If you can tolerate those FODMAPs separately, you likely will be able to tolerate them together.

Lactose group

- Milk, cows, goat, 8 fl. oz.
- Soft cheese, cottage cheese, ricotta

Check the labels for other FODMAP ingredients besides lactose in these foods:

- Ice cream, frozen yogurt
- Pudding
- Yogurt, regular
- Yogurt, Greek

Fructose group

- Agave syrup or nectar, 1 Tbsp.
- Asparagus
- Figs, fresh
- Honey, 1 Tbsp.
- Mango
- Rum, 1.5 oz.
- Sugar snap peas
- Apples. *Note:* Contain fructose and sorbitol.
- Artichokes. *Note:* Canned artichokes have fructose. The Jerusalem artichoke contains fructan and fructose.
- Cherries. *Note:* Contain fructose and sorbitol.
- Juice. *Note:* Contains fructose and sorbitol.
- Pears. *Note:* Contain fructose and sorbitol.
- Products with high-fructose corn syrup. *Note:* Check the labels for other FODMAP ingredients.
- Watermelon. *Note:* Contains fructose, fructan and mannitol.

Fructan group

- Banana, more than ⅓ ripe, with brown spots

- Barley
- Beets, more than 2 slices
- Broccoli, more than 1 cup
- Brussels sprouts, more than ½ cup
- Cabbage, savoy, more than ½ cup
- Dates
- Dried fruit: raisins, cranberries, currants, more than 1 Tbsp.
- Garlic, 1 clove
- Grapefruit
- Inulin and chicory root
- Okra, more than 6 pods
- Onions, shallots, leeks
- Persimmons
- Pistachios, cashews, ¼ cup. *Note:* Contain fructan and galactan.
- Pomegranate, more than ½ small
- Pumpkin, more than ¼ cup
- Rye
- Tea: chamomile, chai, fennel, oolong, 8 fl. oz.
- Wheat-based food: pasta, cereal, crackers, bread, baked goods
- Artichoke. *Note:* The globe artichoke has fructan. The Jerusalem artichoke contains fructan and fructose.
- Nectarine. *Note:* Contains fructan and sorbitol.
- Plums/prunes. *Note:* Contain fructan and sorbitol.
- Watermelon. *Note:* Contains fructan, fructose and mannitol.

Polyol group Candy, gum and medicine sweetened with sugar alcohols:

- Erythritol
- Isomalt

- Maltitol
- Mannitol. *See also* Polyol (mannitol) group.
- Sorbitol. *See also* Polyol (sorbitol) group.
- Xylitol

Polyol (mannitol) group

- Cauliflower
- Celery, more than ¼ stalk
- Mushrooms
- Snow peas, more than 5 pods
- Sweet potato, more than ½ cup
- Butternut squash, more than ½ cup. *Note:* Contains mannitol and galactan.
- Watermelon. *Note:* Contains mannitol, fructose and fructan.

Polyol (sorbitol) group

- Apricots
- Avocado, more than ⅛
- Blackberries
- Peaches, yellow
- Sweet corn, more than ½ cob, more than ⅓ cup of kernels
- Apples/apple juice. *Note:* Contain sorbitol and fructose.
- Asian pears. *Note:* Contain sorbitol and fructose.
- Cherries. *Note:* Contain sorbitol and fructose.
- Nectarines. *Note:* Contain sorbitol and fructan.
- Pears/pear juice. *Note:* Contain sorbitol and fructose.
- Plums/prunes. *Note:* Contain sorbitol and fructan.

Galactan group (GOS)

- Butternut squash, more than ¼ cup. *Note:* Contains galactan and mannitol.
- Chickpeas, also called garbanzo beans, canned, more than ¼ cup
- Coffee, regular or decaffeinated, more than 8 fl. oz.
- Edamame
- Green peas
- Hummus, more than ¼ cup
- Jicama
- Legumes: black beans, kidney beans, pinto beans, baked beans. *Note:* Beans that are canned, rinsed, drained and then cooked will have the lowest amount of FODMAPs.
- Lentils, canned, more than ½ cup
- Nuts: Pistachios and cashews, ¼ cup. *Note:* Contain galactan and fructan.
- Soy milk, 8 fl. oz.
- Tofu, silken
- Veggie/soy burger, 1 serving

THE MAINTENANCE PHASE

The maintenance phase is the eating plan you follow long term. This phase is about eating as many FODMAP foods as you can to enjoy a healthy and varied diet, while avoiding those foods that you learned in the elimination phase trigger your symptoms.

FODMAP tolerances can change over time. So, if there are foods you didn't tolerate well during the reintroduction phase, you might try them again several months later to see if anything has changed.

Many foods that are high in FODMAPs are also foods that are good for you. For your overall health and your digestive health, you want to eat as wide a variety of foods as you can, while avoiding uncomfortable signs and symptoms.

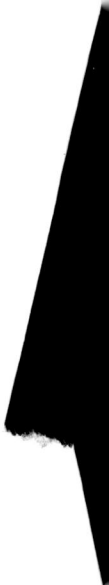

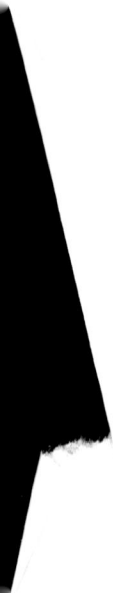

www.ingramcontent.com/pod-product-compliance
Lightning Source LLC
Chambersburg PA
CBHW081758200326
41597CB00023B/4074